Genetic Disorders Sourcebook,
1st Edition
Genetic Disorders Sourcebook,
2nd Edition
Head Trauma Sourcebook
Headache Sourcebook
Health Insurance Sourcebook
Health Reference Series Cumulative
Index 1999
Healthy Aging Sourcebook
Healthy Heart Sourcebook for Women
Heart Diseases & Disorders
Sourcebook, 2nd Edition
Household Safety Sourcebook
Immune System Disorders Sourcebook
Infant & Toddler Health Sourcebook
Injury & Trauma Sourcebook
Kidney & Urinary Tract Diseases &
Disorders Sourcebook
Learning Disabilities Sourcebook
Liver Disorders Sourcebook
Lung Disorders Sourcebook
Medical Tests Sourcebook
Men's Health Concerns Sourcebook
Mental Health Disorders Sourcebook,
1st Edition
Mental Health Disorders Sourcebook,
2nd Edition
Mental Retardation Sourcebook
Obesity Sourcebook
Ophthalmic Disorders Sourcebook
Oral Health Sourcebook
Osteoporosis Sourcebook
Pain Sourcebook, 1st Edition
Pain Sourcebook, 2nd Edition
Pediatric Cancer Sourcebook
Physical & Mental Issues in Aging
Sourcebook
Podiatry Sourcebook
Pregnancy & Birth Sourcebook
Prostate Cancer

Public Health Sourcebook
Reconstructive & Cosmetic Surgery
Sourcebook
Rehabilitation Sourcebook
Respiratory Diseases & Disorders
Sourcebook
Sexually Transmitted Diseases
Sourcebook, 1st Edition
Sexually Transmitted Diseases
Sourcebook, 2nd Edition
Skin Disorders Sourcebook
Sleep Disorders Sourcebook
Sports Injuries Sourcebook
Stress-Related Disorders Sourcebook
Substance Abuse Sourcebook
Surgery Sourcebook
Transplantation Sourcebook
Traveler's Health Sourcebook
Women's Health Concerns Sourcebook
Workplace Health & Safety Sourcebook
Worldwide Health Sourcebook

Teen Health Series

Diet Information for Teens
Drug Information for Teens
Mental Health Information
for Teens
Sexual Health Information
for Teens

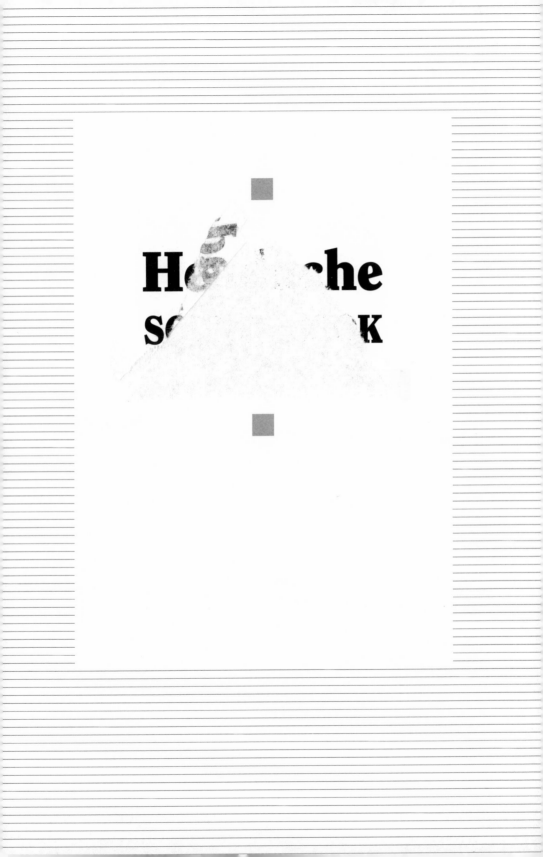

Health Reference Series

First Edition

Headache
SOURCEBOOK

■

Basic Consumer Health Information about Migraine, Tension, Cluster, Rebound, and Other Types of Headaches, with Facts about the Cause and Prevention of Headaches, the Effects of Stress and the Environment, Headaches during Pregnancy and Menopause, and Childhood Headaches

Along with a Glossary and Other Resources for Additional Help and Information

■

Edited by
Dawn D. Matthews

Omnigraphics

615 Griswold Street • Detroit, MI 48226

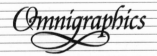

Bibliographic Note

Because this page cannot legibly accommodate all the copyright notices, the Bibliographic Note portion of the Preface constitutes an extension of the copyright notice.

Edited by Dawn D. Matthews

Health Reference Series

Karen Bellenir, *Managing Editor*
David A. Cooke, MD, *Medical Consultant*
Elizabeth Barbour, *Permissions Associate*
Dawn Matthews, *Verification Assistant*
Carol Munson, *Permissions Assistant*
Laura Pleva, *Index Editor*
EdIndex, Services for Publishers, *Indexers*

* * *

Omnigraphics, Inc.

Matthew P. Barbour, *Senior Vice President*
Kay Gill, *Vice President—Directories*
Kevin Hayes, *Operations Manager*
David P. Bianco, *Marketing Consultant*

* * *

Peter E. Ruffner, *President and Publisher*

Frederick G. Ruffner, Jr., *Chairman*

Copyright © 2002 Omnigraphics, Inc.

ISBN 0-7808-0377-X

Library of Congress Cataloging-in-Publication Data

Headache sourcebook : basic consumer health information about migraine, tension, cluster, rebound, and other types of headaches, with facts about the cause and prevention of headaches, the effects of stress and the environment, headaches during pregnancy and menopause, and childhood headaches; along with a glossary and other resources for additional help and information / edited by Dawn D. Matthews.-- 1st ed.
    p. cm. -- (health reference series ; I)
  ISBN 0-7808-0337X
  1. Heacache--Popular works. I. Matthews, Dawn D. II. Series

RC392 .H43 2002
616.8'491--dc21

2002016977

∞

This book is printed on acid-free paper meeting the ANSI Z39.48 Standard. The infinity symbol that appears above indicates that the paper in this book meets that standard.

Printed in the United States

Table of Contents

Part III: Treatment of Headaches

Part IV: Headaches, Hormones, and Other Co-Existing Conditions

Part V: Additional Help and Information

Preface

About This Book

According to the National Institute of Neurological Disorders and Stroke, an estimated 45 million Americans experience chronic headaches. For at least half of these people, the problem is severe and sometimes disabling. It can also be costly. Annually, migraine victims lose 157 million workdays because of headache pain. Although many triggers of headache pain are unknown, others have been identified, including diet, illness, stress, depression, hormonal changes, and environmental factors. Traditional treatment approaches can vary in effectiveness and sufferers sometimes turn to alternative medicine for relief.

This *Sourcebook* contains information about the causes, prevention, and treatment of the most common types of headaches, including migraine, tension, cluster, and rebound headaches. It describes frequently used medications and offers facts about other treatments including acupuncture, biofeedback, relaxation, and oxygen therapy. Special concerns related to headaches in children and women are also addressed. A glossary of related terms and directories of specialized resources provide additional help and information.

How to Use This Book

This book is divided into parts and chapters. Parts focus on broad areas of interest. Chapters are devoted to single topics within a part.

Part I: Types of Headaches provides facts about migraine, tension, cluster, rebound and other common types of headaches. It summarizes the relationship between headaches and other medical conditions and reviews special concerns related to headaches in children.

Part II: Causes and Prevention of Headaches gives helpful information about the effects of stress, depression, diet, and environmental and physical factors on headaches. Advice on how to prevent headaches is also included.

Part III: Treatment of Headaches describes the various techniques used to relieve headache pain, including over-the-counter and prescription medications, acupuncture, biofeedback, oxygen therapy, and experimental treatments.

Part IV: Headaches, Hormones, and Other Co-Existing Conditions provides facts about special concerns among women who may suffer headaches related to monthly hormonal changes, the use of oral contraceptives, pregnancy, or menopause. Other conditions, including sinusitis, stroke, and brain tumors, that may occur with headache pain are also discussed.

Part V: Additional Help and Information includes a glossary of related terms and additional resources for further information, along with a recommended reading list.

Bibliographic Note

This volume contains documents and excerpts from publications issued by the following government agencies: Food and Drug Administration (FDA); National Cancer Institute (NCI); National Center for Complementary and Alternative Medicine (NCCAM); National Institutes of Health (NIH); and National Institute of Neurological Disorders and Stroke (NINDS).

In addition, this volume contains copyrighted articles from the American Council for Headache Education (ACHE); the American Headache Society (AHS); Beth Israel Medical Center; and the National Headache Foundation.

Full citation information is provided on the first page of each chapter. Every effort has been made to secure all necessary rights to reprint the copyrighted material. If any omissions have been made, please contact Omnigraphics to make corrections for future editions.

Acknowledgements

Thanks go to Karen Bellenir, Carol Munson, David Cooke, and Margareta-Erminia Cassani for their help with the many details involved in the production of this book.

Note from the Editor

This book is part of Omnigraphics' *Health Reference Series*. The series provides basic information about a broad range of medical concerns. It is not intended to serve as a tool for diagnosing illness, in prescribing treatments, or as a substitute for the physician/patient relationship. All persons concerned about medical symptoms or the possibility of disease are encouraged to seek professional care from an appropriate health care provider.

Our Advisory Board

The *Health Reference Series* is reviewed by an Advisory Board comprised of librarians from public, academic, and medical libraries. We would like to thank the following board members for providing guidance to the development of this series:

Dr. Lynda Baker, Associate Professor of Library and Information Science, Wayne State University, Detroit, MI

Nancy Bulgarelli, William Beaumont Hospital Library, Royal Oak, MI

Karen Imarasio, Bloomfield Township Public Library, Bloomfield Township, MI

Karen Morgan, Mardigian Library, University of Michigan-Dearborn, Dearborn, MI

Rosemary Orlando, St. Clair Shores Public Library, St. Clair Shores, MI

Medical Consultant

Medical consultation services are provided to the *Health Reference Series* editors by David A. Cooke, MD. Dr. Cooke is a graduate of Brandeis University, and he received his M.D. degree from the University of Michigan. He completed residency training at the University of Wisconsin

Hospital and Clinics. He is board-certified in Internal Medicine. Dr. Cooke currently works as part of the University of Michigan Health System and practices in Brighton, MI. In his free time, he enjoys writing, science fiction, and spending time with his family.

Health Reference Series *Update Policy*

The inaugural book in the *Health Reference Series* was the first edition of *Cancer Sourcebook* published in 1992. Since then, the *Series* has been enthusiastically received by librarians and in the medical community. In order to maintain the standard of providing high-quality health information for the layperson the editorial staff at Omnigraphics felt it was necessary to implement a policy of updating volumes when warranted.

Medical researchers have been making tremendous strides, and it is the purpose of the *Health Reference Series* to stay current with the most recent advances. Each decision to update a volume will be made on an individual basis. Some of the considerations will include how much new information is available and the feedback we receive from people who use the books. If there is a topic you would like to see added to the update list, or an area of medical concern you feel has not been adequately addressed, please write to:

Editor
Health Reference Series
Omnigraphics, Inc.
615 Griswold
Detroit, MI 48226

The commitment to providing on-going coverage of important medical developments has also led to some format changes in the *Health Reference Series*. Each new volume on a topic is individually titled and called a "First Edition." Subsequent updates will carry sequential edition numbers. To help avoid confusion and to provide maximum flexibility in our ability to respond to informational needs, the practice of consecutively numbering each volume has been discontinued.

Part One

Types of Headaches

Chapter 1

Headaches: An Overview

Introduction

For two years, Jim suffered the excruciating pain of cluster headaches. Night after night he paced the floor, the pain driving him to constant motion. He was only 48 years old when the clusters forced him to quit his job as a systems analyst. One year later, his headaches are controlled. The credit for Jim's recovery belongs to the medical staff of a headache clinic. Physicians there applied the latest research findings on headache, and prescribed for Jim a combination of new drugs.

Joan was a victim of frequent migraine. Her headaches lasted two days. Nauseous and weak, she stayed in the dark until each attack was over. Today, although migraine still interferes with her life, she has fewer attacks and less severe headaches than before. A specialist prescribed an antimigraine program for Joan that included improved drug therapy, a new diet and relaxation training.

An avid reader, Peggy couldn't put down the new mystery thriller. After 4 hours of reading slumped in bed, she knew she had overdone it. Her tensed head and neck muscles felt as if they were being squeezed between two giant hands. But for Peggy, the muscle-contraction headache and neck pain were soon relieved by a hot shower and aspirin.

The text in this chapter is from an undated fact sheet titled, "Headache—Hope through Research," from the National Institute of Neurological Disorders and Stroke (NINDS), available online at http://www.ninds.nih.gov/health_and_medical/pubs/headache_htr.htm; cited September, 2001.

An estimated 45 million Americans experience chronic headaches. For at least half of these people, the problem is severe and sometimes disabling. It can also be costly: headache sufferers make over 8 million visits a year to doctor's offices. Migraine victims alone lose over 157 million workdays because of headache pain.

Understanding why headaches occur and improving headache treatment are among the research goals of the National Institute of Neurological Disorders and Stroke (NINDS). As the leading supporter of brain research in the Federal Government, the NINDS also supports and conducts studies to improve the diagnosis of headaches and to find ways to prevent them.

Why Does It Hurt?

What hurts when you have a headache? Several areas of the head can hurt, including a network of nerves which extends over the scalp and certain nerves in the face, mouth, and throat. Also sensitive to pain, because they contain delicate nerve fibers, are the muscles of the head and blood vessels found along the surface and at the base of the brain.

The bones of the skull and tissues of the brain itself, however, never hurt, because they lack pain-sensitive nerve fibers. The ends of these pain-sensitive nerves, called nociceptors, can be stimulated by stress, muscular tension, dilated blood vessels, and other triggers of headache. Once stimulated, a nociceptor sends a message up the length of the nerve fiber to the nerve cells in the brain, signaling that a part of the body hurts. The message is determined by the location of the nociceptor. A person who suddenly realizes "My toe hurts," is responding to nociceptors in the foot that have been stimulated by the stubbing of a toe.

A number of chemicals help transmit pain-related information to the brain. Some of these chemicals are natural painkilling proteins called endorphins, Greek for "the morphine within." One theory suggests that people who suffer from severe headache and other types of chronic pain have lower levels of endorphins than people who are generally pain free.

When Should You See a Physician?

Not all headaches require medical attention. Some result from missed meals or occasional muscle tension and are easily remedied. But some types of headache are signals of more serious disorders, and call for prompt medical care. These include:

- Sudden, severe headache
- Sudden, severe headache associated with a stiff neck
- Headache associated with fever
- Headache associated with convulsions
- Headache accompanied by confusion or loss of consciousness
- Headache following a blow on the head
- Headache associated with pain in the eye or ear
- Persistent headache in a person who was previously headache free
- Recurring headache in children
- Headache which interferes with normal life

A headache sufferer usually seeks help from a family practitioner. If the problem is not relieved by standard treatments, the patient may then be referred to a specialist—perhaps an internist or neurologist. Additional referrals may be made to psychologists.

What Tests Are Used to Diagnose Headache?

Diagnosing a headache is like playing Twenty Questions. Experts agree that a detailed question-and-answer session with a patient can often produce enough information for a diagnosis. Many types of headaches have clear-cut symptoms which fall into an easily recognizable pattern. Patients may be asked: How often do you have headaches? Where is the pain? How long do the headaches last? When did you first develop headaches? The patient's sleep habits and family and work situations may also be probed.

Most physicians will also obtain a full medical history from the patient, inquiring about past head trauma or surgery, eye strain, sinus problems, dental problems, difficulties with opening and closing of the jaw, and the use of medications. This may be enough to suggest strongly that the patient has migraine or cluster headaches. A blood test may be ordered to screen for thyroid disease, anemia, or infections which might cause a headache. A complete and careful physical and neurological examination will exclude many possibilities and the suspicion of aneurysm, meningitis, or certain brain tumors. X-rays may be taken to rule out the possibility of a brain tumor or blood clot.

A test called an electroencephalogram (EEG) may be given to measure brain activity. EEG's can indicate a malfunction in the brain, but they cannot usually pinpoint a problem that might be causing a headache. A physician may suggest that a patient with unusual headaches undergo a computed tomographic (CT) scan and/or magnetic resonance imaging (MRI). The CT scan produces images of the brain that show structures or variations in the density of different types of tissue. The scan enables the physician to distinguish, for example, between a bleeding blood vessel in the brain and a brain tumor, and is an important diagnostic tool in cases of headache associated with brain lesions or other serious disease. MRI uses magnetic fields and radio waves to produce an image that provides information about the structure and biochemistry of the brain.

An eye exam is usually performed to check for weakness in the eye muscle or unequal pupil size. If an aneurysm—an abnormal ballooning of a blood vessel—is suspected, a physician may order a CT scan to examine for blood and then an angiogram. In this test, a special fluid, which can be seen on an X-ray, is injected into the patient and carried in the bloodstream to the brain to reveal any abnormalities in the blood vessels there.

Thermography, an experimental technique for diagnosing headache, promises to become a useful clinical tool. In thermography, an infrared camera converts skin temperature into a color picture or thermogram with different degrees of heat appearing as different colors. Skin temperature is affected primarily by blood flow. Research scientists have found that thermograms of headache patients show strikingly different heat patterns from those of people who never or rarely get headaches.

A physician analyzes the results of all these diagnostic tests along with a patient's medical history and examination in order to arrive at a diagnosis.

Headaches are diagnosed as:

- Vascular
- Muscle contraction (tension)
- Traction
- Inflammatory

Vascular headaches—a group that includes the well-known migraine—are so named because they are thought to involve abnormal function of the brain's blood vessels or vascular system. Muscle contraction headaches appear to involve the tightening or tensing of facial and neck muscles. Traction and inflammatory headaches are symptoms of other disorders, ranging from stroke to sinus infection. Some people have more than one type of headache.

What Are Migraine Headaches?

The most common type of vascular headache is migraine. Migraine headaches are usually characterized by severe pain on one or both sides of the head, an upset stomach, and at times disturbed vision.

Former basketball star Kareem Abdul-Jabbar remembers experiencing his first migraine at age 14. The pain was unlike the discomfort of his previous mild headaches.

"When I got this one I thought, 'This is a headache,'" he says. "The pain was intense and I felt nausea and a great sensitivity to light. All I could think about was when it would stop. I sat in a dark room for an hour and it passed."

Symptoms of Migraine

Abdul-Jabbar's sensitivity to light is a standard symptom of the two most prevalent types of migraine-caused headache: classic and common.

The major difference between the two types is the appearance of neurological symptoms 10 to 30 minutes before a classic migraine attack. These symptoms are called an aura. The person may see flashing lights or zigzag lines, or may temporarily lose vision. Other classic symptoms include speech difficulty, weakness of an arm or leg, tingling of the face or hands, and confusion.

The pain of a classic migraine headache may be described as intense, throbbing, or pounding and is felt in the forehead, temple, ear, jaw, or around the eye. Classic migraine starts on one side of the head but may eventually spread to the other side. An attack lasts 1 to 2 pain-wracked days.

Common migraine—a term that reflects the disorder's greater occurrence in the general population—is not preceded by an aura. But some people experience a variety of vague symptoms beforehand, including mental fuzziness, mood changes, fatigue, and unusual retention of fluids. During the headache phase of a common migraine, a person may have diarrhea and increased urination, as well as nausea and vomiting. Common migraine pain can last 3 or 4 days.

Both classic and common migraine can strike as often as several times a week, or as rarely as once every few years. Both types can occur at any time. Some people, however, experience migraines at predictable times—near the days of menstruation or every Saturday morning after a stressful week of work.

The Migraine Process

Research scientists are unclear about the precise cause of migraine headaches. There seems to be general agreement, however, that a key element is blood flow changes in the brain. People who get migraine headaches appear to have blood vessels that overreact to various triggers.

Scientists have devised one theory of migraine which explains these blood flow changes and also certain biochemical changes that may be involved in the headache process. According to this theory, the nervous system responds to a trigger such as stress by causing a spasm of the nerve-rich arteries at the base of the brain. The spasm closes down or constricts several arteries supplying blood to the brain, including the scalp artery and the carotid or neck arteries.

As these arteries constrict, the flow of blood to the brain is reduced. At the same time, blood-clotting particles called platelets clump together—a process which is believed to release a chemical called serotonin. Serotonin acts as a powerful constrictor of arteries, further reducing the blood supply to the brain.

Reduced blood flow decreases the brain's supply of oxygen. Symptoms signaling a headache, such as distorted vision or speech, may then result, similar to symptoms of stroke.

Reacting to the reduced oxygen supply, certain arteries within the brain open wider to meet the brain's energy needs. This widening or dilation spreads, finally affecting the neck and scalp arteries. The dilation of these arteries triggers the release of pain-producing substances called prostaglandins from various tissues and blood cells. Chemicals which cause inflammation and swelling, and substances which increase sensitivity to pain, are also released. The circulation of these chemicals and the dilation of the scalp arteries stimulate the pain-sensitive nociceptors. The result, according to this theory: a throbbing pain in the head.

Women and Migraine

Although both males and females seem to be equally affected by migraine, the condition is more common in adult women. Both sexes may develop migraine in infancy, but most often the disorder begins between the ages of 5 and 35.

The relationship between female hormones and migraine is still unclear. Women may have "menstrual migraine"—headaches around the time of their menstrual period—which may disappear during pregnancy. Other women develop migraine for the first time when they are pregnant. Some are first affected after menopause.

The effect of oral contraceptives on headaches is perplexing. Scientists report that some women with migraine who take birth control pills experience more frequent and severe attacks. However, a small percentage of women have fewer and less severe migraine headaches when they take birth control pills. And normal women who do not suffer from headaches may develop migraines as a side effect when they use oral contraceptives. Investigators around the world are studying hormonal changes in women with migraine in the hope of identifying the specific ways these naturally occurring chemicals cause headaches.

Triggers of Headache

Although many sufferers have a family history of migraine, the exact hereditary nature of this condition is still unknown. People who get migraines are thought to have an inherited abnormality in the regulation of blood vessels.

"It's like a cocked gun with a hair trigger," explains one specialist. "A person is born with a potential for migraine and the headache is triggered by things that are really not so terrible." These triggers include stress and other normal emotions, as well as biological and environmental conditions. Fatigue, glaring or flickering lights, changes in the weather, and certain foods can set off migraine. It may seem hard to believe that eating such seemingly harmless foods as yogurt, nuts, and lima beans can result in a painful migraine headache. However, some scientists believe that these foods and several others contain chemical substances, such as tyramine, which constrict arteries—the first step of the migraine process. Other scientists believe that foods cause headaches by setting off an allergic reaction in susceptible people.

While a food-triggered migraine usually occurs soon after eating, other triggers may not cause immediate pain. Scientists report that people can develop migraine not only during a period of stress but also afterwards when their vascular systems are still reacting. For example, migraines that wake people up in the middle of the night are believed to result from a delayed reaction to stress.

9

Other Forms of Migraine

In addition to classic and common, migraine headache can take several other forms.

Patients with hemiplegic migraine have temporary paralysis on one side of the body, a condition known as hemiplegia. Some people may experience vision problems and vertigo—a feeling that the world is spinning. These symptoms begin 10 to 90 minutes before the onset of headache pain.

In ophthalmoplegic migraine, the pain is around the eye and is associated with a droopy eyelid, double vision, and other problems with vision.

Basilar artery migraine involves a disturbance of a major brain artery. Preheadache symptoms include vertigo, double vision, and poor muscular coordination. This type of migraine occurs primarily in adolescent and young adult women and is often associated with the menstrual cycle.

Benign exertional headache is brought on by running, lifting, coughing, sneezing, or bending. The headache begins at the onset of activity, and pain rarely lasts more than several minutes.

Status migrainosus is a rare and severe type of migraine that can last 72 hours or longer. The pain and nausea are so intense that people who have this type of headache must be hospitalized. The use of certain drugs can trigger status migrainosus. Neurologists report that many of their status migrainosus patients were depressed and anxious before they experienced headache attacks.

Headache-free migraine is characterized by such migraine symptoms as visual problems, nausea, vomiting, constipation, or diarrhea. Patients, however, do not experience head pain. Headache specialists have suggested that unexplained pain in a particular part of the body, fever, and dizziness could also be possible types of headache-free migraine.

How Is Migraine Headache Treated?

During the Stone Age, pieces of a headache sufferer's skull were cut away with flint instruments to relieve pain. Another unpleasant remedy used in the British Isles around the ninth Century involved drinking "the juice of elderseed, cow's brain, and goat's dung dissolved in vinegar." Fortunately, today's headache patients are spared such drastic measures.

Drug therapy, biofeedback training, stress reduction, and elimination of certain foods from the diet are the most common methods of preventing and controlling migraine and other vascular headaches. Joan, the migraine sufferer, was helped by treatment with a combination of an antimigraine drug and diet control.

Regular exercise, such as swimming or vigorous walking, can also reduce the frequency and severity of migraine headaches. Joan found that whirlpool and yoga baths helped her relax.

During a migraine headache, temporary relief can sometimes be obtained by applying cold packs to the head or by pressing on the bulging artery found in front of the ear on the painful side of the head.

Drug Therapy

There are two ways to approach the treatment of migraine headache with drugs: prevent the attacks, or relieve symptoms after the headache occurs.

For infrequent migraine, drugs can be taken at the first sign of a headache in order to stop it or to at least ease the pain. People who get occasional mild migraine may benefit by taking aspirin or acetaminophen at the start of an attack. Aspirin raises a person's tolerance to pain and also discourages clumping of blood platelets. Small amounts of caffeine may be useful if taken in the early stages of migraine. But for most migraine sufferers who get moderate to severe headaches, and for all cluster headache patients, stronger drugs may be necessary to control the pain.

One of the most commonly used drugs for the relief of classic and common migraine symptoms is ergotamine tartrate, a vasoconstrictor which helps counteract the painful dilation stage of the headache. For optimal benefit, the drug is taken during the early stages of an attack. If a migraine has been in progress for about an hour and has passed into the final throbbing stage, ergotamine tartrate will probably not help.

Because ergotamine tartrate can cause nausea and vomiting, it may be combined with antinausea drugs. Research scientists caution that ergotamine tartrate should not be taken in excess or by people who have angina pectoris, severe hypertension, or vascular, liver, or kidney disease. Patients who are unable to take ergotamine tartrate may benefit from other drugs that constrict dilated blood vessels or help reduce blood vessel inflammation.

For headaches that occur three or more times a month, preventive treatment is usually recommended. Drugs used to prevent classic and common migraine include methysergide maleate, which counteracts blood vessel constriction; propranolol hydrochloride, which stops blood vessel dilation; and amitriptyline, an antidepressant.

Antidepressants called MAO inhibitors also prevent migraine. These drugs block an enzyme called monoamine oxidase, which normally helps nerve cells absorb the artery-constricting brain chemical, serotonin.

MAO inhibitors can have potentially serious side effects—particularly if taken while ingesting foods or beverages that contain tyramine, a substance that constricts arteries.

Several drugs for the prevention of migraine have been developed in recent years, including drugs which mimic the action of serotonin, including serotonin agonists which mimic the action of this key brain chemical. Prompt administration of these drugs is important.

Many antimigraine drugs can have adverse side effects. But like most medicines they are relatively safe when used carefully and under a physician's supervision. To avoid long-term side effects of preventive medications, headache specialists advise patients to reduce the dosage of these drugs and then stop taking them as soon as possible.

Biofeedback and Relaxation Training

Drug therapy for migraine is often combined with biofeedback and relaxation training. Biofeedback refers to a technique that can give people better control over such body function indicators as blood pressure, heart rate, temperature, muscle tension, and brain waves. Thermal biofeedback allows a patient to consciously raise hand temperature. Some patients who are able to increase hand temperature can reduce the number and intensity of migraines. The mechanisms underlying these self-regulation treatments are being studied by research scientists.

"To succeed in biofeedback," says a headache specialist, "you must be able to concentrate and you must be motivated to get well."

A patient learning thermal biofeedback wears a device which transmits the temperature of an index finger or hand to a monitor. While the patient tries to warm his hands, the monitor provides feedback either on a gauge that shows the temperature reading or by emitting a sound or beep that increases in intensity as the temperature increases. The patient is not told how to raise hand temperature, but is given suggestions such as "Imagine your hands feel very warm and heavy."

"I have a good imagination," says one headache sufferer who traded in her medication for thermal biofeedback. The technique decreased the number and severity of headaches she experienced.

In another type of biofeedback called electromyographic or EMG training, the patient learns to control muscle tension in the face, neck, and shoulders.

Either kind of biofeedback may be combined with relaxation training, during which patients learn to relax the mind and body.

Biofeedback can be practiced at home with a portable monitor. But the ultimate goal of treatment is to wean the patient from the machine. The patient can then use biofeedback anywhere at the first sign of a headache.

The Antimigraine Diet

Scientists estimate that a small percentage of migraine sufferers will benefit from a treatment program focused solely on eliminating headache-provoking foods and beverages.

Other migraine patients may be helped by a diet to prevent low blood sugar. Low blood sugar, or hypoglycemia, can cause dilation of the blood vessels in the head. This condition can occur after a period without food: overnight, for example, or when a meal is skipped. People who wake up in the morning with a headache may be reacting to the low blood sugar caused by the lack of food overnight.

Treatment for headaches caused by low blood sugar consists of scheduling smaller, more frequent meals for the patient. A special diet designed to stabilize the body's sugar-regulating system is sometimes recommended.

For the same reason, many specialists also recommend that migraine patients avoid oversleeping on weekends. Sleeping late can change the body's normal blood sugar level and lead to a headache.

Besides Migraine, What Are Other Types of Vascular Headaches?

After migraine, the most common type of vascular headache is the toxic headache produced by fever. Pneumonia, measles, mumps, and tonsillitis are among the diseases that can cause severe toxic vascular headaches. Toxic headaches can also result from the presence of foreign chemicals in the body. Other kinds of vascular headaches include "clusters," which cause repeated episodes of intense pain, and headaches resulting from a rise in blood pressure.

Chemical Culprits

Repeated exposure to nitrite compounds can result in a dull, pounding headache that may be accompanied by a flushed face. Nitrite, which dilates blood vessels, is found in such products as heart medicine and dynamite, but is also used as a chemical to preserve meat. Hot dogs and other processed meats containing sodium nitrite can cause headaches.

Eating foods prepared with monosodium glutamate (MSG) can result in headache. Soy sauce, meat tenderizer, and a variety of packaged foods contain this chemical which is touted as a flavor enhancer.

Headache can also result from exposure to poisons, even common household varieties like insecticides, carbon tetrachloride, and lead. Children who ingest flakes of lead paint may develop headaches. So may anyone who has contact with lead batteries or lead-glazed pottery.

Artists and industrial workers may experience headaches after exposure to materials that contain chemical solvents. These solvents, like benzene, are found in turpentine, spray adhesives, rubber cement, and inks.

Drugs such as amphetamines can cause headaches as a side effect. Another type of drug-related headache occurs during withdrawal from long-term therapy with the antimigraine drug ergotamine tartrate.

Jokes are often made about alcohol hangovers but the headache associated with "the morning after" is no laughing matter. Fortunately, there are several suggested remedies for the pain, including ergotamine tartrate. The hangover headache may also be reduced by taking honey, which speeds alcohol metabolism, or caffeine, a constrictor of dilated arteries. Caffeine, however, can cause headaches as well as cure them. Heavy coffee drinkers often get headaches when they try to break the caffeine habit.

Cluster Headaches

Cluster headaches, named for their repeated occurrence over weeks or months at roughly the same time of day or night in clusters, begin as a minor pain around one eye, eventually spreading to that side of the face. The pain quickly intensifies, compelling the victim to pace the floor or rock in a chair. "You can't lie down, you're fidgety," explains a cluster patient. "The pain is unbearable." Other symptoms include a stuffed and runny nose and a droopy eyelid over a red and tearing eye.

Cluster headaches last between 30 and 45 minutes. But the relief people feel at the end of an attack is usually mixed with dread as they await a recurrence. Clusters may mysteriously disappear for months or years. Many people have cluster bouts during the spring and fall. At their worst, chronic cluster headaches can last continuously for years.

Cluster attacks can strike at any age but usually start between the ages of 20 and 40. Unlike migraine, cluster headaches are more common in men and do not run in families.

Studies of cluster patients show that they are likely to have hazel eyes and that they tend to be heavy smokers and drinkers. Paradoxically, both nicotine, which constricts arteries, and alcohol, which dilates them, trigger cluster headaches. The exact connection between these substances and cluster attacks is not known.

Despite a cluster headache's distinguishing characteristics, its relative infrequency and similarity to such disorders as sinusitis can lead to misdiagnosis. Some cluster patients have had tooth extractions, sinus surgery, or psychiatric treatment in futile efforts to cure their pain.

Research studies have turned up several clues as to the cause of cluster headache, but no answers. One clue is found in the thermograms of untreated cluster patients, which show a "cold spot" of reduced blood flow above the eye.

The sudden start and brief duration of cluster headaches can make them difficult to treat; however, research scientists have identified several effective drugs for these headaches. The antimigraine drug ergotamine tartrate can subdue a cluster, if taken at the first sign of an attack. Injections of dihydroergotamine, a form of ergotamine tartrate, are sometimes used to treat clusters. Some cluster patients can prevent attacks by taking propranolol or methysergide. Investigators have also discovered that mild solutions of cocaine hydrochloride applied inside the nose can quickly stop cluster headaches in most patients. This treatment may work because it both blocks pain impulses and constricts blood vessels.

Another option that works for some cluster patients is rapid inhalation of pure oxygen through a mask for 5 to 15 minutes. The oxygen seems to ease the pain of cluster headache by reducing blood flow to the brain.

In chronic cases of cluster headache, certain facial nerves may be surgically cut or destroyed to provide relief. These procedures have had limited success. Some cluster patients have had facial nerves cut only to have them regenerate years later.

Painful Pressure

Chronic high blood pressure can cause headache, as can rapid rises in blood pressure like those experienced during anger, vigorous exercise, or sexual excitement.

The severe "orgasmic headache" occurs right before orgasm and is believed to be a vascular headache. Since sudden rupture of a cerebral blood vessel can occur, this type of headache should be evaluated by a doctor.

What Are Muscle-Contraction Headaches?

It's 5:00 p.m. and your boss has just asked you to prepare a 20-page briefing paper. Due date: tomorrow. You're angry and tired and the more you think about the assignment, the tenser you become. Your teeth clench, your brow wrinkles, and soon you have a splitting tension headache.

Tension headache is named not only for the role of stress in triggering the pain, but also for the contraction of neck, face, and scalp muscles brought on by stressful events. Tension headache is a severe but temporary form of muscle-contraction headache. The pain is mild to moderate and feels like pressure is being applied to the head or neck. The headache usually disappears after the period of stress is over. Ninety percent of all headaches are classified as tension/muscle contraction headaches.

By contrast, chronic muscle-contraction headaches can last for weeks, months, and sometimes years. The pain of these headaches is often described as a tight band around the head or a feeling that the head and neck are in a cast. "It feels like somebody is tightening a giant vise around my head," says one patient. The pain is steady, and is usually felt on both sides of the head. Chronic muscle-contraction headaches can cause sore scalps—even combing one's hair can be painful. Many scientists believe that the primary cause of the pain of muscle-contraction headache is sustained muscle tension. Other studies suggest that restricted blood flow may cause or contribute to the pain.

Occasionally, muscle-contraction headaches will be accompanied by nausea, vomiting, and blurred vision, but there is no preheadache syndrome as with migraine. Muscle-contraction headaches have not been linked to hormones or foods, as has migraine, nor is there a strong hereditary connection.

Research has shown that for many people, chronic muscle-contraction headaches are caused by depression and anxiety. These people tend to get their headaches in the early morning or evening when conflicts in the office or home are anticipated.

Emotional factors are not the only triggers of muscle-contraction headaches. Certain physical postures that tense head and neck muscles—such as holding one's chin down while reading—can lead to head and neck pain. So can prolonged writing under poor light, or holding a phone between the shoulder and ear, or even gum-chewing.

More serious problems that can cause muscle-contraction headaches include degenerative arthritis of the neck and temporomandibular joint dysfunction, or TMD. TMD is a disorder of the joint between the temporal bone (above the ear) and the mandible or lower jaw bone. The disorder results from poor bite and jaw clenching.

Treatment for muscle-contraction headache varies. The first consideration is to treat any specific disorder or disease that may be causing the headache. For example, arthritis of the neck is treated with anti-inflammatory medication and TMD may be helped by corrective devices for the mouth and jaw.

Acute tension headaches not associated with a disease are treated with analgesics like aspirin and acetaminophen. Stronger analgesics, such as propoxyphene and codeine, are sometimes prescribed. As prolonged use of these drugs can lead to dependence, patients taking them should have periodic medical checkups and follow their physicians' instructions carefully.

Nondrug therapy for chronic muscle-contraction headaches includes biofeedback, relaxation training, and counseling. A technique called cognitive restructuring teaches people to change their attitudes and responses to stress. Patients might be encouraged, for example, to imagine that they are coping successfully with a stressful situation. In progressive relaxation therapy, patients are taught to first tense and then relax individual muscle groups. Finally, the patient tries to relax his or her whole body. Many people imagine a peaceful scene—such as lying on the beach or by a beautiful lake. Passive relaxation does not involve tensing of muscles. Instead, patients are encouraged to focus on different muscles, suggesting that they relax. Some people might think to themselves, "Relax" or "My muscles feel warm."

People with chronic muscle-contraction headaches my also be helped by taking antidepressants or MAO inhibitors. Mixed muscle-contraction and migraine headaches are sometimes treated with barbiturate compounds, which slow down nerve function in the brain and spinal cord.

People who suffer infrequent muscle-contraction headaches may benefit from a hot shower or moist heat applied to the back of the neck. Cervical collars are sometimes recommended as an aid to good posture. Physical therapy, massage, and gentle exercise of the neck may also be helpful.

When Is Headache a Warning of a More Serious Condition?

Like other types of pain, headaches can serve as warning signals of more serious disorders. This is particularly true for headaches caused by traction or inflammation.

Traction headaches can occur if the pain-sensitive parts of the head are pulled, stretched, or displaced, as, for example, when eye muscles are tensed to compensate for eyestrain. Headaches caused by inflammation include those related to meningitis as well as those resulting from diseases of the sinuses, spine, neck, ears, and teeth. Ear and tooth infections and glaucoma can cause headaches. In oral and dental disorders, headache is experienced as pain in the entire head, including the face.

Traction and inflammatory headaches are treated by curing the underlying problem. This may involve surgery, antibiotics, or other drugs.

Characteristics of the various types of traction and inflammatory headaches vary by disorder:

- *Brain tumor.* Brain tumors are diagnosed in about 11,000 people every year. As they grow, these tumors sometimes cause headache by pushing on the outer layer of nerve tissue that covers the brain or by pressing against pain-sensitive blood vessel walls. Headache resulting from a brain tumor may be periodic or continuous. Typically, it feels like a strong pressure is being applied to the head. The pain is relieved when the tumor is treated by surgery, radiation, or chemotherapy.

- *Stroke.* Headache may accompany several conditions that can lead to stroke, including hypertension or high blood pressure, arteriosclerosis, and heart disease. Headaches are also associated with completed stroke, when brain cells die from lack of sufficient oxygen.

  Many stroke-related headaches can be prevented by careful management of the patient's condition through diet, exercise, and medication.

  Mild to moderate headaches are associated with transient ischemic attacks (TIA's), sometimes called "mini-strokes," which result from a temporary lack of blood supply to the brain. The head pain occurs near the clot or lesion that blocks blood flow.

The similarity between migraine and symptoms of TIA can cause problems in diagnosis. The rare person under age 40 who suffers a TIA may be misdiagnosed as having migraine; similarly, TIA-prone older patients who suffer migraine may be misdiagnosed as having stroke-related headaches.

- *Spinal tap.* About one-fourth of the people who undergo a lumbar puncture or spinal tap develop a headache. Many scientists believe these headaches result from leakage of the cerebrospinal fluid that flows through pain-sensitive membranes around the brain and down to the spinal cord. The fluid, they suggest, drains through the tiny hole created by the spinal tap needle, causing the membranes to rub painfully against the bony skull. Since headache pain occurs only when the patient stands up, the "cure" is to remain lying down until the headache runs its course—anywhere from a few hours to several days.

- *Head trauma.* Headaches may develop after a blow to the head, either immediately or months later. There is little relationship between the severity of the trauma and the intensity of headache pain. One cause of trauma headache is scar formation in the scalp. Another is ruptured blood vessels which result in an accumulation of blood called a hematoma. This mass of blood can displace brain tissue and cause headaches as well as weakness, confusion, memory loss, and seizures. Hematomas can be drained to produce rapid relief of symptoms.

- *Arteritis and meningitis.* Arteritis, an inflammation of certain arteries in the head, primarily affects people over age 50. Symptoms include throbbing headache, fever, and loss of appetite. Some patients experience blurring or loss of vision. Prompt treatment with corticosteroid drugs helps to relieve symptoms.

  Headaches are also caused by infections of meninges, the brain's outer covering, and phlebitis, a vein inflammation.

- *Trigeminal neuralgia.* Trigeminal neuralgia, or tic douloureux, results from a disorder of the trigeminal nerve. This nerve supplies the face, teeth, mouth, and nasal cavity with feeling and also enables the mouth muscles to chew. Symptoms are headache and intense facial pain that comes in short, excruciating jabs set off by the slightest touch to or movement of trigger

19

points in the face or mouth. People with trigeminal neuralgia often fear brushing their teeth or chewing on the side of the mouth that is affected. Many trigeminal neuralgia patients are controlled with drugs, including carbamazepine. Patients who do not respond to drugs may be helped by surgery on the trigeminal nerve.

- *Sinus infection.* In a condition called acute sinusitis, a viral or bacterial infection of the upper respiratory tract spreads to the membrane which lines the sinus cavities. When one or more of these cavities are filled with bacterial or viral fluid, they become inflamed, causing pain and sometimes headache. Treatment of acute sinusitis includes antibiotics, analgesics, and decongestants. Chronic sinusitis may be caused by an allergy to such irritants as dust, ragweed, animal hair, and smoke. Research scientists disagree about whether chronic sinusitis triggers headache.

What Causes Headache in Children?

Like adults, children experience the infections, trauma, and stresses that can lead to headaches. In fact, research shows that as young people enter adolescence and encounter the stresses of puberty and secondary school, the frequency of headache increases.

Migraine headaches often begin in childhood or adolescence. According to recent surveys, as many as half of all schoolchildren experience some type of headache.

Children with migraine often have nausea and excessive vomiting. Some children have periodic vomiting, but no headache—the so-called abdominal migraine. Research scientists have found that these children usually develop headaches when they are older.

Physicians have many drugs to treat migraine in children. Different classes that may be tried include analgesics, antiemetics, anticonvulsants, beta-blockers, and sedatives. A diet may also be prescribed to protect the child from foods that trigger headache. Sometimes psychological counseling or even psychiatric treatment for the child and the parents is recommended.

Childhood headache can be a sign of depression. Parents should alert the family pediatrician if a child develops headaches along with other symptoms such as a change in mood or sleep habits. Antidepressant medication and psychotherapy are effective treatments for childhood depression and related headache.

Conclusion

If you suffer from headaches and none of the standard treatments help, do not despair. Some people find that their headaches disappear once they deal with a troubled marriage, pass their certifying board exams, or resolve some other stressful problem. Others find that if they control their psychological reaction to stress, the headaches disappear.

"I had migraines for several years," says one woman, "and then they went away. I think it was because I lowered my personal goals in life. Today, even though I have 100 things to do at night, I don't worry about it. I learned to say no."

Information Resources

The National Institute of Neurological Disorders and Stroke, a component of the National Institutes of Health, is the leading Federal supporter of research on disorders of the brain and nervous system. The Institute also sponsors an active public information program and can answer questions about diagnosis, treatment, and research related to headache.

For information on neurological disorders or research programs funded by the National Institute of Neurological Disorders and Stroke, contact:

National Institute of Neurological Disorders and Stroke (NINDS)
6001 Executive Boulevard Suite 3309
Bethesda, MD 20892- 9531
Tel: 800-352-9424
Internet: http://www.ninds.nih.gov

Private voluntary organizations that offer information and services to those affected by headache include the following:

American Council for Headache Education (ACHE)
19 Mantua Road
Mt. Royal, NJ 08061
Toll Free: 800-255-2243
Tel: 856-423-0258
Fax: 856-423-0082
Internet: http://www.achenet.org
E-Mail: achehq@talley.com

This organization is a nonprofit patient/health professional partnership dedicated to advancing treatment and management of headache and to raising the public awareness of headache as a valid, biologically based illness. ACHE offers headache brochures, a quarterly newsletter, the book *Migraine: The Complete Guide*, assistance through in-person support groups, and support via the Internet and commercial on-line service providers.

National Headache Foundation
428 W. St. James Place
2nd Floor
Chicago, IL 60614-2750
Toll Free: 888-843-2256
Tel: 773-388-6399
Internet: http://www.headaches.org
The foundation promotes research and public education, publishes a newsletter, and offers many publications including a state-by-state list of physician members, a headache chart, a handbook, brochures, and fact sheets.

Chapter 2

Frequently Asked Questions about Headaches

General Information about Headaches

What exactly is a headache?

Headache is a general term used to describe a variety of painful conditions of the head. The symptoms and causes vary widely. Some relate directly to problems within the brain, while others may be due to conditions affecting other parts of the body. However, they can be divided in several general categories:

- *Tension:* the most common form of headache, it is presumed to be due to prolonged contraction of facial, scalp, jaw, and neck muscles. Pain is typically widespread, often involving most of the head. It is often worst in the forehead area and at the base of the skull. Pain is usually described as steady and "tight." It tends to be less severe than other kinds of headaches, but it can be persistent, sometimes lasting for days at a time.

- *Migraine:* a common but poorly understood kind of headaches. It affects women three times as often as men, although it can affect either sex. It is frequently hereditary; many patients with migraines have relatives who are also affected. It is believed that migraines are triggered by abnormal activity within the brain. Migraines are extremely variable in character. However,

"Frequently Asked Questions about Headaches," by David A. Cooke, M.D. © 2001 Omnigraphics, Inc.

they are typically more severe than other types of headache, and may be disabling. Pain is frequently limited to one side of the head, although it need not be. Light and noise is often painful to someone suffering a migraine. Nausea and vomiting is common. Pain is often described as throbbing, pounding, or pulsating. Patients are usually most comfortable lying down in a dark, quiet room during the headache. Some patients may have a warning that they are about to develop a headache, often taking the form of visual disturbances. Migraines usually last for hours, and often resolve with sleep. Occasionally, they may last for days.

- *Cluster:* a less common form of headache. In contrast to migraines, patients with cluster headaches are overwhelmingly likely to be male. These are some of the most severe and intense headaches known. Typically, they will affect one side of the head, with pain centering behind one eye. Frequently, the patient will develop eye redness and have a runny nose on the same side as the pain. These are usually completely disabling, and patients may describe it as though "an ice pick" is being driven into their eye. The headaches are extraordinarily severe, but tend to be short-lived, rarely lasting more than an hour. Interestingly, patients with clusters tend to have the headache occur at the same time of day for several days or weeks at a time. They will then resolve, and may not recur for months or years.

- *Sinus:* headache presumed to be due to congestion and pressure within the sinus cavities of the head. These headaches are usually associated with nasal stuffiness and drainage, such as that occurs with a cold or allergies. Decongestants are usually effective at relieving this kind of headache.

- *Hangover:* a headache related to overindulgence in alcohol. It usually occurs several hours after heavy alcohol consumption, often the following morning. It is often accompanied by a feeling of head fullness and mental clouding. The exact cause is not clear, but is believed to be due to the build-up of byproducts of alcohol metabolism. While "hangover remedies" abound, the most reliable cure for this kind of headache is time.

- *Illness-Related:* almost any illness can be accompanied by headache. This is most often seen during infections and fever. In this case, the headache is believed to be due to the release of substances from active immune cells. These chemicals serve as messengers between different portions of the immune system, and enhance the body's ability to fight infection. However, they also may cause generalized headache, as well as fatigue and muscle soreness.

Are premenstrual headaches different from regular headaches?

Some women tend to get headaches that seem to relate to their menstrual cycle. Usually, they occur during the week before the menstrual period, but some women get them during or even after their periods. They tend to follow a consistent pattern for a given woman.

Such headaches usually relate to the changes in hormone levels that occur during the menstrual cycle. Female hormones such as estrogen and progesterone have effects on the brain and blood vessels, and in some women, this leads to headaches. The majority of such headaches are considered migraine headaches.

How are children's headaches different from adult headaches?

Most of the general headache types that affect adults can also affect children, including migraine headaches. However, they are generally less frequent than adult headaches. A child who has recurrent headaches should probably be seen by a doctor.

Children who get headaches may take medications to relieve them, similar to adults. However, aspirin should not be used to treat headaches in children under twelve years of age. A rare, but often fatal, condition called Reye's Syndrome has been associated with aspirin use in children. Acetaminophen and ibuprofen are generally safer choices.

Can Temporomandibular Joint (TMJ) disorders cause headaches?

Absolutely. TMJ disorders involve excessive stresses on the temporomandibular joint, which is located at the jaw hinge, just in front of the ears. This frequently results in tension-type headaches and pain with chewing, most often on the sides of the head. When these types of headaches occur, referral to a dentist specializing in TMJ disorders is usually necessary.

When should I see a doctor about my headaches?

Virtually everyone gets at least an occasional headache. This is normal, and usually relates to activities and/or illness. However, there are some headaches that require medical attention. Such headaches could be a sign of serious illness, and need more evaluation.

In general, frequent headaches warrant a visit to the doctor. If the cause isn't known, it should be investigated. If the cause is known, changes in treatment should probably be made.

Some examples of headaches that you should see your doctor about include:

- Persistent headaches
- Recurrent severe headaches, when a diagnosis hasn't been established.
- Frequent migraine headaches, occurring more than twice per month.
- Recurrent headaches associated with visual changes, loss or strength, or changes in sensation in one part of the body.
- Headaches which are disabling.

There are also headaches that require emergency assessments. These are discussed in the next section.

When is a headache a medical emergency?

Any patient who is having "the worst headache of my life" needs prompt medical attention. An extraordinarily severe headache, especially if sudden in onset, may be a sign of bleeding in the brain or an impending stroke. If associated with fever or stiff neck, this may also be a sign of meningitis. Such patients should be taken to the nearest emergency immediately, as this can be a life-threatening emergency.

Headache associated with vision changes, weakness in one or more portions of the body, or local sensory changes should be evaluated, if this is the first time this has occurred. While migraine headaches can cause these types of symptoms, any patient with these changes should seek immediate care unless they have an established pattern of similar changes with headaches.

A prolonged, incapacitating headache should be treated in an emergency room if other measures have failed. The vast majority of headaches can be successfully treated at home or in a doctor's office, and most will eventually resolve on their own. However, there is little point to allowing a patient to suffer for long periods of time. Generally speaking, a severe headache that lasts more than twelve hours and has not responded to usual measures should be treated urgently.

Causes of Headaches

Do emotions cause headaches?

Sometimes. Emotional stress may lead to muscle contraction, resulting in a tension headache. Prolonged crying may cause sinus congestion and pressure, leading to a sinus headache. Some individuals with migraine headaches may find that emotional upset can trigger their headaches. Headaches are typically more frequent and severe in patients who suffer from depression. Treating depression may cause improvement in headaches.

Do allergies cause headaches?

Sometimes. Most often, people with moderate to severe respiratory allergies may develop sinus headaches as a result of sinus congestion. Prescription nasal steroid sprays, antihistamines, and decongestants often help.

Do changes in the weather cause headaches?

Sometimes. Certain people appear to be able to sense changes in barometric pressure, presumably via their sinus cavity membranes. Some individuals may get headaches from this, particularly those with a history of sinus problems.

Can exposure to fragrances cause headaches?

Certain fragrances may trigger migraine headaches in susceptible individuals.

Can the air quality in my office be giving me a headache?

Possibly. People with respiratory allergies may develop sinus headaches if their work environment contains large amounts of substances that they are allergic to. Certain industrial chemical fumes can also cause headaches. Typically, patients with this problem will notice that they get headaches during the week, which resolve over weekends, vacations, and holidays, and recur after one or two days back at work.

Can using a computer give me a headache?

Prolonged computer use is a common cause of headaches. There are several reasons for this. Computer use involves looking at a screen at a short distance from the eyes, forcing the eyes to strain to remain focused. Most computer monitors also have some degree of flicker, which adds to the strain. These factors may lead to excessive strain on the eye muscles, which may produce a tension-type headache. Similar headaches may also result from prolonged reading of a book or newspaper.

There are ways to prevent this. One is good lighting. For generations, mothers have warned their children that reading in poor light will damage your eyesight. It won't, but it will make you more likely to get an eyestrain headache. Bright, but not brilliant, lighting reduces the stress on the eye muscles. Taking breaks from prolonged computer use is also important. Taking a minute to look away from the monitor at more distant objects will help prevent eye muscle spasms. Finally, make sure that the monitor is properly positioned. A monitor should not require you to have to look up or down, and should be no closer than 18 inches from your face.

Can some foods cause a headache?

Certain individuals may find that particular foods trigger a headache. This is most commonly true of migraine headaches. Common offenders include wine, alcohol, cheese, and chocolate. The exact reason for this is not known. However, this is highly variable from person to person. Some people may have well-defined headache triggers, while others may not have any identifiable triggers at all. Being aware of common causative foods may be helpful in finding patterns to headaches. However, if a given food does not reliably trigger your headaches, there is no reason to avoid it.

MSG (monosodium glutamate) is a special case. MSG is a commonly used flavor enhancer, especially in Chinese restaurants. While the majority of people have no reaction whatsoever to MSG, certain individuals develop a syndrome of severe, migraine-like headache, flushing, fatigue, and weakness after ingesting it. The cause is not known. Avoidance is the best strategy for people with a past history of MSG sensitivity.

Why does eating ice cream too fast cause a headache?

No one really knows. The diagnosis of "ice cream headache" is a real one, and has been long described in the medical literature. Some believe that rapid cooling of blood in the mouth causes spasm of blood vessels in the head, causing headache.

Headache Treatments

Does ice help? Does heat help?

Some people find either of these remedies helpful. Response is not consistent, but there is no harm in using either if it seems to help.

What is the "best" over-the-counter headache medicine?

Millions of dollars are spent each year by manufacturers of headache remedies to try to convince the public that their product is superior. Scientifically, at least, the answer is less clear. It appears that most over-the-counter (OTC) headache medications do work well. Certain medications will work better for some people than others. However, this isn't consistent from one person to another. For example, one person may find aspirin extremely effective, while another finds acetaminophen to be the only medication that works. As a general rule, the group of medications known as nonsteroidal anti-inflammatory drugs (NSAID's), which includes ibuprofen, naproxen, and ketoprofen, are slightly more effective than acetaminophen as pain relievers. Aspirin tends to be intermediate between the two. However, past experience is probably the best guide when looking for a headache medicine, not advertising.

Are prescription-strength headache medicines available?

Yes. A wide variety of medications for headaches are available by prescription. Most OTC headache remedies are available by prescription in higher doses. A number of additional NSAID's not available OTC are also available by prescription. There are a variety of medications specifically for treating migraine headaches which may be used. Finally, for the most severe, resistant headaches, narcotics are sometimes prescribed.

Why is caffeine used in some headache medications?

Certain types of headaches, particularly migraine headaches, cause temporary changes in stomach function. In some cases, the stomach essentially shuts down during the headache, and ceases digestion. As a result, pills taken by mouth may sit in the stomach, and not reach the bloodstream for prolonged periods of time. Caffeine acts as a gastric stimulant, and improves absorption of headache medications in these situations. Thus, it is part of a number of common headache formulations. Other strategies to deal with this problem have been developed. Some pills are formulated to dissolve on the tongue. Other medications can be given as nasal sprays, rectal suppositories (a very efficient, if unappealing, method of drug delivery), or self-injection kits.

Chapter 3

Migraine Headaches

More than 28 million Americans suffer from migraine, striking three times more women than men. This vascular headache is most commonly experienced between the ages of 15 and 55, and 70% to 80% of sufferers have a family history of migraine.

Many factors can trigger migraine attacks such as alteration of sleep-wake cycle; missing or delaying a meal; medications that cause a swelling of the blood vessels; daily or near daily use of medications designed for relieving headache attacks; bright lights, sunlight, fluorescent lights, TV and movie viewing; certain foods; and excessive noise. Stress and/or underlying depression are important trigger factors that can be diagnosed and treated adequately.

Migraine characteristics include:

- Pain typically on one side of the head

Text in this chapter is from the following documents: "Migraine," © 2000 The National Headache Foundation. Used with permission from the National Headache Foundation. For more information on headache causes and treatments, call the National Headache Foundation at 1-888-NHF-5552 or visit the web site at www.headaches.org. "Migraine Update," National Institute of Neurological Disorders and Stroke (NINDS), 2000; "Migraine Headaches," National Women's Health Information Center (NWHIC), a service of the Office on Women's Health (OWH) in the Department of Health and Human Services (DHHS), 1998. And "Migraineur's Bill of Rights," © 2000 American Council for Headache Education (ACHE), reprinted from the web site of the American Council for Headache Education (http://www.achenet.org); reprinted with permission.

- Pain has a pulsating or throbbing quality
- Moderate to intense pain affecting daily activities
- Nausea or vomiting
- Sensitivity to light and sound
- Attacks last four to 72 hours, sometimes longer
- Visual disturbances or aura
- Exertion such as climbing stairs makes headache worse

Approximately one-fifth of migraine sufferers experience aura, the warning associated with migraine, prior to the headache pain. Visual disturbances such as wavy lines, dots or flashing lights and blind spots as well as disruptions in smell, taste or touch begin from twenty minutes to one hour before the actual onset of migraine. The origin of aura is not well understood. It has been thought to be due to constriction of small arterioles supplying specific areas of the brain. Others believe it to be due to transient changes in the activity of specific nerve cells.

The headache of migraine may have several different factors at play. These include alterations in platelet adhesiveness and release of serotonin, shifting of blood flow from the arteries to the veins through vessels known as "anastomoses" which direct blood flow away from the nutrient capillaries and changes in the function of the nerves of the trigeminal nerve centers and fibers in the brain and on the blood vessels causing local chemical changes that may play a role in inducing the pain of migraine as well as the non infective inflammation which may surround and involve the vessels of the brain during an attack.

Diagnosis of migraine headache is made by establishing the history of the migraine related symptoms and other headache characteristics as well as a family history of similar headaches. By definition in between the attacks of migraine the physical examination of a patient with migraine headache does not reveal any organic causes for the headaches. Tests such as the CT scan and MRI are useful to confirm the lack of organic causes for the headaches.

Treatment

Many factors may contribute to the occurrence of migraine attacks. These factors are known as trigger factors and may include diet, sleep, activity, psychological issues as well as many other factors. The use of a diary to record events that may play a role in causing the headaches can be useful for you and your doctor. Avoidance of identifiable trigger factors reduce the number of headaches a patient may experience. Healthful lifestyles including regular exercise and avoidance of nicotine may also enhance migraine management. Non-pharmacological techniques for control of migraine are helpful to some patients. These include biofeedback, physical medicine, and counseling. These as with most elements of migraine need to be individualized to the patient.

Abortive

Ergotamine preparations are available for oral, rectal or sublingual administration, and Dihydroergotamine (DHE) may be used for self-injection. A four-day hiatus between days of use must be maintained for the ergotamine preparations and DHE. This medication is also available as the nasal spray Migranal. A combination product containing isometheptene (Midrin®) may be used for those unable to tolerate the ergotamine preparations.

The use of the anti-inflammatory agents such as aspirin, naproxen sodium or ibuprofen may be effective for some migraines. These agents may have gastrointestinal side effects, which limit their use since larger than normal doses may be required to treat the migraine attack.

Sumatriptan (Imitrex®), a 5-HT agonist, is available in self-injectable, nasal spray and tablet forms. Other 5-HT agonists are naratriptan (Amerge®) and zolmitriptan (Zomig®). Both are available as tablets. Rizatriptan (Maxalt®) is the newest approved medication for migraine. The orally disintegrating tablet can be taken without water. It also comes in regular tablet form.

Some attacks may not be eliminated by abortive therapy, yet the patient requires pain-relieving measures. Due to the severity of the headaches, some patients may require a narcotic analgesic, but if the patient is experiencing frequent migraine attacks habituating analgesics should be avoided.

Butorphanol (Stadol®) is available for intranasal administration and is not typically associated with dependency problems, but may result in dependency if used regularly for pain relief.

Alternative medical treatments with medications belonging to the group known as the Phenothiazines have proven useful as non-analgesic alternatives for treating severe migraine headaches. Patients with prolonged migraine attacks lasting more than 24 hours are experiencing status migraine, and corticosteroids may be used in these cases due to their anti-inflammatory effects.

The FDA has approved three over-the-counter products to treat migraine. Excedrin® Migraine (a combination of aspirin, acetaminophen and caffeine) is indicated for migraine and its associated symptoms. Advil® Migraine and Motrin® Migraine Pain, both ibuprofen medications, are approved to treat migraine headache and its pain.

Preventive

If patients have frequent migraine attacks, if the attacks do not respond consistently to migraine specific acute treatments, if the migraine specific medications are ineffective or contraindicated because of other medical problems, then preventative medications should be given to reduce the migraine frequency and improve the response to the acute migraine medicines. Cost considerations also may lead to increased use of preventative medications, this is an important consideration in this age of cost effective medicine.

The Food and Drug Administration (FDA) has approved four drugs for migraine prevention. These include methysergide, propranolol, timolol and divalproex sodium. These have had many years of use and make up the majority of the items considered "first line" therapy for migraine prevention. Methysergide should be reserved for special situations because of the problems it may have with the kidneys. Amitryptyline, which is an anti-depressant, may also be very effective as a migraine preventative. All migraine preventative medications require that adequate doses of the medicine be given for a sufficient length of time to determine the effectiveness. Titration of the does may be needed to reduce adverse effects to medicines.

There are a host of alternative choices for patients whose headaches do not respond to the first line medications. These include calcium channel blockers, NSAIDs, a variety of anti-depressants and several miscellaneous medications.

Biofeedback

As an alternative to drug therapy, this training uses special equipment that monitors physical tension to teach the patient how to control the physical processes that are related to stress. Once familiar with this technique, people can use it, without the monitoring equipment, to stop an attack or reduce its effects. Self-hypnosis exercises are also taught to control both muscle contraction and the swelling of blood vessels. This patient-directed therapy, with the clinician serving as a guide or teacher, should be practiced daily. Children have an excellent response to biofeedback training, since they are open to new methods, learn quickly and have not become firmly entrenched in a chronic pain pattern.

Migraine Update

Despite the fact that 1 in 4 households in the United States have someone affected by migraine headaches, migraine is still not considered by many employers and insurers to be a legitimate medical problem. Migraine, however, can cause significant disability and costs the American taxpayers $13 billion in missed work or reduced productivity annually.

On June 8-9, 2000, leading migraine experts from around the world gathered together in Bethesda, Maryland for 21st Century Prevention and Management of Migraine Headaches, a scientific meeting designed to develop practice guidelines for migraine management. The National Institute of Neurological Disorders and Stroke presented the meeting in cooperation with the American Academy of Neurology, the American Headache Society, and the National Headache Foundation. Thomas Jefferson University, Philadelphia, and Gardiner-Caldwell SynerMed jointly sponsored the program.

For many years, scientists believed that migraines were linked to the dilation and constriction of blood vessels in the head. Investigators now believe that migraine is caused by inherited abnormalities in certain cell populations in the brain. Using new imaging technologies, scientists can see changes in the brain during migraine attacks. Scientists believe that there is a migraine pain center located in the brainstem, a region at the base of the brain. As neurons fire, surrounding blood vessels dilate and become inflamed, causing the characteristic pain of a migraine. In order to keep this process in check, prompt treatment is of the essence.

What causes migraine? Though the causes are not precisely known, it is clear that migraine is a genetic disorder. For some forms of migraine, specific abnormal genes have been identified. People with migraine have an enduring predisposition to attacks triggered by a range of factors.

What triggers migraine? Lack of food or sleep, exposure to light, or hormonal irregularities in women, can set off a migraine attack in individuals with the disorder. Anxiety, stress or relaxation after stress, and fatigue are also triggers.

Medications for migraine may be taken on a daily basis to prevent attacks. Some medications developed for epilepsy and depression may prove to be effective treatment options. Medicines can also be used to relieve pain and restore function during attacks. The most promising of these are drugs called triptans. For some women suffering from migraines, hormone therapy may help. Stress management strategies, such as exercise, relaxation, biofeedback and other therapies designed to help limit discomfort, may also have a place in the migraine treatment arsenal.

Some Frequently Asked Questions

How do migraine headaches differ from tension headaches?

Tension headaches are usually described as a continuous pressure pain or tightness of varying severity over the entire head, whereas migraine headaches are a severe, throbbing pain over one or both temples, or behind one eye or ear, and are often accompanied by nausea and vomiting. A migraine often starts on waking up in the morning, but can occur later in the day and can last hours to one or two days. In individuals with a form of migraine called classic migraine, visual symptoms described as blurriness, dazzling zigzag lines, blind spots or sensitivity to light occur just before and sometimes during the headache. While fatigue and stress can sometimes bring on both tension and migraine headaches, bright lights, noise and alcohol are specific factors that can trigger a migraine.

Are women more prone to migraine headaches?

Yes. In fact, 20 million women in the U.S. suffer from headaches; 9 million of whom suffer debilitating migraines. Over a quarter of women are affected by migraines during their life. Although these headaches are common among both men and women, there are important differences. The prevalence of migraine is 2-3 times higher in women. The character of the headaches also differs. Women tend to report higher levels of pain, longer duration of headaches, and more associated symptoms, such as nausea and vomiting. Visual symptoms are also less common in women.

There is a long recognized association between ovarian hormones and migraine. Over half of women with migraine report an association between their headaches and their menstrual cycle. The frequency and severity of migraine is increased commonly with the use of oral contraceptive pills and during the menopause. In addition, changes in the levels of ovarian hormones and prolactin during pregnancy and breast-feeding may modify the course of a migraine. A better understanding of these changes is leading to better treatment of migraine.

How do you treat a migraine at home?

Sometimes at the onset of a migraine, lying down in a dark room with a cold compress can bring relief, along with over-the-counter drugs including acetaminophen or aspirin with caffeine. You may want to talk with your doctor about ways to prevent future migraines.

What if home remedies don't work?

Women with moderate migraines may need prescription drugs for relief. These could include agents that affect neurotransmitters (the chemicals that are the messengers in the brain) such as sumatriptin and various antidepressants. Other drugs might include agents that dilate blood vessels in the brain. In some cases, doctors prescribe painkillers.

Some drugs can be given intranasally, through a transdermal patch (on the skin), oxygen inhalation, and laser therapy to the maxillary nerve.

Because migraine is affected by hormonal fluctuation, estrogen use during the premenstrual period is sometimes helpful. However, ironically, estrogen may also trigger migraines. Women should discuss with their physicians use of estrogen such as oral contraceptives and hormonal therapy for migraines.

To help your doctor find the right treatment for you, keeping a "headache calendar" is important, documenting the time of day, point in your menstrual cycle, your location (at work, at home, at the park, etc.) and your activity when the migraine started.

Is there anything I can do to prevent a migraine?

Because stress often triggers migraines, women who are habitual sufferers should learn relaxation and stress management techniques. These are especially helpful in aborting headaches when warning signs are felt. Massage, relaxation exercises of the neck, shoulder, and jaw muscles may all be helpful. Rest in a dark room with cool compresses can prevent the headache. Foods such as alcohol, aged cheeses, chocolate, fermented or marinated foods, MSG, artificial sweeteners such as aspartame, and caffeine all may trigger headaches; diet should be monitored to reduce or eliminate intake of these. Nicotine may cause migraine—yet another good reason to give up smoking! In summary, each woman's migraine pain, her triggers, and her "headache calendar" (when headaches tend to occur) are unique. Treatments are also unique for each case. Women need to consider their individual triggers, lifestyle issues such as stress level and eating habits, and their own preferences for medication as they and their physicians choose treatments.

Migraineur's Bill of Rights

1. I have a right to be taken seriously by my physician when I go for treatment of my headaches.

2. I have a right to complete and thorough medical examination, including a medical history and complete neurological evaluation.

3. I have a right to appropriate diagnostic testing, including neuro-diagnostics, CT scans and MRI scans, if necessary, when my headache is first evaluated, and when the headache pattern or severity changes.

4. I have the right to be referred to a specialist—for example, a neurologist, a headache specialist, or a headache clinic if my headaches do not respond to my primary physician's treatment, or if my primary physician feels a specialist's care is needed.

5. I have the right to receive specific headache therapy, if needed, instead of non-prescription drugs, narcotics, or combination analgesics that may increase the problem.

6. I have the right to ask for a comprehensive, written treatment plan that will tell me exactly how to use my preventive medications and non-drug preventives and, complete instructions on what to do when a headache occurs.

7. I have the right to return for additional help whenever my treatment plan seems to be inadequate to control my headache.

8. I have the right to be treated courteously and responsibly in emergency room, if a severe headache fails to respond to my usual treatment plan.

9. I have the right to expect my insurance company to recognize migraine as a legitimate medical illness as any other illness such as diabetes, arthritis, etc.

10. I have the right to expect those around me—family, friends, co-workers, and others who come in contact with me to make an effort to understand my illness and to cooperate with me in my efforts to live a full, rich life.

Note: "The Migraineur's Bill of Rights" is reprinted with permission from the web site of the American Council for Headache Education (www.achenet.org).

Chapter 4

Tension-Type Headaches

Tension-type headache is a nonspecific headache, which is not vascular or migrainous, and is not related to organic disease. The most common form of headache, it is caused by muscle tightening in the back of the neck and/or scalp. There are two general classifications of tension-type headache, episodic and chronic, differentiated by frequency and severity of symptoms. Both are characterized as dull, aching and non-pulsating and affect both sides of the head.

Symptoms for both types are similar and may include:

- Muscles between head and neck contract
- A tightening band-like sensation around the neck and/or head which is a "vice-like" ache
- Pain primarily occurs in the forehead, temples or the back on head and/or neck

Episodic

Episodic tension-type headache occurs randomly and is usually triggered by temporary stress, anxiety, fatigue or anger. They are what

Text in this chapter is from the following documents: "Tension-Type Headache," © 2000 The National Headache Foundation. Used with permission from the National Headache Foundation. For more information on headache causes and treatments, call the National Headache Foundation at 1-888-NHF-5552 or visit the web site at www.headaches.org. And, "Tension-Type Headache," © 2000 Beth Israel Medical Center; reprinted with permission. More information is available online at http://www.StopPain.org.

most of us consider "stress headaches." It may disappear with the use of over-the-counter analgesics, withdrawal from the source of stress or a relatively brief period of relaxation.

For this type of headache, over-the-counter drugs of choice are aspirin, acetaminophen, ibuprofen or naproxen sodium. Combination products with caffeine can enhance the action of the analgesics.

Chronic

Chronic tension-type headache is a daily or continuous headache, which may have some variability in the intensity of the pain during a 24-hour cycle. It is always present. If a sufferer is taking medication daily or almost daily and is receiving little or no relief from the pain, then a physician should be seen for diagnosis and treatment.

The primary drug of choice for chronic tension-type headache is amitriptyline or some of the other tricyclic antidepressants. Antidepressant drugs have analgesic actions, which can provide relief for headache sufferers. Although a patient may not be depressed, these drugs may be beneficial. Selecting an antidepressant is based on the presence of a sleep disturbance. Other classes of antidepressants may be effective but have not been as thoroughly studied as the tricyclic compounds.

The use of propranolol is sometimes helpful as a singular drug, particularly when there is a mild chronic anxiety state. Biofeedback techniques can also be helpful in treating tension-type headaches.

For the patient with chronic tension-type headaches, habituating analgesics must be strictly avoided.

Chronic tension-type headache can also be the result of either anxiety or depression. Changes in sleep patterns or insomnia, early morning or late day occurrence of headache, feelings or guilt, weight loss, dizziness, poor concentration, ongoing fatigue and nausea commonly occur. One should seek professional diagnosis for proper treatment if these symptoms exist.

The Diagnosis of Tension-Type Headache

The diagnosis of a tension-type headache is only based upon the patient's description of the headache along with a normal neurological examination. The International Headache Society (IHS) criteria include:

1. At least 10 previous attacks that fulfill Items 2-4 following.

2. Headache attacks last 30 minutes to 7 days (untreated or unsuccessfully treated)

3. At least two of the following:

   - bilateral (both sides of the head)

   - pressing/tightening quality

   - mild or moderate intensity (may inhibit but does not prohibit activities) not made worse by walking stairs or similar routine physical activity

4. During headache, both of the following:

   - no nausea or vomiting

   - photophobia (sensitivity to light) and phonophobia (sensitivity to sound) are absent, or one but not the other is present

5. History, physical and neurologic examination do not suggest a brain tumor, infection, or blood vessel abnormality (very rare)

Although neurological examination is normal, the majority of patients with tension-type headache have tight muscles in their temples, neck and shoulders. Some have poor movement of the neck.

The Causes of Tension-Type Headache

The causes of tension-type headache are controversial. Prior to 1998, when the International Headache Society's (IHS) new classification schema was developed, this headache syndrome was called muscle contraction headache because most experts believed that the underlying cause of this headache was tight and spastic muscles in the shoulders, neck, and head. Today some experts continue to believe that muscle spasm causes the pain, but others believe that brain chemicals and stress/psychological problems may also play a role. Importantly, the name tension-type headache does not imply that the headache is thought to be due to primarily a psychological problem.

Tension-type headache is much more common than migraine headache. It is thought that up to 60-70% of people suffer from a tension-type headache every year.

All tests are normal in tension-type headache. Like migraine, there is no reason to have a brain MRI or CT scan if the history and examination are consistent with uncomplicated tension-type headache.

Drug Therapy

Drug therapy is often recommended for tension-type headache. Drugs for headache are divided into two types:

- abortive/symptomatic medications

- prophylactic medications

Unlike migraine headache, however, many patients with tension-type headache do not experience excellent pain relief from drugs. For these patients, non-drug therapy may be more important.

Abortive/symptomatic medications are those drugs that are taken at the onset or during a headache attack in the hopes of stopping the headache from occurring or decreasing associated symptoms. When prescribing abortive/symptomatic medications, it is very important to remember the following points:

- Each patient is different; it is not possible to predict whether a particular person will respond favorably to a drug.

- If abortive/symptomatic medication is used excessively, the development of Rebound Headache Syndrome can result. (Rebound headache means headache that is actually worsened by the overuse of short-acting abortive medication). Some authorities recommend that a patient take no more than 10 doses of abortive/symptomatic headache medication per month. Others allow more but become very concerned when abortive/symptomatic drugs are needed more than a few times each week.

Abortive/symptomatic headache medications include:

- over-the-counter analgesics (such as aspirin, acetaminophen, ibuprofen, naproxen, etc.)

- prescription nonsteroidal anti-inflammatory drugs (such as diclofenac, ketorolac, etc.)

- barbiturates (such as butalbital)

- ergots (such as ergotamine or dihydroergotamine)

- antiemetics (such as prochlorperazine)

- "muscle relaxants" (such as Flexeril, Soma, etc.). (Note that these drugs do not actually relax skeletal muscles directly, but rather are analgesic [pain-relieving] drugs that act on a patient's brain.)

- opioids (such as meperidine, morphine, etc.)

Prophylactic headache medications are those drugs that are taken every day, regardless of whether a headache is being experienced, in the hopes of preventing headache attacks. These daily medications should only be prescribed when patients have frequent headaches (e.g., three or more times per month) that are significantly interfering with quality of life.

When prescribing prophylactic headache medication, it is very important to remember the following points:

- every tension-type headache patient is different; response to a drug cannot be predicted

- only one drug should be prescribed at a time

- most drugs should have careful dose adjustment. The first dose is relatively low, and the dose is gradually increased if a headache occurs and if no intolerable side effects are experienced by the patient.

Prophylactic medications for tension-type headache include:

- antidepressants (such as amitriptyline, nortriptyline, desipramine, doxepin, venlafaxine, etc.) These drugs act on headache independent of their effects on depression. They typically work for headache at lower doses than are needed to treat affective disorders; the tricyclic antidepressant drugs also may improve sleep, which is often disturbed in headache patients.

- alpha-2 adrenergic agonists (such as tizanidine)

- opioids

- some physicians try gabapentin for these headaches

Nondrug Therapy

Biofeedback

Many studies have shown biofeedback to be very effective treatment for tension-type headache.

Acupuncture

Some patients may obtain benefit from acupuncture.

Physical Therapy

Studies have shown that aerobic conditioning (getting in shape) can reduce the amount and intensity of tension-type headaches. Also, some patients find that techniques that may reduce the degree of muscle tension in the neck and shoulder musculature can reduce the frequency of headache; methods include trained stretching exercises, osteopathic manipulation, and craniosacral manipulation.

TENS (Transcutaneous Electrical Nerve Stimulation)

Some patients report that applying a transcutaneous nerve stimulation device on their neck and shoulder muscles helps with tension-type headache.

Stress Management

Many studies have found that stress is a common trigger for tension-type headache (in over 60% of patients). Techniques that help relieve stress, such as relaxation, imagery, and even yoga, have been shown in studies to be very effective.

Trigger Point Injections

Some patients report benefit from trigger point injections. A needle is inserted directly into a specific tender site within a muscle. A variety of trigger point injection techniques are used; some doctors just insert a needle, others inject local anesthetic (like Novocaine), and others inject a safe form of botulinum toxin.

Headache / Pain Clinic Treatment

Most often, tension-type headache patients can be successfully managed by one physician, without the need for a comprehensive pain clinic treatment. However, some patients with severe headaches that fail to respond to routine measures may need a multidisciplinary approach involving several headache specialists, which may be provided in headache and pain clinics.

Chapter 5

Cluster Headaches

Cluster headache refers to the characteristic grouping or clustering of attacks. Cluster headaches may also be known as histamine headache, red migraine, Horton's headache, cephalalgia or spenopalatine neuralgia. The headache periods can last several weeks or months, then disappear completely for months or years leaving considerable amounts of pain-free intervals between series.

Cluster is one of the least common types of headache, and the cause is unknown. It is vascular in nature, and the pain is caused by blood vessel swelling in the head. Although rare, it is possible for someone with cluster headache to also suffer from migraine headache.

Cluster headache starts suddenly, and a minimal type of warning of the oncoming headache may occur, including a feeling of discomfort or a mild one-sided burning sensation. The pain is of short duration, generally 30 to 45 minutes. However, the headache may last anywhere from a few minutes to several hours and will disappear only to recur later that day. Most sufferers get one to four headaches per day during a cluster period. They occur regularly, generally at the same time each day. Cluster headaches often awaken the sufferer in the early morning or during the night and have been called "alarm clock headaches."

Text in this chapter is from "Cluster Headache," © 2000 The National Headache Foundation. Used with permission from the National Headache Foundation. For more information on headache causes and treatments, call the National Headache Foundation at 1-888-NHF-5552 or visit the web site at www.headaches.org.

Typical cluster headache characteristics include:

- pain almost always one-sided

- pain remains on the same side during a series

- pain can occur on the opposite side when a new series starts

- pain is localized behind the eye or in the eye region and may radiate to the forehead, temple, nose, cheek or upper gum on the affected side

- the affected eye may become swollen or droop and the pupil may contract

- the nostril on the affected side of the head is often congested

- nasal discharge and tearing of the eye is on the same side as the pain

- excessive sweating

- face may become flushed on the affected side

Cluster headaches are not associated with the gastrointestinal disturbances or sensitivity to light that are found in other vascular headaches, such as migraine.

The pain of cluster headache is generally intense and severe and often described as a burning or piercing sensation. It may be throbbing or constant, the scalp may be tender and the arteries often can be felt increasing their pulsation. The pain is so intense that most sufferers cannot sit still and will often pace during an acute attack. Cluster headaches generally reach their full force within five or ten minutes after onset. The attacks are usually very similar, varying only slightly from one attack to another.

The cluster headache sufferer has considerable amounts of pain-free intervals between series. Sufferers are generally affected in the spring or autumn, and, due to their seasonal nature, cluster headaches are often mistakenly associated with allergies or business stress. The seasonal relationship is individual for each sufferer.

Substances that cause blood vessel swelling can provoke an acute attack during a series period. Nitroglycerin or histamine, smoking or minimal amounts of alcohol can precipitate or increase the severity of the attacks as the sufferer's blood vessels seem to change and become susceptible to the action of these substances. The blood vessels are not sensitive to these substances during headache-free periods.

Hormonal influences in women do not appear to be a factor in cluster headaches.

Some patients will note that the series of headaches are continuous, not separated by periods of remission. About 20% of cluster sufferers' attacks are chronic, occurring throughout the year, thus making the control of these headaches more difficult. These chronic cluster headaches vary from episodic cluster headaches as the periods are continuous, and the patients do not respond to conventional forms of cluster therapy.

Treatment

The patient with episodic cluster headaches should be started on prophylactic therapy as early as possible in the series in order to curtail the length of the cluster period and decrease the severity of the headaches. The agent of choice in cluster prophylaxis is methysergide (Sansert®). The corticosteroids are often used concomitantly with methysergide. These agents are slowly tapered and then discontinued as the headaches decrease and disappear. For patients with chronic cluster headaches, other agents may be employed such as lithium or calcium channel blockers. Histamine desensitization and surgical intervention may be considered for chronic cluster headache patients who have not responded to other forms of standard therapy.

Because of the brief duration of an acute cluster attack, the abortive treatment of these headaches is difficult. Often, the acute headache has disappeared before the patient arrives at the emergency department or physician's office to receive treatment. Oxygen inhalation by facial mask can be used at the first signs of a cluster attack and has been successful in aborting an acute cluster headache. The cluster patient may respond to ergotamine preparations, if used immediately at onset of symptoms. Some patients have gained some relief with the use of intranasal applications of a local anaesthetic agent, such as lidocaine. Sumatriptan (Imitrex®), a 5 HT agonist, is indicated for the abortive therapy of cluster headaches. It is available in injectable, nasal spray and tablet forms, although the latter is the least effective because of the time it takes before the onset of action. Any of these treatments should be used under the direction of a physician familiar with cluster headache therapy.

Chapter 6

Rebound Headaches

Symptoms

Symptoms of rebound headache include:

- daily or nearly daily headache

- pain on both sides of the head

- pressing/tightening quality ("like a tight belt around my head")

- perhaps a mild degree of photophobia (sensitivity to light) or phonophobia (sensitivity to sound)

- tight and tender neck and shoulder muscles

- the patient is regularly taking symptomatic/abortive pain medication

It is important to realize that Rebound Headache is a SYNDROME and is NOT one particular type of headache that a patient suffers.

Text in this chapter is from the following documents: "Rebound Headache," © 2000 Beth Israel Medical Center; reprinted with permission. More information is available online at http://www.StopPain.org. And, "Analgesic Rebound Headaches," © 2000 The National Headache Foundation. Used with permission from the National Headache Foundation. For more information on headache causes and treatments, call the National Headache Foundation at 1-888-NHF-5552 or visit the web site at www.headaches.org.

How to Make a Diagnosis of Rebound Headache

Rebound headache most often develops in a migraine patient. Typically, the migraine headaches gradually become more and more frequent over several months with a gradual change in the type of headache: The migraine headache happens less often and is replaced by a tension-type headache, which becomes a daily occurrence.

A common scenario in rebound headache patients is the following:

- for some reason (sometimes increased stress), the migraine worsens;

- the patient ingests more and more of their symptomatic/abortive migraine headache medication;

- eventually, the patient's medication becomes less and less effective;

- gradually, a daily or near daily tension-type headache develops often accompanied by periodic, severe migraine headache.

The Causes of Rebound Headache

Abnormalities in the body that cause rebound headache are not known. Up to 40-70% of patients seeking care at headache or pain clinics are thought to be suffering from this syndrome. It probably is a rather common problem, but it is under-recognized by doctors.

What Drugs Can Cause Rebound Headache?

Many headache specialists believe that any abortive/symptomatic headache medication can cause rebound headache; the most common culprits are actually the over-the-counter medications!

What Is Too Much Symptomatic/Abortive Medication?

The number of times a person with a history of migraine can ingest symptomatic/abortive medication is not clear. Many authorities now suggest that migraine patients take no more than a total of 10 doses of symptomatic/abortive medication per month. Others allow more but become concerned about rebound when abortive therapy is needed more than a few times per week.

Analgesic Rebound Headaches

Analgesic agents are prescription or over-the-counter medications used to control pain including migraine and other types of headaches. When used on a daily or near daily basis, these analgesics can perpetuate the headache process. They may decrease the intensity of the pain for a few hours; however they appear to feed into the pain system in such a way that chronic headaches may result. If under these circumstances the patient does not completely stop using these analgesics, despite any other treatment undertaken, the chronic headache is likely to continue unabated.

Usually when analgesics are discontinued the headache may get worse for several days and the sufferer may experience nausea or vomiting. However, after a period of three to five days, sometimes longer, these symptoms begin to improve. For those patients willing to persevere, the headaches will gradually improve as response to more appropriate medication occurs. Most patients are able to stop he use of analgesics at home under physician supervision, but some find in difficult and may require hospitalization, as many suffers have been using analgesics several times a day for many years.

Treatments for Rebound Headache

Stop the Culprit Drug

If patients with rebound headache stop taking the drug(s) that are causing the syndrome, in 4-8 weeks 80% note dramatic improvement—without doing anything else! However, for many patients, the initial few weeks may result in a worsening of their headache.

If the culprit medication is not stopped, additional treatments often will have very limited benefit. Studies have shown that a prophylactic headache medication often will not have a beneficial anti-headache effect when given to a patient that is rebounding. Therefore, when a rebound headache patient tells the doctor that he/she "has tried every headache medication known to man," more likely than not the prophylactic medications were prescribed while the patient was in the rebound cycle, and thus the drugs were not given an adequate drug trial.

Prophylactic Headache Medication

In addition to stopping the symptomatic/abortive drugs, some patients may benefit from addition of a prophylactic medication, such as an antidepressant.

Stress Management

An important element in treating rebound headache is helping the patient rid him/herself of the knee-jerk reaction to take a medication at the first sign of head pain. Techniques such as relaxation, imagery, and biofeedback can be helpful.

Biofeedback

Biofeedback may be an effective treatment for rebound headache.

Physical Therapy

Aerobic conditioning, neck and shoulder muscle stretches, craniosacral manipulation, and massage may help.

Headache/Pain Clinic Treatment

Rebound headache patients are often difficult to treat and require a multidisciplinary approach, including strict medication management, stress management training, and physical therapy modalities, all of which can be provided in a headache or pain clinic.

Chapter 7

Other Causes of Headache Pain

Abdominal Migraine

Abdominal migraine is one of the variants of migraine headache. It is also known by other terms including "periodic syndrome." This variant most typically occurs in children. They usually have a family history of migraine and go on to develop typical migraine later in their life.

The attacks are characterized by periodic bouts of abdominal pain lasting for about two hours. Along with the abdominal pain they may have other symptoms such as nausea and vomiting, flushing or pallor. Tests fail to reveal a cause for the pain. Occasionally there may be EEG findings suggestive of epilepsy but this is rarely related to seizures. Medications that are useful for treating migraine work to control these attacks in most children.

Information in this chapter is from "Abdominal Migriane," "Alcohol and Headaches," "Early Morning Awakening Headache," "Epilepsy," "Exertional Headaches," "Fumes and Headache," "Hypertension (High Blood Pressure," "Migraine Equivalents or Migraine Variants," "Sinus Headache," "Teeth Grinding (Bruxism), "TMJ and MPD," "Headaches Caused by Viral Infection," and "Weekend Headache," © 2000 The National Headache Foundation. Used with permission from the National Headache Foundation. For more information on headache causes and treatments, call the National Headache Foundation at 1-888-NHF-5552 or visit the web site at www.headaches.org. And, "Pseudotumor Cerebri Information Page," an undated fact sheet from the National Institute of Neurological Disorders and Stroke (NINDS), available online at http://www.ninds.nih.gov; cited September, 2001.

Alcohol and Headaches

Alcohol, which is consumed in beverages such as liquor, wine and beer, is a chemical called ethanol. Ethanol may cause headaches by several means. First, it is a direct vasodilator; in some individuals vasodilation may cause a headache. Second, ethanol is a natural diuretic; this leads to excretion of salt, vitamins and minerals from the body through the kidneys. Excess consumption of ethanol may produce dehydration and chemical imbalances in the body. Except in "moonshine" we consume ethanol in beverages that contain other chemicals. These chemicals are called congeners. Congeners impart the specific tastes and flavors that make each beverage unique. These congeners also have a variety of effects that can cause headaches and alter other chemicals in the body, which if consumed in excess may cause the hangover effect. Fructose, the naturally occurring sugar from fruits helps return portions of the body's chemical balance back to normal following ethanol consumption.

Early Morning Awakening Headaches

Cluster, migraine and tension-type headaches may produce a headache that awakens an individual in the early morning hours (usually after 4 AM), or is present upon awakening. Those individuals with chronic tension-type headache are most likely to be awakened in the early morning hours due to headache. This headache also tends to be at its worst severity at that time of day. A variety of causes may account for this early-morning pattern to the headaches.

Depression is most often associated with chronic tension-type headaches. Additionally, withdrawal effects from pain medications, ergots and caffeine, often produce this pattern. Several important physiological changes, which occur during these early morning hours, can influence migraine and tension-type headache, as well as symptoms other than headache.

Between about 4 AM and 8 AM, the body tends to produce less of its natural painkillers, the endorphins and enkephalins, than at other times of the day. Adrenalin is released in larger quantities during the early morning hours. Since adrenalin affects blood pressure and the regulation of dilation or contraction of the blood vessels, it may play a role in migraine attacks.

Rarely, serious diseases may cause early morning awakening headaches. These diseases may include brain tumors, sleep apnea, and severe high blood pressure.

Epilepsy

Epilepsy has been linked to migraine headaches. They are comorbid conditions, which means if you have one of them, there is a greater likelihood of the other being there. In most cases, however, it is a matter of a patient with two different neurologic conditions with occasional overlapping of symptoms. Patients with epilepsy may at times have a "postictal" or "post-seizure" headache. This headache is diffuse, throbbing, and moderate and subsides over a number of hours.

The diagnosis of epilepsy or seizure disorder is partially based on the results of electroencephalography (EEG). EEGs may also be ordered in the workup of migraine patients, particularly in children with headaches or those patients experiencing basilar artery migraine. Occasionally, mild abnormalities in the brain wave patterns may be observed on EEG. These changes are not characteristic of epilepsy.

Antiepileptic drugs, such as phenobarbital and phenytoin, have been used previously as agents in migraine treatment. The results have been insignificant, although a rare patient may respond to this form of therapy. Recently, interest has grown in the antiepileptic medication valproic acid and its derivatives as a viable treatment for migraine and cluster headaches. Although some positive results with this agent have been demonstrated, side effects may limit its usefulness for many patients. Other antiepileptic drugs like gabapentin and toprimate are also sometimes used.

Exertional Headaches

Exertional headaches are a group of headache syndromes which typically have a very short onset-to-peak intensity time and are associated with some physical activity. With exercise, the muscles of the head, neck and scalp require more blood and this causes a swelling of vessels or vasodilation which can cause head pain. Exertional headaches can, in some instances, be a sign of organic disease, and anyone who develops a severe headache following running, coughing, sneezing, bowel movement, or other exertions should certainly be checked to rule out any organic cause.

Among those more frequently seen are the benign orgasmic headache (sex headache), straining headache and jogger's headache. While these may occur in isolation, they are most commonly associated with patients who have inherited susceptibility to migraine.

It has been found that most exertional headaches are benign and respond to usual headache therapy. Some are particularly responsive to indomethacin, an anti-inflammatory agent. However, exertional headaches should be evaluated to exclude significant organic disease.

Fumes and Headache

Certain fumes and vapors can cause the blood vessels of the susceptible person to swell and dilate, triggering a migraine headache. Carbon monoxide poisoning from a poorly ventilated environment can provoke a headache. Faulty furnaces in winter can be responsible for such fumes.

The nitrites used in explosives can trigger a headache in susceptible persons who are employed in munitions plants. Smoking can provoke or intensify a headache. It can cause biological changes in the blood and blood vessels. Just being in a smoke-filled environment can provoke a headache in susceptible persons. Strong perfume and loud and irritating noises can also precipitate migraine headaches in some migraine sufferers. This may be associated with stress as well as change in environmental conditions.

Hypertension (High Blood Pressure)

High blood pressure can cause headache, but in general is not the cause of recurring headaches. Blood pressure usually has to be quite elevated. Studies show that headaches have been precipitated by blood pressures of 200/110 or higher. A physician should determine whether or not an elevated blood pressure is responsible for a patient's headache.

Some high blood pressure medications can also cause headache.

Migraine Equivalents or Migraine Variants

This term applies to migraine that exhibits itself in a form other than head pain. A diagnosis of migraine equivalent is determined by a previous history of migraine attacks, no evidence of organic lesions, and the replacement of normal headaches by an equivalent group of symptoms. It is important that these patients be evaluated thoroughly, with attention to past and family migraine histories. Characteristically, drugs used to treat migraine usually help the equivalent symptoms.

Although not common, the most prevalent migraine equivalent is "abdominal migraine," which is characterized by recurrent episodes of vomiting and abdominal pain without headache. The bouts of pain can last for hours and occur more frequently in female children. Patients characteristically show other symptoms of migraine such as yawning, listlessness, and drowsiness during their attacks. A migraine equivalent may also be characterized by visual symptoms such as blind spots, partial vision, neurologic deficits, or psychic disturbances without headache.

Pseudotumor Cerebri

Pseudotumor cerebri, also called benign intracranial hypertension, literally means "false brain tumor." It is caused by increased pressure within the brain and is most common in women between the ages of 20 and 50. Symptoms of pseudotumor cerebri, which include headache, nausea, vomiting, and pulsating intracranial noises, closely mimic symptoms of brain tumors, possibly because of the abnormal buildup of pressure within the brain.

Treatment for pseudotumor cerebri is generally symptomatic. Pressure may be controlled by removing excess fluid with repeated spinal taps or by shunting. Steroids may be prescribed to reduce swelling of brain tissue. Drugs to reduce cerebrospinal fluid production or hyperosmotic drugs may be used to reduce fluid buildup.

Once the diagnosis is made and the disorder is treated, pseudotumor cerebri generally has no serious consequences. If visual loss occurs, however, it may be permanent regardless of treatment. In some cases, pseudotumor cerebri recurs.

Sinus Headache

Whether the symptoms of headache are referable to sinus disease should be determined through an examination by a physician.

The headache of sinus origin or acute sinusitis is usually associated with constant pain and tenderness over the affected sinus, a deep dull ache, and exaggerated by head movements or straining. Nasal symptoms are prominent, including sinus pain, which is usually accompanied by other symptoms of sinus disease such as nasal discharge, ear sensations or fullness, and facial swelling. Allergic reactions and tumors in the sinuses also can produce inflammation, swelling, and blockage of the sinuses. However, vascular headaches can cause similar symptoms. The vast majority of people who think they are experiencing "sinus" problems are actually suffering from a vascular type of headache. When sinus disease is the cause of the headache, an accompanying fever is often present, and x-rays will indicate some sinus blockage. One or both nostrils are blocked and the pain extends over the cheek or forehead. The area is tender to the touch.

Therapy is usually directed toward relief of infection or accompanying allergy. Symptomatic relief includes analgesics and nasal vasoconstrictors. The use of local corticosteroids may offer the allergic individual added relief where nasal symptoms are prominent. Therapy of the symptomatic type is similar in both cases where sinus and nasal symptoms are prominent, but the acute sinusitis requires the added therapy directed toward the offending organism or allergy. The migrainous individual requires the added therapy directed toward the basic migraine disorder.

Teeth Grinding (Bruxism)

Many people grind or clench their teeth, either by day or night, without being aware of what they are doing. This can be triggered by a dental malocclusion, stress, or worry. This muscular over-activity sometimes gives rise to muscle spasm and headache. Most often, these headaches are classified as tension-type. A dentist often can ease those symptoms by fitting a small appliance to the upper teeth, which is worn during sleep. Medications and other stress reduction techniques sometimes are utilized.

In recent years, the growing awareness of dental causes of puzzling facial and head pain has enabled many individuals to benefit from appropriate dental treatment.

TMJ and MPD

Dull, aching pain in the area where the skull meets the jaw (the temporomandibular joint), is a common symptom which may vary greatly in intensity. It is a pain that may radiate to the back of the head, side, or down into the neck. Chewing, talking or any use of the jaw may increase the pain, as will excessive talking or yawning. There may be clicking, popping or grating sounds. The pressure around the head can be either tension-type or migraine-like. Vertigo, dizziness, and ringing in the ears are also complaints of this disorder.

While the symptoms are common in this area, the diagnosis of TMJ requires that there be a triad of symptoms including a painful clicking or popping of the joint, abnormal motion of the joint and disorders of the bite. Conservative treatment should be used including rest, heat, physical therapy, bite plates, and simple analgesics before aggressive therapy involving surgery of the jaw or the joint is entertained.

TMJ was the term formerly used for this condition, which is now called myofascial pain dysfunction (MPD) syndrome.

Headaches Caused by Viral Infections

Anyone who has suffered from influenza has probably experienced the headache that accompanies this infection. Many viral infections can either directly or indirectly cause headache.

The headache related to these viral infections appears to be related to the fever, the body's production of interferon, and other elements of the immune system in combating the viral infection. Headache may also be associated with those viral infections that affect the upper respiratory tract, such as the common cold virus, the Rhinovirus. This particular infection may produce intense congestion in the nasal passages, which at times causes a blockage of the sinus drainage passages, and can also cause headaches. Headache may also result from viral infections that specifically attack the brain and its coverings, such as encephalitis and meningitis.

Chronic viral infections have been identified as a cause of headache and other conditions, such as the chronic fatigue syndrome. There is scant evidence and substantial medical research that negates this theory.

Regardless of the role of chronic viral infections in these disorders, there is considerable evidence that suggests antidepressant medications may be helpful in controlling these conditions. Sometimes a benign viral infection may set off a cycle of chronic daily headaches that do not have typical features of migraine or tension-type headache.

Weekend Headache

Those migraineurs who experience "weekend" headaches or headaches precipitated by oversleeping should try to awaken at the same time on weekends as they do during the week and to maintain a regular sleep pattern throughout the entire week. Moreover, it is essential for the migraine sufferer to get enough sleep, as fatigue can provoke a headache. In fact, fatigue is one of the most common triggers of migraine headaches.

A sudden wearing off of the effect of caffeine can lead to abrupt vasodilation and a "caffeine withdrawal" headache. Caffeine is also a stimulant, which can add a letdown feeling after the effect wears off.

This kind of headache is common in heavy coffee drinkers. One of the factors contributing to "weekend" or "holiday" headaches may be caffeine withdrawal. If a person normally consumes large amounts of caffeine-containing substances during the week, a withdrawal, rebound headache may result on weekends or holidays if similar amounts are not consumed. The pain-producing mechanism of the headache is the vasodilation of cranial arteries. The headache may be a persistent, generalized one that lasts for weeks. A gradual withdrawal from caffeine-containing substances can help to bring these headaches under control.

Chapter 8

Childhood Headaches

Like adults, children and adolescents suffer from headaches. Most often, their headaches are not serious, and they are not the result of any life-threatening disease. Research shows that more than half of school age children have had headaches, and as many as 10% have severe or frequent headaches.

As children get older, they are more likely to have headaches. Before puberty, headaches affect both boys and girls about the same. After puberty, though, girls are two to three times more likely to suffer from headaches than boys.

Frequent or severe headaches can interfere with a child's daily life, and may keep her from school or play. There are many different reasons a child may have headaches. If headaches are severe, are getting worse over time, or are accompanied by other symptoms (like vision changes or vomiting), the doctor should be consulted. Sometimes a specific cause for the headaches can be found, but more often the cause is not any other disease—the only problem is the headache itself. Doctors can recommend treatments to help with headache pain experienced by children and adolescents, no matter what the reason is for the pain.

Information in this chapter is from "Headache in Children," © 2000 The National Headache Foundation. Used with permission from the National Headache Foundation. For more information on headache causes and treatments, call the National Headache Foundation at 1-888-NHF-5552 or visit the web site at www.headaches.org. And, "Pediatric Headache," © 2000 Beth Israel Medical Center; reprinted with permission. More information is available online at http://www.StopPain.org.

Headache is a frequent symptom in children but deciding whether it is organic or functional can be a difficult task, even for the most experienced physician. A detailed history, physical examination, and appropriate tests are essential in determining the correct diagnosis. Fortunately, the large majority of children complaining of headache do not have any organic disease as a basis for their complaints. When taking a history, which is the most important factor in making an accurate diagnosis, it is necessary to question both children and parents to elicit signs of emotional friction that may provide a clue to reasons for the headache. Equally important is a thorough and complete neurological examination to identify any variations from normal. As in adults, headache in children can be classified into three types: vascular, tension-type and organic.

Some headaches occur only once, and these are called acute headaches. Acute headaches might be due to infection or trauma.

Infection: There are many infections that may cause headaches in children. For instance, the flu commonly starts with headache and fever. Children with ear infections or sinus infections also often have headache symptoms. In very rare instances, headache may be due to more severe infections, such as meningitis or encephalitis. If serious infection is suspected, the child must be brought to a doctor promptly.

Trauma: A short-lasting headache after a bump to the head is common in children. If there is any doubt about the condition of a child after a head injury, call a doctor or go to the emergency room right away. If the child was unconscious, does not remember the fall or bump, is nauseated or throwing up, is acting irritable or confused, is dizzy or has trouble seeing, or has a headache serious enough to interfere with sleep or play, see a doctor immediately.

Some children have chronic or recurrent headaches. Parents might worry that long-lasting headaches in children or repeated headaches might be caused by a brain tumor. This is very uncommon. Actually, headaches that children and adolescents get repeatedly are usually migraine headaches or tension headaches.

Migraine Headaches: It is thought that about 5 to 10% of children have migraine headaches. Migraines differ from child to child, but usually children experience many of the following:

- The child has headache pain that is moderate to severe.
- The child has headache pain that is throbbing or pounding.

- The child has headache pain that is worse on one side of the head, or pain that is on both sides of the head in the forehead area.

- The child feels nauseated or vomits.

- The child shows a sensitivity to light, sound or smells, or has tenderness of the scalp.

- The child goes to a darkened, quiet room and tries to sleep. Children with migraines rarely want to move around, watch TV, read or listen to music, because these all tend to make the headache worse.

Migraine headaches may occur only once in a while, or may occur more than once a week. Headaches may last anywhere from a few hours to several days. Between headaches, the child feels fine.

Some children with migraines have "auras" before the headache begins, when their vision may blur or they may see flashing lights, spots or colored zig-zag lines. Less common auras include weakness in an arm or leg, funny feelings (tingling, pins and needles) in an arm or leg, speech difficulty, or abdominal pain. Headaches usually start during the aura or shortly after the aura stops.

If your child complains of any of these symptoms for the first time, it is important to take him to a doctor. The doctor will make sure that the child is experiencing an aura (which does no permanent damage and goes away completely between headaches) and not anything more serious. Doctors and researchers don't know exactly what causes migraine headaches. Some migraines do have "triggers," however:

- *Stress:* Parents should ask children suffering from migraines if they are worried, upset or anxious about anything. Stress for children usually originates from school or the home. Any known sources of stress (i.e., a recent divorce) should be discussed with the child's doctor.

- *Hunger:* In some children, missing meals or not eating enough at meals can trigger migraine headaches.

- *Diet:* Doctors think that a diet plays an important role in migraines for some children. Foods that might trigger migraines are cheeses, chocolate, caffeine, citrus fruits and food preservatives. It is unknown why foods can cause migraine headaches to start.

- *Exercise:* Hard exercise can bring about migraines in some children. Eating before and after exercise may help prevent these attacks.

- *Motion sickness:* Children who experience motion sickness while riding in a car, boat or plane may later develop a migraine headache.

- *Sleep deprivation:* Not getting enough sleep or poor sleeping habits can trigger migraine headaches in children. Good sleeping habits, including going to bed and getting up at about the same time every day, may help control some headaches.

- *Environment:* Bright lights, flickering lights, noise, strong smells or weather changes can sometimes cause migraines to start.

Vascular Headaches

Migraine is one-sided and throbbing and is almost always accompanied by nausea and vomiting. Periodic vomiting without headache is viewed as a migraine variant and may indicate migraine in later years. Children exhibiting car or motion sickness, especially if there is a history of migraine in the family, will often develop migraine later.

Fortunately, the symptoms will disappear in the majority of children with migraine in a period of five to seven years after their appearance. Migraine will occur in about one-quarter of migraine sufferers before the age of five and in about half before the age of 20.

It is important to realize that migraine may occur after head injury, especially after injury sustained in sporting activities such as football and baseball. The outcome is generally full recovery over varying time periods.

Tension-Type Headaches

This is the most common type of headache in children, and emotional factors are the most likely cause. The pain is described as diffuse, sometimes like a tight band around the head and is usually not associated with nausea and vomiting.

These headaches are almost always related to stress situations at school, competition, family friction or excessive demands by parents. Examination of child and parents is required to determine whether anxiety or depression may be present.

Doctors and researchers don't know much about the causes of tension-type headaches. In some children, they seem to be associated with stress. For these children, tension headaches might start when the child is feeling stressed or anxious; for instance, before going to school. Tension headaches usually hurt on both sides of the head, with a steady, non-throbbing pain that may feel like a pressure or tightness in the head. The child does not usually feel nauseated. While the child may want to sit quietly during a headache, movement, lights, watching TV, reading or listening to music usually do not make the headaches any worse.

Tension headaches last anywhere from a half hour to many days. It is possible for a new tension headache to start every day for a long period of time.

Organic

Headache associated with traction or inflammation of pain-sensitive structures of the head may occur in children. If fever is present, meningitis or encephalitis should be suspected. Traction on large arteries and veins causes pain, which may be accompanied by such symptoms as nausea, vomiting, muscular incoordination, weakness, seizures, personality changes and lethargy.

A first priority is to rule out increased pressure in the brain and surrounding tissues, which may be due to tumors, infection or blood clots. It is important to remember that restlessness and irritability may be the only signs of head pain in young children unable to express themselves adequately.

Treatment

Treatment is individualized depending on the age and reliability of the child and the frequency and severity of attacks. Interestingly, many have fewer and less distressing attacks after they are reassured that no serious abnormality exists. In children younger than age 14 years with infrequent attacks, analgesics, antiemetics and sedatives are useful at the time of the attack. Narcotic analgesics should be avoided. Young children cannot be relied on to carry their own medication and take it at the start of the headache. If attacks occur more than once a month or are particularly distressing, prophylaxis should be considered.

If a child has frequent or severe headaches, she should be seen by a doctor. The doctor will first take a careful history, which will involve asking the child and parents questions that will help the doctor understand why the child is having headaches. The doctor may ask questions about past illnesses or injury, when the child had her first headache and what her headaches have been like since then. The doctor will probably also ask the parents many questions about the child's recent headaches, such as:

- How often has she had the headaches?

- How severe have the headaches been?

- How long have the headaches lasted?

- What time of the day or night does she usually get headaches?

- Where is the pain?

- How does the child act when she has the headaches? What does she do?

- What causes the headaches or makes them worse (stress, hunger, exercise, bright light, etc.)?

- What makes the headaches better?

- What treatments have been tried and how well have they worked?

- Has she missed school or other activities because of the headaches?

- Do headaches make it hard for the child to sleep, or does the pain wake her up during the night?

- Is there a history of headache in the family?

Depending on the age of the child, the doctor may also ask her to answer each of these questions. Often, the doctor wants to speak with the child alone. It is important for the doctor to hear the child describe her symptoms in her own words. Also, talking to the child alone ensures that the she feels free to discuss aspects of her headache that she may not be comfortable discussing in front of her parents.

The doctor may want the parents and/or child to keep a record of the headaches (sometimes called a "headache diary"). This involves writing down how often the child has the headaches, how bad the headaches are, how long the headaches last, what medications were given and whether or not they helped, and anything that makes the headaches begin, get worse, or get better.

Once important information about the headaches has been gathered, the doctor may do a physical exam. Sometimes, the doctor wants to do some tests. These tests might include blood tests, a cranial computed tomography (CT), or a magnetic resonance imaging (MRI) study.

If the child is found to have an infection or other disease, treatment might be available for that condition. If the doctor can find no cause for the headaches, this does not mean that there is no treatment. Remember, doctors do not know the cause for the common tension-type headaches or migraine headaches. But there are treatments they can offer to help with the headache symptoms.

For migraine and tension-type headaches, treatment might begin with good sleep and nutrition habits. Things that trigger the headaches, if identified, can be avoided. For some children, these simple changes can make a big difference in how often they suffer from headaches, how bad the pain is and how long the headaches last.

Drug Treatment

Doctors often first recommend acetaminophen (like Tylenol®) for headaches in children. If this does not stop the pain, it is important to let the doctor know—NEVER give more medicine to a child than the doctor recommends. Even though acetaminophen is available without a prescription, it can still be dangerous to a child if too much is given.

There are many other medications that the doctor can try for the headaches. The more information the child and parents are able to give the doctor about the headaches, the easier it will be for the doctor to find the best medication for that child. However, even with good information about the headaches, it might take trials of several different medications before the most effective one is found. This is because each child reacts differently to medications—if two children with exactly the same headache symptoms are given the same medication, one may feel better and one may not.

Also, medication may be prescribed for the child's nausea, vomiting or diarrhea, if these symptoms are present.

Preventive Treatment ("Prophylactic" Treatment)

These are medications given to the child daily to help prevent headaches from starting. Preventive treatments may be prescribed by a doctor if the child's headaches are severe and occur often. Sometimes children and adolescents who have very bad headaches, and their parents, choose not to use preventive treatments. This is usually because they do not want to take medications every day. This is a choice that each child and his parents must make based on how hard it is for the child to cope with the headaches and how well medications work if taken after the headaches start. There are many preventive medications that can be tried.

Nondrug Treatment

Some nondrug treatments, like biofeedback and relaxation therapies, can be helpful, particularly in older children. These techniques are taught to the child, who can practice and then use them to cope with headache pain as it starts. Also, if the techniques are practiced every day, they may even help prevent headaches from starting. Biofeedback machines measure electrical impulses or heat from the child's skin and show these measurements on a TV screen, a flashing light bulb, or a beeper. The feedback from their own bodies can help the child to practice relaxation and make internal adjustments that help relieve the headache pain.

Because stress and anxiety play a part in many childhood headaches, it might be helpful for some children to see a mental health specialist, like a psychologist. Mental health specialists can help children with the relaxation techniques described above, and also help them deal with the stress and anxiety they are feeling.

Summary

Like adults, children suffer from headaches. Headaches may result from infection or injury, but most repeated headaches have no clear cause. These are usually migraine headaches or tension-type headaches. Doctors may be able to offer medication and nondrug treatments to help control pain in migraine or tension-type headaches.

Part Two

Causes and Prevention of Headaches

Chapter 9

Prevention of Migraine Headaches

Do You Need Migraine Prevention?

Migraine patients do not want to suffer from an attack, so prevention is important, even if they suffer from only one attack a year. Those who suffer from frequent attacks will need more aggressive prevention strategies that sometimes include medication. This decision is made by discussing treatment and management options with your physician. Additionally, nonpharmacological prevention may help if you have:

1. poor tolerance for specific pharmacological treatments,

2. medical contraindications for specific acute pharmacological treatments,

3. insufficient or no response to pharmacological treatment,

4. history of long-term, frequent, or excessive use of pain medications (analgesics) or acute medications that make headaches worse (or lead to decreased responsiveness to other pharmacotherapies), or

5. high stress levels or difficulty coping with stress.

"Prevention of Migraine Headaches: What Every Patient Should Know," © 2000 American Council for Headache Education, available online at http://www.achenet.org; reprinted with permission.

Goals of Preventive Therapy

Migraine prevention is intended to reduce the suffering and disability associated with attacks. Unfortunately, preventive treatment strategies rarely eliminate migraine, but they can reduce the frequency and severity of attacks. Ideally, migraine sufferers should learn how to gain a sense of control over their attacks. This will lead to a better sense of well being and improved quality of life.

The ultimate goals of migraine preventive therapy are to:

1. reduce frequency, severity, and duration of attacks,

2. improve responsiveness to treatment of acute attacks, and

3. reduce level of disability.

These goals can be achieved through a combination of education, lifestyle changes, and therapies (pharmacological [drug] and nonpharmacological [nondrug]). Specifically, learning about your specific migraine "triggers" may help you reduce the frequency of attacks.

Using a headache diary will help identify items that are associated with triggering migraine that you may have not been aware of such as menstruation, red wine, and caffeine, among others. The information collected in a headache diary also will allow your physician to review the severity, frequency, disability, and triggers associated with your attacks. A complete understanding of these details will help you and your doctor design a successful treatment plan.

Avoiding Triggers

"Triggers" are specific factors that may increase your risk of having a migraine attack. The migraine sufferer has inherited a sensitive nervous system that under certain circumstances, can lead to migraine.

Triggers do not "cause" migraine. Instead, they are thought to activate processes that cause migraine in people who are prone to the condition. A certain trigger will not induce a migraine in every person; and, in a single migraine sufferer, a trigger may not cause a migraine every time. By keeping a headache diary, you will be able to identify some triggers for your particular headaches.

Once you have identified triggers, it will be easier for you to avoid them and reduce your chances of having a migraine attack.

Table 9.1. Common Triggers

Categories	Triggers	Examples
Dietary	Skipping meals/ fasting Food Items	MSG (monosodium glutamate), Chocolate, Processed meats (containing nitrates), Aged cheese, Alcohol/red wine, Too much caffeine
	Medications	Nitroglycerine
Chronobiology	Change in sleep patterns	Napping, Oversleeping, Too little sleep
Environmental	Weather changes	Extreme heat or cold
	Bright lights	Office lighting
	Odors/pollution	Smog, perfumes, chemicals, Flashing lights or screens
Hormonal	Estrogen level changes (rapid fluctuations in estrogen levels)	Menstruation, Hormone replacement therapies, Birth control pills Around the time of menopause
Stress	Work	Unrealistic timelines
	Home	Financial issues
	Family	Job changes, Moving, Childbirth, Marriage, Death/Loss
Stress Letdown	Discontinuation of work	Weekends, Vacations, Ending a project or stressful task (such as a presentation)
Physical	Injuries	Marathon running
	Over-exertion	Exercising when out of shape, Exercising in heat

Table 9.2. Tracking Your Triggers

Dietary Factors

alcoholic beverages
foods containing tyramine:
    aged cheeses
    Chianti wine
    pickled herring
    dried smoked fish
    sour cream
    yogurt
    yeast extracts
chocolate
citrus fruits
dairy products
onions
nuts
beans
caffeine (excess, withdrawal)
fatty foods
food additives:
    nitrites (e.g., in hot dogs, lun-
    cheon meats)
    monosodium glutamate (MSG)
    aspartame artificial sweetener
    (NutraSweet, Equal)

Environmental Factors

bright light
flickering light sources
fluorescent lighting
perfumes
strong odors
fumes from industrial complexes
air pollution
secondhand cigarette smoke
motion
travel
complex visual patterns (e.g., checks,
    zig-zag lines)
weather changes

Lifestyle Factors

stress
disrupted sleep patterns
"letdown"
fatigue
irregular eating habits
cigarette smoking

Medications

blood vessel dilating drugs (e.g., ni-
    troglycerin)
drugs for high blood pressure (e.g.,
    hydralazine, reserpine)
diuretics
anti-asthma medications (e.g., ami-
    nophylline)
too-frequent use of analgesics, er-
    gotamine

Physical Factors

head trauma
invasive medical tests (adverse effect)
exertion (e.g., sports, sexual orgasm)
disorders of the neck

Hormonal Factors

onset of puberty in girls
menstruation
menopause
pregnancy
delivery
birth-control pills
estrogen replacement therapy

Source for Table 9.2: Excerpted from "Heading Off Migraine Pain," by Tamar Nordenberg, *FDA Consumer*, U.S. Food and Drug Administration (FDA), May-June 1998.

Common Triggers

The science linking triggers to migraine is not yet clearly established. Nonetheless, patients commonly report that they have migraine triggers.

Lifestyle Changes

Migraine is not a predictable disorder for all people. Simple things like changes to a normal routine can lead to a severely disabling migraine attack. Understanding how lifestyle impacts the severity and frequency of attacks can be a large part of successful migraine prevention.

It is an unrealistic to expect anyone to completely change a certain life style. However, certain things are relatively easy to do. For example:

- Maintain regular sleep patterns. Go to sleep and wake up at the same time each day.

- Exercise regularly. For example, aerobic exercise for at least 30 minutes three times a week will help reduce frequency or severity of migraine.

- Eat regular meals, do not skip meals, and eat a good, healthy breakfast.

- Reduce stress. Limit stress by avoiding conflicts and resolving disputes calmly. Some people find it helpful to take a daily "stress break."

- Avoiding known triggers.

Establishing daily routines that help reduce migraine attacks is important for long-term migraine prevention. For example:

- Schedule a relaxation period that includes relaxation strategies such as:

  Take slow, deep breaths

  Focus the mind on a relaxing image or scene

  Try soft relaxing lighting and sounds

  Exercise on a regular basis, even if your daily routine changes (such as when traveling, when you have houseguests, or when your workload increases).

- Maintain the medication treatment plan designed by you and your physician. Early intervention may help prevent the migraine from progressing into a severe, disabling attack.

Nonpharmacological Strategies

You can do certain things that do not involve medications. Others involve techniques employed by trained practitioners. Many different kinds of "nonpharmacological techniques" are available, including behavioral and physical treatments.

Some examples of behavioral treatments are:

- biofeedback therapy
- relaxation training
- cognitive-behavioral training (also known as stress-management training)
- hypnosis

Some examples of physical treatments are:

- acupuncture
- massage
- cervical manipulation

Biofeedback Therapy

Biofeedback is a technique where people learn to gain control of their body's internal functions. Specifically, biofeedback involves learning to sense changes in the body's activity, and using relaxation and other techniques to control the body's responses.

Biofeedback requires specific training sessions with a trained biofeedback therapist. This training usually takes one to two months of weekly 30-45 minute sessions, although many books and audiotapes are available to teach these techniques at home.

Biofeedback is monitored by measuring skin temperature and muscle tension. Changes in skin temperature and muscle tension indicate the level of activation of the patient's nervous system. Learning to control body functions, such as body temperature, is achieved by first learning to relax the skeletal muscles (muscles that support the bones). This relaxation is achieved through relaxation, visualization, and breathing techniques. Most important, though, is the daily practice of these techniques. The practice sessions can be only a few seconds or minutes long, but they need to be done frequently. A conscious effort is required in the first few weeks of training, but gradually, self-monitoring and very brief relaxation techniques become a subconscious habit.

Biofeedback allows many headache sufferers to lower tension throughout the body, which results in fewer headaches. Children adapt especially well to biofeedback. They can often learn to prevent a headache in four to five sessions, and also they can learn to stop the headache once it begins.

Biofeedback therapy may be coupled with relaxation therapy. Relaxation therapy teaches a variety of relaxation strategies for reducing tension and stress throughout the body.

Cognitive-Behavioral Training (Also Known As Stress-Management Training)

This technique often is done with the help of a psychologist, psychiatrist, or other therapist. This training focuses on teaching migraine sufferers coping skills and other "cognitive" (thinking) strategies for managing stressful parts of their life.

Hypnosis

Hypnosis is now being studied in clinical trials for treatment of a variety of conditions including pain management. Little has been done so far about its use in preventing migraine.

Acupuncture

The ancient method of acupuncture recently received a boost in popularity because of the consensus statement released by a panel convened by the National Institutes of Health. This statement strongly suggests that acupuncture is in fact a legitimate therapy proven to be effective for some conditions, and acupuncture deserves additional studies for other conditions. The panel concluded that nausea and acute dental pain clearly respond to acupuncture. Many painful conditions, including headaches, may respond to acupuncture, but additional studies are needed.

Acupuncture treatment is done using very thin disposable needles, which cause very little discomfort or pain. For patients with chronic headaches, treatment involves 10 or more weekly 20-minutes sessions. Electric simulation of the needles is frequently used instead of the traditional manual twirling of the needles. Issues of cost, convenience, and patient preference should be taken into account when deciding whether to try this mode of treatment. Some insurance plans may cover this form of therapy.

Massage

Many migraine sufferers have tight, stiff, tender muscles in the back of the head, neck, and shoulders. If you feel these muscles, they often have tight bands or knots that are tender to pressure. Pressure on these points in the muscle may cause pain in the head, which is similar to the pain of a migraine. These points are often called trigger points. Massaging these trigger points can reduce the pain and tightness in the muscles and can decrease head pain and migraine in some sufferers.

Massage therapy is a healthy maneuver to reduce stress and tension. Its value in treating migraine, however, is not fully determined. Massage initially can be done once to twice a week for 4 to 6 weeks. Stretching and strengthening exercises should be continued even after therapy sessions have ended. Massage techniques can be taught to a spouse or significant other.

The likelihood of behavioral techniques working as preventive treatment for migraine depends upon appropriate training and discipline for the person using the technique. Headache sufferers must be willing to try these techniques and must be committed to maintaining the training programs designed by technicians and other professionals in order for them to be successful.

Preventive Medications

Preventive medications are taken daily to prevent the onset of migraine. They are not intended for use during a migraine attack.

Many different preventive medications are available, and the choice of medication depends on many factors such as co-existing conditions including high blood pressure, diabetes, or pregnancy (among others). Therefore, choosing medications for preventive therapy can be a complex process.

Before starting to take medications, several basic principles need to be considered:

1. The choice of a preventive medication needs to be tailored to meet each person's individual needs.

2. Co-existing medical conditions, drug side effects, other medications being taken, and individual patient needs will help determine which medication a physician chooses.

When deciding on preventive therapies, it is important to review with your doctor several important management principles:

- Low doses are used at first and gradually increased to higher doses as needed. Therefore, you may need to increase medication dose until the desired response is achieved.

- It may take 2 to 3 months before you notice a decrease in the frequency or severity of attacks.

- Treatment may be required for 6 to 12 months or longer.

- All medications have potential side effects so any unusual symptoms should be reported to your physician. It is important to discuss potential side effects, since some medications may be better tolerated than others.

- Side effects can often be limited by using low doses, increasing the dose slowly, or allowing time to adjust to the medication. If you are not tolerating the medication and if you start to have side effects, contact your doctor to discuss changes to the treatment plan.

- You should not suddenly stop taking preventive medications because of the risk of rebound headache or other side effects. Preventive medications need to be gradually tapered off after a period of sustained benefit.

Assessing Disability from Migraine

Disability caused by migraine can come from the pain of the attack itself or from non-headache symptoms associated with the attack, such as nausea or sensitivity to light and sound. Whether pain, nausea, or vomiting is the primary disabling feature, migraine prevents people from continuing with their daily routines. The goal of migraine prevention is to eliminate disability through pain management and treatment of associated symptoms. Disability created by migraine attacks can lead to:

- Time lost from school
- Time lost from work

Table 9.3. Commonly Used Preventive Medications

Type of Medication	Medication Class	Generic Name	Side Effects
Blood pressure medications	Beta-Blockers	Propranolol, Timolol, Metoprolol	Fatigue, Depression, Nausea, Insomnia, Dizziness
	Calcium channel blockers	Verapamil, Diltiazem, Nimodipine	Weight gain, Constipation, Dizziness, Low blood pressure
Antidepressants	Tricyclic antidepressants	Amitriptyline, Nortriptyline, Imipramine	Dry mouth, Sedation, Decreased libido (sex drive), Low blood pressure
	Selective Serotonin Reuptake Inhibitors (SSRIs)	Fluoxetine, Paroxetine, Sertraline	Weight gain or loss, Decreased libido
Anticonvulsants		Divalproex sodium, Gabapentin, Topiramate	Weight gain or loss, Sedation, Skin rash
Serotonin antagonists		Methysergide, Methylergonovine	Blood vessel spasm, Abdominal scarring (very rare),
Unconventional treatments	Magnesium salts	Magnesium oxide, magnesium diglycinate, magnesium chloride slow release	Diarrhea
	Vitamins	Riboflavin	Urine discoloration
	Feverfew		

- Time lost from household activities
- Reduced productivity and work performance
- Time lost from social activities and family activities
- Unemployment
- Strain in relationships with spouse or children

The fear of future migraine attacks can be just as disabling as the actual attack. For some people the fear of having another attack keeps them from taking part in activities such as vacations, parties, or having visitors.

Migraine also affects the sufferer's spouse, children, family, and friends. Coworkers are affected by a colleague's migraine because work plans may suddenly change, meetings may be canceled, work may not be done, responsibilities may be shifted, or the quality of work may be reduced.

The ultimate impact of a migraine disability may be underestimated and, in general, this information is poorly communicated between headache sufferers and their physicians. Measuring the total impact of migraine on your life will help you understand the severity of your illness and it will affect your physician's assessment of your need for treatment.

Several disability tools are available to assess the impact of migraine on your life. One such instrument is the MIDAS Questionnaire (Migraine Disability Assessment) which measures days missed or days with lower capacity to function due to migraine. Your physician can use this information to decide on need and choice of medications or other treatment strategies. Other disability assessment tools include IMPACT, PACE, and HDI. Importantly, prevention of migraine should be aimed at reducing disability and limiting disruption of your daily routine.

Monitoring Headaches

To fully understand the impact of migraine, it is important to keep track of your migraine attacks. Filling out a headache diary gives you and your physician an accurate picture of the frequency, severity, and disability of your attacks. It also provides a way to identify patterns, such as the association with the menstrual cycle.

Some reasons to use a headache diary include:

- *Triggers:* migraine triggers may become more apparent as you monitor your migraines using a daily diary form.

- *Track progress:* diary forms also are an excellent way to track success, or failure, of treatment. For example, you may be thinking that your headaches are not getting better, but long-term improvement may only be detected by comparing regular reports of severity, frequency, duration, and disability from attacks.

Table 9.4. Headache Help

In 1993, migraine sufferer and artist Michael Coleman founded an organization called "MAGNUM" (Migraine Awareness Group: A National Understanding for Migraineurs), which uses art as a vehicle to help educate people about migraine. You can contact MAGNUM at:

Migraine Awareness Group
113 South Saint Asaph Street, Suite 300
Alexandria, VA 22314
Tel: 703-739-9384
Internet: http://www.migraines.org

Other groups that specialize in headache:

American Council for Headache Education
19 Mantua Road
Mount Royal, NJ 08061
Toll Free: 800-255-ACHE (800-255-2243)
Internet: http://www.achenet.org

National Headache Foundation
428 West Saint James Place, 2nd Floor
Chicago, IL 60614
Toll Free: 800-843-2256
Internet: http://www.headaches.org

National Institutes of Health Neurological Institute
P.O. Box 5801
Bethesda, MD 20824
Tel: 301-496-5751
Internet: http://www.ninds.nih.gov

Source for Table 9.4: Excerpted from "Heading Off Migraine Pain," by Tamar Nordenberg, *FDA Consumer*, U.S. Food and Drug Administration (FDA), May-June 1998.

Talk to Your Doctor

Three simple steps to taking better care of you and your migraine

1. Keep monthly headache calendars.

2. Fill out a disability questionnaire.

3. Make an appointment to specifically talk with your doctor about your headaches. Many patients do not discuss migraine with their doctors and may suffer unnecessarily. Plan on discussing migraine as the main reason for the visit. You should not try and "squeeze" in a quick discussion about your headaches when your doctor has not scheduled enough time for a thorough headache evaluation. Designing a specific treatment plan that meets your individual needs will take additional time.

When going to the doctor's office remember to take with you

*   a list of all prescription medications you use.

*   a list of all over-the-counter medications you use.

*   a list of all dietary supplements you take, including vitamins, herbal therapies, and other nontraditional remedies.

*   your completed headache diary.

*   your completed MIDAS Questionnaire or other disability assessment tool, if you have one.

Remember

1. Be honest about the number of medications you use and how often you take them. This will help your physician determine how to properly treat your migraines, especially regarding your need for preventive therapies. Medication overuse is a common consequence of out-of-control migraine, not drug addiction.

2. Agree to a treatment plan that is appropriate to your specific needs. This includes assessing migraine severity and disability. Take into account your lifestyle, health, and any other issues that may affect the medications you take. For example:

    type of delivery (oral, nasal, liquid, tablet, suppository, injection), frequency of dosing (once, twice, three times or four times a day),

other existing health conditions (high blood pressure, depression, fatigue), and

other health concerns (such as weight gain, drowsiness, desire to get pregnant).

3. Be sure that you understand your treatment plan when you leave the office.

    Taking medications incorrectly will decrease their effectiveness and could lead to additional side effects. Be sure the plan is written out. If it is not clear, ask to have it explained again or call back and ask to have it clarified.

    Changes in the treatment plan MUST be discussed with your doctor. Make sure you have a follow-up appointment when you leave the office, and be sure and keep the appointment, even if your headaches are doing better.

    Bring your completed diary to your follow-up visit. Treatment plans often require modifications and adjustments so do not give up if one particular plan is not working.

Remember, migraine can be effectively managed and treated. Patients do not need to "live with their migraine." A large number of medications and non-pharmacological treatment strategies are effective for treatment of migraine. Consult with you physician regularly to make sure you are getting the best possible care.

Chapter 10

Headaches, Stress, and "Moods"

Stress and Headaches

Stress is by far the most common headache "trigger." Both female and male headache sufferers report that headaches are more likely to occur during or after periods of stress. Major life-changing events like marriage, birth of a child, or career changes all are sources of stress. However, research has found that it is actually the day-to-day stress or chronic "hassles" that are important in triggering headache. Compared to men, women often experience more of the types of stress that provoke headache.

Identifying the Most Common Stresses

Multiple-Role Stress: Women are likely to have "multiple-role" which is stress due to managing many different roles and responsibilities. Common roles include being a mother, wife, professional working woman, and caretaker of the home. Often these important roles conflict with one another, and women are forced to make tough choices between competing demands.

Sometimes, women overextend themselves trying to do it all. Other times, women suffer disappointment and guilt if they are not able to meet all of the demands of family, home, and work.

Text in this chapter is from the American Council for Headache Education (ACHE) © 2000. Reprinted from the web site of the American Council for Headache Education (www.achenet.org); reprinted with permission.

Women that overextend themselves might find it helpful to actually schedule time for themselves (yes, mark it on the calendar, and put it in the daily planner...). One easy way to do this is to make an appointment with "yourself," and show up on time as one would with any other appointment. Should someone ask for "this or that," the answer is "I am sorry, I have an appointment." Women with migraine do not need to make themselves more important than anyone else, but they need to consider themselves at least as important as everyone else.

Workplace Stress: The majority of women in America today work outside the home. Although some women hold high-status and powerful positions, many more women have jobs with high demands and low control. These jobs can lead a woman to feel "helpless" in the workplace. Helplessness worsens the physical and emotional effects of stress, and also prevents individuals from even trying to improve their situation.

Financial Stress: Women on average earn less money than men and have a lower overall standard of living. Therefore, women often feel pressures from inadequate housing, poor access to healthcare, and fear of unexpected expenses. In such cases, women also have fewer opportunities for recreation and escape from day-to-day stress.

Caregiver Stress: Women are likely to be the primary caretaker in the family. Though many men are taking active roles in parenting, women still provide the majority of childcare. There are great joys in parenting, but it can also be a physically and emotionally taxing responsibility. Women also are more likely to be the primary caregiver for aging parents and ill family members. Providing family care does not end at the close of a 40-hour workweek. Instead, the caretaker sometimes needs to provide 24-hours care on a daily basis.

Stress Management

Headache sufferers can learn skills to identify the stress that triggers their headaches. Sometimes the stress can be removed or resolved. In cases where the stress is uncontrollable, a woman can learn to change her own physical and emotional reactions to stressful situations. Individuals learn to recognize and change their own reactions to stress through a variety of stress-management techniques. Techniques such as biofeedback and relaxation training are effective in reducing headache frequency and pain in many sufferers.

Other techniques can help cope with headaches while they are occurring such as taking charge of headache. This involves keeping track of headaches, monitoring success and failure of therapies, identifying and monitoring things that may "trigger" headache, and making and keeping appointments with health care providers.

The Impact of Mood on Headaches

Headache and Psychological Symptoms

Personality: Headache is not a psychological disorder, and the majority of headache sufferers do not have significant psychological problems. Physicians in the 1800s and early 1900s suggested that headaches were related to a particular personality pattern. Headache researchers have now collected over 200 scientific studies examining the personality and behavior of headache sufferers. In most studies, headache sufferers tend to have increased daily stress, more difficulty coping with stress, and more mild symptoms of depression. However, there is no good evidence for a particular headache-prone personality.

Depression: Women have a higher risk for depression than men. In fact, women are three times more likely to experience an episode of depression than men are. The reason for the increased risk is not entirely clear, but may relate to a combination of biological (such as hormones, pregnancy, genetic predisposition) and environmental factors (stress, allergies, sleep).

Depression also is known to occur more often in headache sufferers than non-headache sufferers. The stress of coping with a chronic painful medical condition, like headache, increases the risk of depression. Even low levels of depression can reduce the effectiveness of medication and behavioral (biofeedback or relaxation training) or cognitive (behavioral) treatments for headache. Therefore, it is very important to recognize the signs of depression and discuss them with the physician. This information can help the physician select treatments that can relieve symptoms of both headache and depression.

Symptoms of possible depression:

- Sad, depressed, or irritable mood
- Loss of interest or pleasure in activities
- Weight loss (when not dieting) or weight gain
- Sleep disturbance (insomnia, early morning awakenings, increased sleeping)

- Feeling agitated or feeling sluggish
- Feelings of worthlessness
- Inability to concentrate
- Recurrent thoughts of death or suicide

Anxiety: As with depression, women are at a greater risk than men are for anxiety. Anxiety involves a state of tension or fear that occurs without clear cause. Anxiety can lower one's threshold to stress so that even small amounts of stress can be difficult for these sufferers to manage. Anxiety also can increase the level of pain or reduce the pain tolerance threshold during a headache that can undermine the effectiveness of traditional headache treatments. For some sufferers, it is necessary to treat both the anxiety and the headaches in order to get both under control.

Symptoms of possible anxiety:

- Feeling restless, keyed up, or on edge
- Being easily fatigued
- Difficulty concentrating, or mind going blank
- Muscle tension
- Sleep disturbance (difficulty falling asleep or staying asleep)

Chapter 11

Depression and Headaches

It is well known that the patient having a mild tension headache which can be relieved by aspirin is rarely seen by the physician for this condition. However, if the headache occurs daily, is present when the patient awakens, remains for most of the day and has been occurring for months or even years, the patient becomes an important therapeutic problem. These are the patients seen by the practicing physician because of the continuous headache, which does not usually respond to the common analgesic drugs.

In 1964, this type of headache was described by the author as being a major symptom in patients with depressive reactions. The presence of depression is often subtle and the diagnosis is often missed. Probably most physicians are able to recognize the classically depressed patient. This is the patient who walks into the office with a certain look of sadness, speech and movements are slow, exhibits little interest in anything, and sighs frequently. However, since the majority of depressed patients do not fit the classic mode, diagnosis will require some detective work on the part of the physician. The physician must obtain a thorough history from the patient, which should include a detailed psychiatric history including the patient's marital relations, occupation, social relationships, life stresses, personality traits, habits, methods of handling tense situations, and sexual problems. Two basic questions are often helpful in providing insight for a possible depression. First, inquiries should be made about family, personal history of prior depression, or if the patient had similar symptoms previously. Second, the patient should be questioned about the onset of his/her symptoms or any precipitating events.

The depressed patient often presents with a wide variety of complaints that can be categorized as physical, emotional, and psychic. The physical complaints include chronic pain and headaches, sleep disturbances, severe insomnia and early awakening, appetite changes, anorexia and rapid weight loss, and a decrease in sexual activity, ranging at times to impotence in males and amenorrhea or frigidity in females. Emotional complaints including feeling "blue," anxiety, and rumination over the past, present, and future. Finally, psychic complaints may include such statements as "morning is the worst time of day," suicidal thoughts, and death wishes. A headache secondary to depression is usually considered a tension-type (muscle contraction) headache.

Tension-type (muscle contraction) headache is believed to be due to sustained and/or tightened muscle contraction of the scalp and neck muscles. Sustained voluntary contraction of skeletal muscles may cause pain after variable periods. The pain may intensify if compression of small vessels causes ischemia or accumulation of noxious metabolites occurs in the affected muscles.

Although evidence regarding the cause of pain is conflicting, a recent study showed that voluntary contraction or decreased circulation in exercising temporalis muscle resulted in pain. A combination of exercise and ischemia markedly shortened the onset of pain.

An earlier study suggested that in susceptible persons contraction of skeletal muscles of the head, together with extracranial vasoconstriction caused by circulating constrictor agents, could produce tension-type (muscle contraction) headaches. The investigator believed that both responses occur concomitantly in anxiety-producing situations. In a later study, researchers observed increased blood flow to the scalp muscles during tension headache. However, this increased blood flow did not rule out decreased circulation, since metabolic demands may have exceeded the observed flow in actively contracting muscles.

Recent studies have questioned the role of muscle in tension headache. They argue that most patients do not manifest increased muscle activity during tension-type (muscle contraction) headache. However, the muscle model should not be dismissed and may be useful in a limited group of patients. The muscle contraction concept is still worthwhile, although evidence is conflicting. Increased muscle contraction and scalp muscle ischemia are probably essential to head pain, central pain mechanisms may also lead to headache. Chronic tension-type (muscle contraction) headaches may conceal a serious emotional disorder, such as depression. The patient will present with a persistent and vague headache, for which no organic cause can be determined. For the patient, the physical symptoms are more socially acceptable than the anxiety or depressive symptoms; many patients are certain there is a somatic basis for their pain.

People with depressive illness may develop bodily symptoms, and conversely people with painful organic diseases tend to become depressed. It should be noted that too little attention is given to the depressive aspects of chronic pain and its treatment. The physical complaints dominate the situation so that the underlying depression tends to be overlooked. Certain details about the headache may indicate an underlying depression. These headaches usually appear at regular intervals in relation to daily life, occurring on weekends, Sundays, or holidays, and on the first days of vacation or after exams. The greatest incidence of "nervous-type" headache occurs from 4:00 p.m. to 8:00 p.m. and from 4:00 a.m. to 8:00 a.m. These are usually the periods of the greatest and sometimes the most silent family crisis. This headache consists of a steady, nonpulsatile ache, often distributed in a band-like pattern around the head. It may be described as vise-like, a steady pressure, a weight, a soreness or a distinct cramp-like sensation. They follow no definite pattern as to location, although the occipital portion of the skull is frequently affected. Their duration is a distinguishing feature. A depressed person will describe his/her headache as lasting for years or throughout life. A depressive headache is usually dull and generalized, characteristically worse in the morning and in the evening.

In making the diagnosis of depressive headache, we must be certain to rule out organic causes. These include cervical arthritis, discogenic bony anomalies of the occipitocervical joints, basilar invagination, chronic mastoiditis, malocclusion of the temporomandibular joint and possibly a posterior fossa lesion in the brain.

The most popular biologic theories of depression hold that the disorder is associated with depletion of brain monoamine neurotransmitters such as serotonin and norepinephrine. Determining the most important substance in depression is controversial. Evidence is available to support both the norepinephrine and serotonin hypotheses. Other neurotransmitters, such as dopamine and endorphin, may also be involved in depression. The discovery of endogenous, opiate-like substances in the brain, the endorphins and enkephalins, has significantly advanced our understanding of pain.

The current treatment of tension-type (muscle contraction) headache often focuses on the underlying depression and includes the use of the antidepressant agent. Biofeedback also has been demonstrated as useful in the treatment of tension-type (muscle contraction) headaches. Some scientists have reported a reduction of the levels of depression in patients with tension-type (muscle contraction) headache following the use of biofeedback. However, in their work, the categorizing of the depression was unclear.

There may also be a relationship between depression and migraines. Researchers have reported a weak but significant relationship between migraine and depression. They noted a high correlation between depression and migraine in relation to weakness, sensory disturbance, difficulty with speech and loss of consciousness. They postulated about a possible subgroup of patients in whom depression and migraine are linked and who are characterized by the presence of those focal neurological signs previously mentioned.

It has been proposed that the antimigraine effect of amitriptyline is independent of its antidepressant effect, but it is undetermined if this effect is due to blocking of the re-uptake of serotonin and, to a lesser degree, norepinephrine at the nerve endings, or due to its anticholinergic, antihistaminic and antiserotonergic actions. Further investigation is warranted in this possible link.

In summary, depression is a widespread affliction that can be treated, but first it must be unmasked. The physician should be cognizant that although the headache may be secondary to depression, the pain is very, very real. The patient should be reassured that he/she can be helped but it is not going to happen immediately and it will require time and complete cooperation.

The tricyclic antidepressants, the selective serotonin re-uptake inhibitors, and the monoamine oxidase inhibitors are agents of choice in the treatment of headaches associated with depression. These drugs must be prescribed by a physician.

Chapter 12

Environmental and Physical Factors

The environmental factors that can provoke a migraine are extremely variable and affect only a small proportion of migraine sufferers. Environmental factors that can trigger a migraine include a change in climate or weather (such as a change in humidity or temperature), a change in altitude or barometric pressure, high winds, traveling, or a change in routine. Other environmental triggers include a bright or flickering light (sunlight reflections, glare, fluorescent lighting, television, or movies), extremes of heat and sound, and intense smells or vapors.

Weather changes can cause biological changes in the body's chemical balance and thus precipitate a migraine headache in some sensitive people. Weather conditions also can increase the severity of a headache induced by other factors. Extremes cold as well as very humid weather conditions have been known to trigger migraine headaches. A very dry and dusty atmosphere also can precipitate a migraine. When too many electrically charged dust particles are inhaled, it is thought that certain vasoactive chemicals are released, thus triggering a headache. These particles also may provoke the migraine headaches associated with certain winds and storms or with crowding in a stuffy room. A change in barometric pressure can trigger a

Text in this chapter is from "Environmental and Physical Factors," © 2000 The National Headache Foundation. Used with permission from the National Headache Foundation. For more information on headache causes and treatments, call the National Headache Foundation at 1-888-NHF-5552 or visit the web site at www.headaches.org.

migraine headache. The reduction of oxygen causes the blood and blood vessels to compensate. The scalp arteries swell, as they are extremely sensitive to the pressure of oxygen in the blood, especially to sudden changes, such as those that occur with flying in an airplane or sea diving. People living or traveling at high elevations can experience similar headaches.

Any change in a migraineur's environment that involves adjustment and adaptation can provoke a headache. Changing schools or jobs requires a great deal of adaptation, resulting in difficulty for the migraine sufferer. Travel may provoke migraine headaches because of the change in routine or diet as well as the new environmental and atmospheric conditions.

Many migraineurs are sensitive to travel and seasickness. The jarring motion of a car, train, or boat can trigger a headache. A change in sleep pattern or activity level may change the frequency of migraine attacks. Many migraine sufferers are very sensitive to light, especially to glare. Bright lights are more likely to trigger migraine headaches when they are of a "flickering" quality, and a slow flicker is usually more irritating than a more rapid one. It is believed that some people have more excitable brain cells in response to light than others. A dazzling, flicker type of light can be found in light reflected on snow, sand, or water, or through clouds. Some fluorescent lighting or the light that flickers from television and movie screens may have a similar effect. The use of polaroid lenses in these glaring conditions can be helpful.

Certain fumes and vapors can cause the blood vessels of the susceptible person to swell and dilate, triggering a migraine headache. Carbon monoxide poisoning from a poorly ventilated environment can provoke a headache. Faulty furnaces in winter can be responsible for such fumes. The nitrites used in explosives can trigger a headache in susceptible persons who are employed in munitions plants. Smoking can provoke or intensify a headache. It can cause biological changes in the blood and blood vessels. Just being in a smoke-filled environment can provoke a headache in susceptible people. Loud and irritating noises also can precipitate migraine headaches. This may be associated with stress as well as change in environmental conditions.

Many physical factors also can trigger migraine headaches, including overexertion such as bending, straining, or lifting; high blood pressure; toothache; or localized head or neck pains.

Chapter 13

Diet and Headaches

Can food allergies cause headache? Should certain foods be avoided?

There is very little evidence that food allergies have anything to do with headaches. Certain foods do contain substances called amines that may affect the brain and trigger migraines in susceptible or headache-prone individuals, but not through an allergic mechanism. Cheese, chocolate, and citrus, the "three Cs," are the most common offending foods, but only a minority of headache sufferers are affected. Some headache patients can eat these potential troublemakers when their lives are running smoothly, but during times of stress or fatigue, or at certain times of the menstrual cycle, these same substances may trigger attacks.

It's generally thought that a hereditary chemical imbalance in the brain causes susceptibility or proneness to headaches. This chemical imbalance involves serotonin, one of the neurotransmitters, or chemicals that transmit messages from one cell to another. Factors such as fatigue, irregular sleep patterns, stress, or hormone changes associated with the menstrual cycle may change the level or threshold of headache susceptibility or proneness, so that certain food "triggers" can set an attack in motion. Alcohol, especially red wine, is often mentioned by migraine sufferers as a trigger, especially when other factors have "set the stage."

Text in this chapter is from the American Council for Headache Education (ACHE) ©2000. Reprinted from the web site of the American Council for Headache Education (www.achenet.org); reprinted with permission.

What about food additives?

Nitrites, which are found in cured or processed meats such as tur-key, ham, hot dogs, and sausage, can cause problems for some people, and so can monosodium glutamate, or MSG, which is found in Ac-cent®, meat tenderizers, canned meats and fish, and some Chinese restaurant food. This common food additive sometimes masquerades under a variety of other names, such as "textured protein" or "natu-ral flavoring." New food labeling requirements will make it harder to conceal MSG.

Eating salty snack food has been linked to headache attacks by some studies. Use of aspartame (Nutrasweet®, Equal®) has been as-sociated with a high frequency of headache in some studies, but not in others. Until this issue is settled, headache sufferers, especially those with migraine, should avoid this artificial sweetener.

Even though the foods and beverages mentioned don't cause prob-lems for all headache sufferers, avoiding them for awhile to see if this helps is worth trying. If you think diet may be an important factor in your attacks, a dietitian who has a special interest in this subject can be helpful.

Keeping a headache diary can also help you spot troublesome foods or beverages, but remember that there may be a "lag period," com-monly 3-12 hours but occasionally as long as a day, between the time a particular food or beverage is used and onset of the headache. It's also good to remember that some headaches may be triggered by a combination of foods. For example, you may be able to eat cheese by itself, but not in a pizza with pepperoni, which has cured meat con-taining nitrites and may also be a headache trigger.

I've heard that caffeine can sometimes cause headache, but caffeine is also used in some painkillers. How can you explain this?

Sometimes it's easy to forget that caffeine is a drug. It's found not only in coffee but also in tea and many soft drinks. Caffeine is a stimu-lant that can speed up the heart, raise blood pressure, and interfere with relaxation. A good rule is to drink no more than two caffeinated beverages per day, or less if headaches are frequent. Strangely, once a headache has begun, caffeine can be helpful. This is because caf-feine is an "adjuvant"—it enhances the effects of pain medicine. That's why caffeine is added to many over-the-counter medications used to treat headache.

Like some other drugs, caffeine can cause headache if overused by a rebound mechanism once the body comes to depend on it. This is the reason why it's probably not a good idea to avoid caffeine altogether on the weekend if you are accustomed to having one or more cups per day. If you decide to cut down on caffeine, it's best to do so very gradually.

What other diet factors are important?

Skipping meals, which can allow blood sugar levels to drop, seems to be one of the most common triggers mentioned by migraine patients. Anyone prone to frequent headaches should avoid skipping meals. A better idea is to have meals at regular intervals during the day, and to eat some protein at least three times during each day.

Chapter 14

Caffeine and Headaches

Here are some of the most important facts about caffeine and its relationship to headaches.

- Most people feel the effects of caffeine within 30 minutes.

- Generally, the effects of caffeine last 3 to 5 hours.

- The average American consumes about 200-300 mg of caffeine daily, or the equivalent of about 2-3 cups of coffee.

- People who get headaches should clearly understand how caffeine affects their headaches.

Caffeine in Headache Medications

Adding 130 mg of caffeine to a regular, two-tablet dose of common ingredients found pain relievers (aspirin and acetaminophen) makes them relieve headache pain about 40% better than they do without caffeine. Caffeine also helps your body absorb these medications, allowing you to get back to your daily life faster.

Because analgesics work better when they have caffeine added, you may be able to take less medicine when you have a headache. And

Text in this chapter is from "Caffeine and Headaches," © 2000 The National Headache Foundation. Used with permission from the National Headache Foundation. For more information on headache causes and treatments, call the National Headache Foundation at 1-888-NHF-5552 or visit the web site at www.headaches.org.

because even non-prescription medications are real medicine with the potential for side effects, taking less reduces the risks associated with inappropriate use.

Caffeine and "Rebound" Headaches

"Rebound headache" is a serious problem that develops from taking too many headache medications too often.

Rebound headache is constant—it won't go away until you completely stop taking the drugs that are causing the problem.

Any headache medicine can cause rebound headache—taking caffeine-containing headache medications doesn't appear to increase the risk.

Rebound headache is rare; in fact, less than 2% of the general population is reported to suffer from rebound headache due to over use of pain relievers.

Addiction or Dependence

According to both the World Health Organization and the American Psychiatric Association, caffeine is considered safe, and in no way resembles other addictive or habit-forming drugs that lead to severe physical and social consequences.

Significant caffeine abuse has not been reported by any culture in the world.

When used according to label directions, headache medicines with caffeine pose no risk of addiction or dependence.

Caffeine Withdrawal Headaches

Technically, a person needs to use caffeine every day and reach a monthly total of at least 15 grams before they will experience caffeine withdrawal headache.

Withdrawal symptoms occur when people consume 500 mg (about 5 cups of coffee) or more daily, but they have been reported after long-term, daily intake of 100 mg or less per day.

Part Three

Treatment of Headaches

Chapter 15

The Best Medicine for Headaches

New headache drugs are coming onto the market every six months, with many more in the research and development pipeline. People with headache have never had so many options for controlling their attacks. But which option is right for you? Is newer better, or is older safer? How do you choose?

Each medicine has a different profile of benefits, side effects and other tradeoffs, but often it isn't possible to predict which will work best for a given individual with headache. All the same, it is possible to make an informed decision about which drug or which type of drug to try first. Several considerations can help you and your doctor select the type of medication most likely to be helpful:

- Do you have symptoms other than pain with the attack, such as nausea or vomiting, that might interfere with your ability to use oral medication (pills or capsules)?

- Are these associated symptoms severe or annoying to the point that they need to be treated too?

- Do your headaches develop gradually or are they sudden and severe, requiring a fast-acting medication?

"What's the Best Medicine for My Headaches?" ©2000 American Headache Society (AHS), available online at http://www.ahsnet.org; reprinted with permission.

- Do your headaches tend to come back a few hours after the first dose of your current medication?

- Do you have other medical conditions that contraindicate the use of a particular drug?

- Do you have special preferences that need to be considered (for example, a non-sedating drug that may allow you to continue to work)?

Pill, Spray, Suppository or Needle?

Medications can be administered and absorbed by a number of different routes. Drugs taken in the form of pills and capsules are absorbed through the gastrointestinal tract. Sublingual tablets that dissolve in the mouth are usually absorbed faster than medication that is swallowed. The same is true of suppositories that are absorbed through the membrane of the rectum. Nasal sprays enter the bloodstream more quickly by being absorbed through the membrane lining the nose. Self-administered injections under the skin or into muscle are still quicker acting. Drugs injected directly into the bloodstream act very rapidly but are generally used only in the doctor's office or the emergency room. Medications for headache are available using all of these routes of administration. The choice involves balancing the need for quick pain relief with other treatment considerations as well as convenience and personal preference.

Pills and Capsules

Many people find oral medicines the most convenient to take, as well as the most portable. Because they take longer to act, however, they are not the best option for people whose severe headache pain peaks rapidly, within a few minutes or a half hour. Also, nausea and vomiting during a migraine attack can seriously interfere with the effectiveness of oral medications. Oral medications are a good choice for people who have tension-type headache, migraine without nausea and vomiting, or migraine attacks that come on slowly, allowing early treatment.

Sublingual tablets or lozenges that are held under the tongue to dissolve are another approach. They are absorbed through the membrane lining the mouth and may be a little quicker to act compared to conventional tablets that must pass through the stomach and small intestine before they enter the bloodstream.

Nasal Sprays and Suppositories

Nasal sprays may be quicker to act than oral drugs and they are easier to use than injection drugs, so they are good options for people who need quick relief or who have significant nausea and vomiting with their attacks. Depending on the product, they may require a little practice for effective use, since the position of the head during administration can affect the efficacy. DHE and sumatriptan are two highly effective headache medications that are available as nasal sprays.

Lidocaine nasal drops are sometimes used as a treatment for severe migraine or cluster headache. Since the development of nasal spray medications for headache, suppositories are less often used, but also provide relatively quick pain relief and are good choices for people who have nausea and vomiting with their headaches.

Self-Injection

Injected drugs generally provide the most rapid pain relief. The disadvantages are discomfort, "hassle," and any embarrassment over using an injection in public. When the headaches are rapid and severe, injection drugs may offer the most effective treatment or the only effective treatment. Side effects may be more intense with injections.

Understanding Your Medication Options

Route of administration is one important consideration in selecting the medication most likely to provide good headache control. There are different classes of headache drugs, which have different mechanisms of action in providing headache relief. Within each class of drugs, the available medications vary in their profile of benefits and side effects, so a person who had a poor result to one triptan or ergot drug, for example, might still do well with another.

Ads, package inserts and published drug profiles give information not only on safety, side effect profile, and overall efficacy, but may also give the rate of headache recurrence and the speed of action. This type of information is very useful in selecting the medicine most likely to suit your specific situation. However, bear in mind that everyone is different and may respond differently to medication. Also, one headache may be different from another. You may get results that are better or worse than those reported in studies.

Simple Analgesics

Simple analgesics include the familiar over-the-counter (OTC) pain relievers such as aspirin (Bufferin, Bayer) and acetaminophen (Tylenol), as well as ibuprofen (Advil, Motrin, Nuprin), ketoprofen (Orudis), and naproxen (Naprosyn, Aleve). These last three belong to a class of drugs called nonsteroidal anti-inflammatory drugs (NSAIDs).

There are also several OTC combination drugs that contain caffeine, which can help relieve migraine when taken in small, well-timed doses. Extra Strength Excedrin and Excedrin for Migraine combine acetaminophen and aspirin with caffeine. Aspirin-Free Excedrin contains acetaminophen plus caffeine, and Anacin combines aspirin and caffeine. It's important to remember that too much caffeine can actually cause headache. Most people with frequent headache are advised to limit their daily intake of caffeine in coffee, tea and soft drinks.

Over-the-counter analgesics are a good choice for milder migraine headaches or for tension-type headaches. If the headache does not respond to these drugs, taking multiple doses won't help and can hurt. These medications can cause stomach irritation and are contraindicated for people with ulcers.

There are also stronger prescription NSAIDs that may be used for headache. Ketorolac (Toradol) is a prescription NSAID that is given by injection and is sometimes used as an emergency room treatment for severe headache.

The Ergot Drugs

The ergot drugs are a family of migraine medications that originally derived from a fungus that grows on rye. They have been available by prescription since the 1920s. Among other effects, they interact with receptors for the brain chemical serotonin, which regulates mood, pain awareness, and blood vessel tone. Ergot drugs reduce inflammation and have powerful effects on blood vessels, causing them to constrict. This vasoconstrictive property helps relieve the throbbing pain of migraine, but it also means these drugs are contraindicated for people with high blood pressure, heart disease, or peripheral vascular disease (for example, Raynaud's disease). Alert your doctor if you experience symptoms of blood vessel constriction after taking ergotamine, such as temporary numbness or tingling sensations, muscle cramps, or cold fingers or toes.

Ergotamine tartrate is available in several different brands and formulations. Combinations containing caffeine in addition to ergotamine are available in tablets (Wigraine) and suppository (Ercaf). Ergomar is a sublingual tablet that is allowed to dissolve under the tongue for somewhat quicker results than conventional tablets. Bellergal-S combines ergotamine with belladonna and phenobarbital. Ergotamine may produce nausea as a side effect. Patients who have good headache control with an ergotamine drug may find that taking an anti-nausea drug beforehand is effective in controlling any nausea.

Dihydroergotamine (DHE) is related to ergotamine but has a less powerful effect on blood vessel constriction, making it somewhat safer to use. It has a low rate of headache recurrence compared to the triptan family of headache medicines. Common side effects such as nausea seem to be milder with DHE compared to ergotamine. DHE is available as a self-injection drug (DHE-45) and as a nasal spray under the brand name Migranal. For best results, your doctor should instruct you in the proper head position for using Migranal. Because they enter the bloodstream more rapidly than pills or tablets, both DHE-45 and Migranal are good choices for people with relatively severe, rapid-onset headaches.

The Triptans

The triptans target specific groups of serotonin receptors that are known to play a role in migraine and in other types of headache. They have similar side effects to the ergot drugs, but the side effects tend to be less severe. As with the ergot drugs, the triptans are used with caution, or not at all, in patients with uncontrolled high blood pressure, heart disease or peripheral vascular disease. Any chest pain or discomfort should be reported to your physician for evaluation. Dosing strategies can sometimes help minimize any problems with headache recurrence, which sometimes happens to people who have prolonged migraine attacks, or a second medication can be prescribed for the recurrences. Four triptans are currently available in the U.S.: sumatriptan (Imitrex), naratriptan (Amerge), zolmitriptan (Zomig), and rizatriptan (Maxalt). Sumatriptan is available in three formulations, as a tablet, a subcutaneous ("under the skin") injection, and a nasal spray.

Rizatriptan can be prescribed as either a conventional tablet or a specially formulated tablet (Maxalt-MLT) that dissolves in the mouth. The dissolving tablet can be taken without water but does not provide faster headache relief than the tablet. Zolmitriptan and naratriptan are available as tablets only. At least three more triptans may become available in the near future; they are eletriptan, frovatriptan, and almotriptan.

While these drugs all act on the nervous system in similar ways, there are some differences in typical side effects, speed of action, and headache recurrence rate. A person who has an unsatisfactory response with one triptan may still do well with another drug in this class. The triptans are usually non-sedating and are often good choices for people who need to stay active and alert during a headache attack. Some people will experience fatigue, drowsiness or dizziness so the medication should be tried at home first.

Isometheptene (Midrin)

Isometheptene is available under the brand name Midrin as a capsule that also contains acetaminophen and dichloralphenazone, a mild sedative. It is a useful treatment for migraine that is often chosen for patients who cannot tolerate ergot drugs.

Combination Analgesics

Combination analgesics contain acetaminophen or aspirin combined with a barbiturate or opioid (narcotic) drug. These drugs are potentially habit-forming and are usually prescribed in limited quantities with strict controls on refills. Since many other migraine medications are contraindicated for people with heart disease or uncontrolled high blood pressure, combination analgesics may be an important option for these patients. They can also be appropriate choices for someone who has infrequent but severe migraine attacks.

Phrenilin combines acetaminophen with butalbital, a barbiturate. Fioricet contains acetaminophen, butalbital and caffeine, while Fiorinal is aspirin, butalbital and caffeine. Both Fioricet and Fiorinal are also available with codeine as an added analgesic. These drugs are all taken by mouth. The narcotic butorphanol is available as a nasal spray under the brand name Stadol. Like all drugs in this category, its use must be limited and closely monitored to avoid the potential for overuse and dependency.

Not Just the Headache: Treating Other Symptoms

For migraine sufferers, the associated symptoms such as sensitivity to light and sound and any nausea or vomiting can often be just as disruptive to normal functioning as the headache itself. An effective headache treatment should address the associated symptoms as well as the head pain.

There are several effective drugs for migraine-related nausea and vomiting. Metoclopramide (Reglan) is an anti-nausea or anti-emetic drug that is taken orally. Promethazine (Phenergan) and prochlorperazine (Compazine) are available as oral drugs or as suppository. Prochlorperazine is effective in relieving headache in addition to nausea. Both promethazine and prochlorperazine are sedating, which may be a benefit if the migraine sufferer is home and able to rest. Metoclopramide is generally preferable for daytime or workplace use. On rare occasions ondansetron (Zofran) may be necessary. It is most often used as an intravenous injection to treat the nausea and vomiting associated with cancer chemotherapy, but is available as a tablet.

Communicating with Your Doctor

Family practice physicians, internists, neurologists and gynecologists can all be skilled in treating headache. However, doctors who do not treat a large number of headache patients may not be aware of all the options for effective treatment, or how these options should be matched to the individual's preferences and needs. They may decide to start with the most familiar or best-studied drug, figuring they can always try something else if that doesn't work out. If your doctor does not ask you about symptoms and headache characteristics that might influence the choice of medication, you should volunteer that information.

For example, depending on your situation, you might say:

- "I'm so nauseous during the headache that I don't think I could keep a pill down. Are there other choices besides oral drugs?"

- "The headache comes on really fast. Can you give me something that will give quicker pain relief?"

- "I operate machinery at work—will this drug make me drowsy or dizzy?"

- "The medication you gave me last time works, but the headache always comes back. Is there something else we could try to prevent recurrence?"

- "The medicine I'm on now sometimes works and sometimes doesn't. Is there a second medication I could use for the more severe headaches that don't respond to my usual treatment?"

What's Important to You?

Remember that you are unlikely to find a 100% effective, side-effect-free treatment for all your headaches. Before you see your doctor, you might want to take some time to think about your priorities and goals in seeking treatment, so you can be clear about what is most important to you in evaluating your medication options. You may have no bothersome side effects with one drug but find that recurrence of your severe headaches is a problem. If you have prolonged, moderate-intensity headaches, speed of action may not be essential, but a drug that leaves you feeling sleepy or light-headed may be unsatisfactory. You can use the following checklist to help you evaluate your preferences for effective treatment.

Rate the following treatment preferences from 0 (not important at all) to 5 (very important). An effective headache medication should:

- Provide quick pain relief

- Decrease pain

- Decrease headache recurrence

- Decrease nausea

- Decrease light sensitivity

- Not cause nausea

- Not cause drowsiness

- Be easy to administer

- Allow me to return to normal functioning

Prevention for Frequent or Severe Headache

The medicines discussed here are all for occasional use and are known as acute or abortive treatments for headache, since they are used to stop a headache attack in progress. If you find you are using your medications more than three times a week on average, you should see your doctor to discuss trying a daily medication to prevent or reduce headache occurrence. Or, if you have three or more severe, hard-to-treat attacks per month, preventive medication should be considered. For people who have predictable patterns to their headache attacks-for example, with menstrual migraine or seasonal cluster headache-it's often possible to control the headaches by taking preventive medications just before and during the headache-prone times.

Preventive medications for headache include beta blockers such as propranolol (Inderal) and timolol (Blocadren); divalproex (Depakote); antidepressants such as amitriptyline (Elavil/Endep) and nortriptyline

(Pamelor); calcium channel blockers such as verapamil (Calan/Isoptin SR); and methysergide (Sansert), among others. Methysergide requires special prescribing and monitoring precautions to avoid rare complications. Otherwise, these drugs have an excellent safety record and are preferable to overuse of the abortive medications described in this brochure.

Avoiding Overuse

A number of analgesic drugs that act to relieve headaches when taken as directed can actually make the headaches worse if overused. In this situation, overuse of headache medication (for example, more than three or four times per week) results in a type of chronic daily headache called drug rebound headache. The headache returns as each dose of medication wears off, prompting the individual to take another dose of medication. This results in a vicious cycle of headache—pain medicine—return of headache—more pain medicine—more headache. The only treatment for drug rebound headache is stopping the medication. Unfortunately, the headache becomes worse when the medication is withdrawn and does not improve significantly for weeks or even months. Most people will see a definite improvement in their headaches, such as a return to the frequency they had before the daily headaches developed.

Many different headache medications can result in a drug rebound headache if overused either singly or in combination with similar drugs. Excessive caffeine alone can produce drug rebound headache in susceptible individuals, even if pain medicine is not being overused. Limit your consumption of caffeine-containing coffee, teas and soft drinks if you are prone to frequent headaches.

Although there are other types of chronic daily headache, drug rebound headache appears to be the most common. While you should not hesitate to take an effective headache medicine as directed, be cautious about too frequent dosing, particularly if you find you are using your medication more than three or four times a week. If you do find you are taking medication several days a week, discuss your situation with your doctor. A combination of preventive and abortive medications may be safer and more effective. Non-drug approaches, such as biofeedback, relaxation therapy, and exercise, can also be helpful in reducing both headache frequency and need for medication.

Chapter 16

Opioid Drugs for Headaches

What Are Opioids?

As the name suggests, opioids are drugs that act on the body and brain in the same basic ways as opium and its many derivatives. Opioids can offer relief from severe, unresponsive pain, can bring sleep to the weary and, unfortunately, can also result in drug dependency if overused or abused.

Opium is an extract of the seeds of the oriental poppy and contains morphine and codeine along with many other active compounds. For decades, researchers have sought to develop new opium-like compounds that might offer the pain relief of the natural narcotics with fewer of their risks and side effects. Oxycodone, methadone, and butorphanol are examples of synthetic or semisynthetic opioids.

Opium-like substances do not come only from poppies and pharmaceutical companies. The body produces its own pleasure-giving and pain-relieving chemicals, such as the endorphins. Opium and opioid drugs work because they act on the same sites in the brain and nervous system as the endorphins. Problems in the body's own opioid system may be a factor in some cases of migraine, although the evidence to support this theory is still limited.

Opioid drugs do not all act in exactly the same way on the brain, however. For example, oxycodone and methadone act primarily on one

"When Are Opioid Drugs Appropriate for Headaches?" ©2000 American Headache Society (AHS), available online at http://www.ahsnet.org; reprinted with permission.

class of opioid receptor (a "gatekeeper" molecule that triggers responses within brain cells), while butorphanol targets a different class of receptor. Effects and side effects can vary accordingly.

When Are Opioids Used to Treat Headache?

There is a growing number of non-narcotic medications available to stop a migraine attack or blunt its pain. These range from over-the-counter Excedrin Migraine to DHE-45 and the triptans. Some patients cannot take either the triptans or the ergot drugs (ergotamine or DHE-45) because of contraindications such as a past heart attack or uncontrolled high blood pressure. A few patients with severe, prolonged headaches may not achieve adequate pain relief with any of the standard treatments. In these situations, physicians will occasionally prescribe short-acting opioids for use when other treatments fail and the headache is severe.

Several prescription pain relievers combine moderate doses of a short-acting opioid with aspirin, acetaminophen and/or caffeine. Codeine combinations are the opioids most often prescribed for relieving severe, unresponsive headache. These include Fioricet with codeine, Tylenol with codeine and Fiorinal with codeine. (Fioricet and Fiorinal also contain butalbital, a barbiturate). Propoxyphene combinations (Darvocet, Darvon) and oxycodone combinations (Percocet, Percodan) can also be used with caution and strict rationing. Physicians often set a limit on use for all these opioid medications, allowing only a specified number of tablets per month, with non-refillable prescriptions.

These are short-acting opioids—they are generally prescribed for "breakthrough" headaches—for use after a non-narcotic analgesic has failed to be effective. Because they produce sedation and drowsiness, many people find they cannot take them at work or school. Also, the individual should not drive a car or operate dangerous machinery for at least one hour after taking the dose. Alcohol use should be avoided.

Butorphanol (Stadol) nasal spray is a viable alternative to the opioid combinations that are taken by mouth. Stadol's primary advantage over opioids taken by mouth is its onset of action—often within 15 minutes. When properly used with patient education and strict limits on refills, to prevent overuse, butorphanol is a reasonable choice for controlling severe headaches. For patients who have vomiting or significant nausea with their migraine attacks, a nasal spray offers advantages over drugs taken by mouth.

Meperidine (Demerol) and hydromorphine (Dilaudid) are other opioids effective for acute pain. In general, these drugs are considered to have a higher risk of drug dependence or severe side effects and would only be used with careful monitoring if other medications were ineffective or contraindicated. Meperidine is frequently given by injection in the emergency room for treatment of severe headache.

How Are Opioids Used to Prevent Headache?

Sufferers who have four or more severe headaches per month are often given a trial of a prophylactic (preventive) medication. Preventive treatments are generally taken daily to reduce the number or severity of the headaches. Patients with seasonal cluster headaches or menstrual migraine can often limit use to their headache-prone times.

A number of different medications have been shown to be effective in reducing headache frequency or severity, including beta blockers, several antidepressants, and divalproex (Depakote). None of these drugs will work for all patients, and a few may find their headaches are resistant to standard preventive approaches. In these instances, long-acting opioids may be tried as a daily preventive.

Steady use of short-acting opioids heightens the potential for drug dependency. Long-acting opioids offer more prolonged pain control, reducing the need for dosing to one to two administrations a day in carefully selected and monitored patients. These drugs are formulated so that the opioid enters the bloodstream relatively slowly, lessening the side effects and reducing the risk of tolerance.

Several long-acting opioids have been used as preventive treatments for severe, treatment-resistant daily headache. These include methadone, oxycontin, fentanyl, levorphanol, and MS Contin, which is a controlled release formulation of morphine.

The use of long-acting opioids for prevention of chronic daily headache is controversial. The safety and efficacy of this approach are still being studied with small groups of patients at major headache referral centers. Currently, patients receiving long-term opioid therapy are a tiny minority—one or two out of a thousand—of all the patients referred to these centers for difficult-to-treat headache conditions.

What Are the Risks and Side Effects?

Opioids have significant side effects. Although the side effect profile of each drug is different, there are a number of common effects, such as constipation, sedation, itching, drowsiness, lightheadedness, dizziness, and mood changes. Sedation can be a benefit for individuals who also have problems getting a good night's rest, if they can take the medication before bed. Sedation and drowsiness tend to improve as therapy is continued, often after the first few days. Some degree of constipation may persist throughout treatment.

These drugs should not be used by someone with emphysema, severe asthma, sleep apnea, or other significant respiratory problems since they also cause respiratory depression (breathing becomes slower and more shallow, as it does during sleep). Alcohol and a number of other drugs can magnify this effect so it's important to review all medication for possible drug interactions. Depending upon the opioid selected for treatment, you will be told to limit alcohol use or avoid alcohol altogether.

This side effect is not dangerous with normal dosing in healthy adults. With overdoses, respiratory depression can be fatal. Many physicians advise their patients to have someone with them when taking an opioid for the first time, in case some undetected health condition or drug interaction results in more serious respiratory depression.

With the exception of meperidine, the opioids suppress the cough reflex. Opioids can also cause the release of histamine, which triggers an inflammatory reaction in the skin and other tissues, and can cause itching as a possible side effect.

Some migraine sufferers will find that the nausea or vomiting they experience with their attacks is relieved by opioid treatment. Because opioids have complex effects on the gastrointestinal system, they can also produce nausea or vomiting as side effects.

The mood changes caused by opioid medication are not all enjoyable. While some drugs do cause euphoria (a pleasant state of consciousness), they can also bring on negative, restless or anxious feelings (called dysphoria, the opposite of euphoria). Either mood change can potentially interfere with thinking and concentration on tasks. For some the mood changes will be minor and improve as therapy continues.

Could I Become Addicted?

The most important concern for both doctors and patients is the fear of becoming addicted to the drugs. In general, pain patients who have no history of drug abuse and who use their opioid medication as directed are at very low risk for true addiction.

Both doctors and patients often misunderstand addiction and misuse the term. Addiction is best defined as psychological dependence. Someone who is psychologically dependent becomes obsessed with obtaining the drugs, uses them for recreation not pain control, and shows an overall loss of control over drug use. Usually their relationships and work performance have deteriorated as a result of their obsession with drug use.

It's important not to confuse addiction with two other potential effects of continued opioid treatment: tolerance and physical dependence. Tolerance means that ever-higher doses are needed to achieve an effect. Some degree of tolerance usually develops after the first few opioid doses but should not escalate if the drug is used properly. Physical dependence involves changes in the nervous system that create withdrawal symptoms if drug use is abruptly stopped. Withdrawal symptoms can include restlessness, sweating, cramping, diarrhea, weakness, anxiety, depression and increased pain—none of them pleasant, but all times—limited and reversible. It is possible to develop physical dependence and to have withdrawal symptoms when treatment is stopped without being addicted.

Patients who take opioids as prescribed to control pain have a very low risk of significant tolerance, physical dependence or psychological dependence. Responsible patients who take opioids only occasionally for their most severe headaches are not at risk. If preventive opioids are appropriately prescribed and used, only slight tolerance develops and physical dependence should not be a problem. The individual who discontinues the medication under medical supervision by gradually tapering doses will generally experience mild or no symptoms of withdrawal, even after long-term use.

Signs of psychological dependence can develop with the opioids, or with any pain medication. Headache patients often come to fear headache and become preoccupied with avoiding and relieving pain. They may then become anxious or agitated if their doctor limits their supply of narcotic medication. This behavior is often called pseudoaddiction. The individual is not abusing drugs recreationally but fear of pain is expressed in drug-seeking behavior. Behavioral therapy can help the individual understand the fear and learn better coping strategies.

When Do Doctors Decide Opioids Are Indicated?

Responsible physicians must be conservative in electing to use opioid drugs for chronic pain conditions such as headache. The risk of physical or psychological dependency with overuse is one major concern. Also, the sedation or drowsiness and the mood changes produced by opioids can interfere with normal activities. The physician and the headache sufferer must be convinced that the standard non-narcotic treatments are unsatisfactory after being tried at the appropriate dosage and for an appropriate length of time.

This is not always simple to do. Many preventive drugs may need adjustments in dosage and a trial of two to three weeks before they will begin to show an effect. Sometimes combinations of different acute and preventive treatments produce much better results than any one drug used alone. Most importantly, some headache sufferers who have failed to get relief from many different medications are actually experiencing rebound headache from medication overuse.

Drug rebound headache is a form of chronic daily headache that is triggered by daily or near-daily use of pain relief medicines, either prescription or over-the-counter analgesics, including short-acting opioids. Caffeine in coffee, tea or sodas can also contribute to drug rebound headache in some people. Some evidence suggests that tolerance to common non-narcotic analgesics can develop, with withdrawal symptoms (including headache) when their use is stopped.

In most instances, patients who develop drug rebound headache have been taking more frequent doses or larger doses than the labeling for the medications advise. However, a few susceptible individuals may develop a chronic daily headache in response to moderately heavy use of analgesics and caffeine.

Drug rebound headache can only be treated by stopping all the pain medications under a physician's supervision. Other preventive medications, including opioids, will not work until the analgesics have been discontinued. Unfortunately, stopping analgesics will bring on more severe headaches and other withdrawal symptoms. It may take up to two months for the headaches to improve, although some people will note improvement within two or three weeks.

How Can I Work with My Doctor to Evaluate My Options?

Physicians vary greatly in their comfort level with prescribing potentially addictive drugs for chronic pain. To avoid emergency room visits for severe unresponsive attacks, they may elect to prescribe limited quantities of codeine combination tablets to responsible patients. If the patient is taking large quantities of non-narcotic medications to obtain unreliable pain relief, the physician may feel that careful use of opioid combinations would actually be a safer alternative. Before prescribing more potent opioids or preventive use of opioids, headache physicians will often consult a colleague for a second opinion, to be certain that there isn't a non-narcotic treatment approach that should still be tried.

Many physicians will require the patient to sign a contract or agreement that states their mutual obligations in using opioids safely. This agreement may specify strict limits on monthly supply, no over-the-phone authorization of refills, and frequent follow-up appointments. A psychological assessment may be used to ensure the individual has no risk factors for poor compliance or drug dependency. The spouse or significant other may also be asked to meet with the doctor to be sure the family understands the purpose of the therapy and the limits on its use.

Before trying opioids for chronic daily headache, the doctor and the headache sufferer should rule out the possibility of drug rebound headache. If you have constant or near-constant pain, it is easy to lose track of how much medication you take, particularly if you are using a number of different over-the-counter and prescription drugs. A headache calendar can be a vital tool for assessing the possibility of analgesic overuse. Use the calendar to record the doses of all pain relievers and any other medication you take for any purpose. Note your daily caffeine intake as well, including coffee, tea, caffeinated drinks and chocolate.

It is important to realize that preventive opioid therapy is not always effective, and the side effects may prove difficult to tolerate. One headache clinic has reported results on 42 patients with severe, treatment-resistant chronic daily headache who were treated with methadone for six months. Between 60% and 86% reported significant improvement in quality-of-life indicators such as relationships and work performance. All reported moderate to excellent relief from their severe chronic daily headaches. However, another 106 patients in the same clinic discontinued methadone treatment because of side effects or ineffectiveness. While long-acting opioids have significant risks and limitations, they can improve quality of life for a small minority of patients whose severe daily or near-daily headaches do not respond to other treatments.

Glossary

Analgesia: The state of lowered pain awareness or pain sensitivity without loss of consciousness. (Anesthesia involves loss of consciousness with loss of pain awareness.)

Analgesics: Pain-relieving drugs, ranging from aspirin to morphine.

Endorphins: Specific substances occurring naturally in the brain and nervous system that relieve pain in the same ways as the opioid drugs do.

Morphine: A drug originally derived from opium and used to relieve severe pain. A schedule II drug considered to have high potential for abuse.

Narcotics: A term for opium—derived and opium-like drugs, or for drugs that cause sedation, stupor, and numbness similar to morphine; often used more loosely to refer to any drug or controlled substance, such as cocaine, that has the potential to produce dependence or addiction.

Opiates: Drugs such as morphine and codeine that are derived from opium. The term is sometimes used to refer to an opium-like narcotic drug.

Opioids: Drugs that act similarly to opium or to morphine or codeine. Usually these are synthetic drugs designed to minimize some of the side effects and addictive potential of the natural opium compounds.

Opium: The extract of the poppy plant, Papaver somnipherus, containing a number of pharmacologically active compounds, including morphine and codeine.

Respiratory depression: A state in which breathing becomes slower and shallower, as during sleep.

Scheduled drugs: Drugs subject to restrictions on their use and distribution because of their potential for producing physical and/or psychological dependence. The FDA classifies these drugs according to their potential for abuse and for dependence as either: Schedule I (heroin); Schedule II (codeine, meperidine, methadone, oxycodone, hydromorphone, etc.); Schedule III (hydrocodone); Schedule IV (butorphanol, pentazocine, propoxyphene); or Schedule V (buprenorphine). Schedule I drugs have the highest abuse potential and Schedule V have the lowest.

Sedation: A lowering of alertness and responsiveness, usually accompanied by drowsiness or sleep.

Stupor: A state of reduced consciousness or profound sedation such that the person can only be aroused by shaking, etc.

Chapter 17

Guide to Over-the-Counter Pain Relievers

Headaches can be managed with proper medication, diet, exercise, and lifestyle modification. When headaches occur occasionally (one time a week), over-the-counter medications, a "time out" for relaxation, or a short nap will likely provide pain relief. In fact, most people with occasional headaches will select a nonprescription "over-the-counter" (OTC) pain reliever from their pharmacy or supermarket shelves.

Medication

Available without prescription, OTC pain relievers contain powerful, effective ingredients. There are several different groups of OTC pain relievers including combination products:

- Aspirin products

- Acetaminophen products

- NSAIDs such as ibuprofen and naproxen sodium products

- Combination products such as those that contain OTC pain relievers and caffeine

Each group has specific advantages and side effects. The most appropriate way to select a medication or combination of medications

©2000 American Headache Society (AHS), available online at http://www.ahsnet.org; reprinted with permission.

123

Table 17.1. Components of Selected OTC Pain Relievers

Product	Active Ingredients	Relieve Pain	Reduce Fever	Forms Available
Aspirin Products				
Bayer®	Aspirin	•	•	Caplet, tablet
Bufferin®	Buffered aspirin	•	•	Caplet, tablet
Ecotrin®	Aspirin	•	•	Caplet, tablet
Acetaminophen Products				
Excedrin PM®*	Acetaminophen, diphenhydramine citrate	•	•	Caplet, tablet, LiquiGel
Tylenol®	Acetaminophen	•	•	Caplet, tablet, gelcap, geltab
Tylenol PM®*	Acetaminophen, diphenhydramine HCl	•	•	Caplet, tablet, gelcap, geltab
Other NSAIDs				
Advil®	Ibuprofen	•	•	Caplet, tablet
Aleve®	Naproxen sodium	•	•	Caplet, tablet
Motrin IB®	Ibuprofen	•	•	Caplet, tablet, gelcap
Nuprin®	Ibuprofen	•	•	Caplet, tablet
Actron®	Ketoprofen	•	•	Tablet
Orudis KT®	Ketoprofen	•	•	Tablet
Combination Products				
Excedrin®, Extra Strength	Aspirin, acetaminophen, caffeine	•	•	Caplet, geltab
Excedrin®, Aspirin Free	Acetaminophen, caffeine	•	•	Caplet, geltab
Anacin®	Aspirin, caffeine	•	•	Caplet, tablet

*For pain with accompanying sleeplessness.

is to weigh the desired effect against potential side effects. Most OTC pain relievers are available in tablets, caplets and geltabs. While all forms of a medication are equally effective, some may be easier to swallow than others.

Note: If you take medications for any other medical condition (such as high blood pressure, arthritis, diabetes, ulcer or even acne), be sure to check with your physician or pharmacist before taking an OTC pain reliever. Make certain that adding a pain reliever to the medicines you already take will not result in undesirable drug interactions.

What's in Frequently Used OTC Pain Relievers

Table 17.1 gives you a quick overview of the ingredients in selected OTC pain relievers often used for the relief of headache pain. Each product consists of an ingredient or combination of ingredients that has been demonstrated safe and effective for use as directed. For most people, the beneficial effects outweigh side effects. Aspirin, ibuprofen, naproxen sodium, and acetaminophen all may cause different side effects in different people.

What You Need to Know about Combination Products

Pain relief products with a combination of aspirin, acetaminophen, and caffeine have been shown to provide greater pain relief than single ingredient aspirin or acetaminophen products. In fact, to get the same relief found with a single dose of the aspirin-acetaminophen-caffeine combination you would have to increase the equivalent dose of aspirin or acetaminophen by almost 40%. If you are sensitive to caffeine, however, you should check with your doctor.

Guidelines for Use of Nonprescription Pain Relievers

Nonprescription pain relievers have been demonstrated to be safe when used as directed on the package. The following precautions, however, are important:

- Know the active ingredients in each product. Be sure to read the entire label.

- Do not exceed recommended dosage on the package.

- Carefully consider how you use pain relievers and all medications; it is easy to escalate from appropriate use to overuse.

125

Check with your doctor before taking products that contain aspirin, ibuprofen, or naproxen sodium if:

- You have a bleeding disorder or hemophilia

- You have asthma

- You have recently had surgery or dental surgery, or are about to have surgery

- You are pregnant, especially during the last three months of pregnancy

- You have ulcers, kidney or liver damage

- You take any arthritis drugs or nonsteroidal anti-inflammatory medications such as ibuprofen, naproxen sodium, piroxicam, etc.

- Check with your doctor before taking acetaminophen-containing products if you suffer from kidney or liver damage.

The Risk of OTC Overuse: Rebound Headache

Rebound headache may result from taking prescription or nonprescription pain relievers daily or almost every day, contrary to directions on the package label. If prescription or nonprescription pain relievers are overused, headache may "rebound" as the last dose wears off, leading one to take more and more medication.

"Try This at Home" Prevention Tips

Exercise

Regular aerobic exercise, including brisk walking, swimming, and bicycling, helps many people handle stress and may help avoid headaches.

- Exercise may help get rid of a headache. So if your headache is mild and is not the kind that requires medical attention, go ahead and exercise! You may be glad you did.

- Migraine sufferers, too, remark that the frequency of their headaches decreases when they exercise regularly.

Diet

Some people with headaches find that certain foods, alcohol, and preservatives trigger headaches.

- Keep a diary that lists what you eat and when your headaches occur. Symptoms can develop between 1 and 24 hours after eating.

- A review of these notes will help you determine whether foods are likely headache triggers.

- A generally healthful diet may help, too. Eating regularly scheduled meals three times a day is especially important. Most people find what works by experimentation.

Guidelines for Managing Your Headaches

1. Know when to consult your doctor.

2. Don't hesitate to ask your pharmacist about headache pain relievers.

3. Choose an appropriate pain reliever. All OTC pain relievers can be effective. When selecting a pain reliever, you should consider any existing medical problems that could be adversely affected by any of the ingredients. Follow all package directions carefully.

4. To reduce risk of rebound headache, do not take pain relievers daily and be sure to follow package directions when you do take them.

5. Eat a healthful diet, and get enough exercise.

Chapter 18

Acupuncture

Acupuncture is one of the oldest, most commonly used medical procedures in the world. Originating in China more than 2,000 years ago, acupuncture became widely known in the United States in 1971 when *New York Times* reporter James Reston wrote about how doctors in Beijing, China, used needles to ease his abdominal pain after surgery. Research shows that acupuncture is beneficial in treating a variety of health conditions.

In the past two decades, acupuncture has grown in popularity in the United States. In 1993, the U.S. Food and Drug Administration (FDA) estimated that Americans made 9 to 12 million visits per year to acupuncture practitioners and spent as much as $500 million on acupuncture treatments.[1] In 1995, an estimated 10,000 nationally certified acupuncturists were practicing in the United States. By the year 2000, that number is expected to double. Currently, an estimated one-third of certified acupuncturists in the United States are medical doctors.[2]

The National Institutes of Health (NIH) has funded a variety of research projects on acupuncture that have been awarded by its National Center for Complementary and Alternative Medicine (NCCAM), National Institute on Alcohol Abuse and Alcoholism, National Institute of Dental Research, National Institute of Neurological Disorders and Stroke, and National Institute on Drug Abuse.

From "Acupuncture Information and Resources," National Center for Complementary and Alternative Medicine (NCCAM), 1999.

Acupuncture Theories

Traditional Chinese medicine theorizes that the more than 2,000 acupuncture points on the human body connect with 12 main and 8 secondary pathways, called meridians. Chinese medicine practitioners believe these meridians conduct energy, or qi, between the surface of the body and internal organs.

Qi regulates spiritual, emotional, mental, and physical balance. Qi is influenced by the opposing forces of yin and yang. According to traditional Chinese medicine, when yin and yang are balanced, they work together with the natural flow of qi to help the body achieve and maintain health. Acupuncture is believed to balance yin and yang, keep the normal flow of energy unblocked, and restore health to the body and mind.

Traditional Chinese medicine practices (including acupuncture, herbs, diet, massage, and meditative physical exercises) all are intended to improve the flow of qi.[3]

Western scientists have found meridians hard to identify because meridians do not directly correspond to nerve or blood circulation pathways. Some researchers believe that meridians are located throughout the body's connective tissue;[4] others do not believe that qi exists at all.[5,6] Such differences of opinion have made acupuncture a source of scientific controversy.

Preclinical Studies

Preclinical studies have documented acupuncture's effects, but they have not been able to fully explain how acupuncture works within the framework of the Western system of medicine.[7,8,9,10,11,12]

Mechanisms of Action

Several processes have been proposed to explain acupuncture's effects, primarily those on pain. Acupuncture points are believed to stimulate the central nervous system (the brain and spinal cord) to release chemicals into the muscles, spinal cord, and brain. These chemicals either change the experience of pain or release other chemicals, such as hormones, that influence the body's self-regulating systems. The biochemical changes may stimulate the body's natural healing abilities and promote physical and emotional well-being.[13] There are three main mechanisms:

1. *Conduction of electromagnetic signals:* Western scientists have found evidence that acupuncture points are strategic conductors of electromagnetic signals. Stimulating points along these pathways through acupuncture enables electromagnetic signals to be relayed at a greater rate than under normal conditions. These signals may start the flow of pain-killing biochemicals, such as endorphins, and of immune system cells to specific sites in the body that are injured or vulnerable to disease.[14,15]

2. *Activation of opioid systems:* Research has found that several types of opioids may be released into the central nervous system during acupuncture treatment, thereby reducing pain.[16]

3. *Changes in brain chemistry, sensation, and involuntary body functions:* Studies have shown that acupuncture may alter brain chemistry by changing the release of neurotransmitters and neurohormones in a good way. Acupuncture also has been documented to affect the parts of the central nervous system related to sensation and involuntary body functions, such as immune reactions and processes whereby a person's blood pressure, blood flow, and body temperature are regulated.[3,17,18]

Clinical Studies

According to an NIH consensus panel of scientists, researchers, and practitioners who convened in November 1997, clinical studies have shown that acupuncture is an effective treatment for nausea caused by surgical anesthesia and cancer chemotherapy as well as for dental pain experienced after surgery. The panel also found that acupuncture is useful by itself or combined with conventional therapies to treat addiction, headaches, menstrual cramps, tennis elbow, fibromyalgia, myofascial pain, osteoarthritis, lower back pain, carpal tunnel syndrome, and asthma; and to assist in stroke rehabilitation.[19]

Increasingly, acupuncture is complementing conventional therapies. For example, doctors may combine acupuncture and drugs to control surgery-related pain in their patients.[20] By providing both acupuncture and certain conventional anesthetic drugs, doctors have found it possible to achieve a state of complete pain relief for some patients.[16] They also have found that using acupuncture lowers the need for conventional pain-killing drugs and thus reduces the risk of side effects for patients who take the drugs.[21,22]

Outside the United States, the World Health Organization (WHO), the health branch of the United Nations, lists more than 40 conditions for which acupuncture may be used.[23] Table 18.1 lists these conditions.

Table 18.1. Conditions Appropriate for Acupuncture Therapy

Digestive

Abdominal pain
Constipation
Diarrhea
Hyperacidity
Indigestion

Emotional

Anxiety
Depression
Insomnia
Nervousness
Neurosis

Eye-Ear-Nose-Throat

Cataracts
Gingivitis
Poor vision
Tinnitis
Toothache

Gynecological

Infertility
Menopausal symptoms
Premenstrual syndrome

Miscellaneous

Addiction control
Athletic performance
Blood pressure regulation
Chronic fatigue
Immune system tonification
Stress reduction

Musculoskeletal

Arthritis
Back pain
Muscle cramping
Muscle pain/weakness
Neck pain
Sciatica

Neurological

Headaches
Migraines
Neurogenic bladder dysfunction
Parkinson's disease
Postoperative pain
Stroke

Respiratory

Asthma
Bronchitis
Common cold
Sinusitis
Smoking cessation
Tonsillitis

Source:

World Health Organization, United Nations. *"Viewpoint on Acupuncture."* 1979 (revised).[23]

Currently, one of the main reasons Americans seek acupuncture treatment is to relieve chronic pain, especially from conditions such as arthritis or lower back disorders.[24,25] Some clinical studies show that acupuncture is effective in relieving both chronic (long-lasting) and acute or sudden pain, but other research indicates that it provides no relief from chronic pain.[27] Additional research is needed to provide definitive answers.

FDA's Role

The FDA approved acupuncture needles for use by licensed practitioners in 1996. The FDA requires manufacturers of acupuncture needles to label them for single use only.[28] Relatively few complications from the use of acupuncture have been reported to the FDA when one considers the millions of people treated each year and the number of acupuncture needles used. Still, complications have resulted from inadequate sterilization of needles and from improper delivery of treatments. When not delivered properly, acupuncture can cause serious adverse effects, including infections and puncturing of organs.[1]

NCCAM-Sponsored Clinical Research

Originally founded in 1992 as the Office of Alternative Medicine (OAM), the NCCAM facilitates the research and evaluation of unconventional medical practices and disseminates this information to the public. The NCCAM, established in 1998, supports nine Centers, where researchers conduct studies on complementary and alternative medicine for specific health conditions and diseases. Scientists at several Centers are investigating acupuncture therapy.

Researchers at the NCCAM Center at the University of Maryland in Baltimore conducted a randomized controlled clinical trial and found that patients treated with acupuncture after dental surgery had less intense pain than patients who received a placebo.[20] Other scientists at the Center found that older people with osteoarthritis experienced significantly more pain relief after using conventional drugs and acupuncture together than those using conventional therapy alone.[29]

Researchers at the Minneapolis Medical Research Foundation in Minnesota are studying the use of acupuncture to treat alcoholism and addiction to benzodiazepines, nicotine, and cocaine. Scientists at the Kessler Institute for Rehabilitation in New Jersey studied acupuncture to treat a stroke-related swallowing disorder and the pain associated with spinal cord injuries.

The OAM, now the NCCAM, also funded several individual researchers in 1993 and 1994 to conduct preliminary studies on acupuncture. In one small randomized controlled clinical trial, more than half of the 11 women with a major depressive episode who were treated with acupuncture improved significantly.[30]

In another controlled clinical trial, nearly half of the seven children with attention deficit hyperactivity disorder who underwent acupuncture treatment showed some improvement in their symptoms. Researchers concluded that acupuncture was a useful alternative to standard medication for some children with this condition.[31]

In a third small controlled study, eight pregnant women were given a type of acupuncture treatment, called moxibustion, to reduce the rate of breech births, in which the fetus is positioned for birth feet-first instead of the normal position of head-first. Researchers found the treatment to be safe, but they were uncertain whether it was effective.[32] Then, researchers reporting in the November 11, 1998, issue of the *Journal of the American Medical Association* conducted a larger randomized controlled clinical trial using moxibustion. They found that moxibustion applied to 130 pregnant women presenting breech significantly increased the number of normal head-first births.[33]

Acupuncture and You

The use of acupuncture, like many other complementary and alternative treatments, has produced a good deal of anecdotal evidence. Much of this evidence comes from people who report their own successful use of the treatment. If a treatment appears to be safe and patients report recovery from their illness or condition after using it, others may decide to use the treatment. However, scientific research may not substantiate the anecdotal reports.

Lifestyle, age, physiology, and other factors combine to make every person different. A treatment that works for one person may not work for another who has the very same condition. You, as a health care consumer (especially if you have a preexisting medical condition); should discuss acupuncture with your doctor. Do not rely on a diagnosis of disease by an acupuncturist who does not have substantial conventional medical training. If you have received a diagnosis from a doctor and have had little or no success using conventional medicine, you may wish to ask your doctor whether acupuncture might help.

Finding a Licensed Acupuncture Practitioner

Doctors are a good resource for referrals to acupuncturists. Increasingly, doctors are familiar with acupuncture and may know of a certified practitioner. In addition, more medical doctors, including neurologists, anesthesiologists, and specialists in physical medicine, are becoming trained in acupuncture, traditional Chinese medicine, and other alternative and complementary therapies. Friends and family members may be a source of referrals as well. In addition, national referral organizations provide the names of practitioners, although these organizations may be advocacy groups for the practitioners to whom they refer.

Check a practitioner's credentials. A practitioner who is licensed and credentialed may provide better care than one who is not. About 30 states have established training standards for certification to practice acupuncture, but not all states require acupuncturists to obtain a license to practice. Although proper credentials do not ensure competency, they do indicate that the practitioner has met certain standards to treat patients with acupuncture.

The American Academy of Medical Acupuncture can give you a referral list of doctors who practice acupuncture. The National Acupuncture and Oriental Medicine Alliance lists thousands of acupuncturists on its Web site and provides the list to callers to their information and referral line. The Alliance requires documentation of state license or national board certification from its listed acupuncturists. The American Association of Oriental Medicine can tell you the state licensing status of acupuncture practitioners across the United States as well.

Check treatment cost and insurance coverage. Reflecting public demand, an estimated 70 to 80 percent of the nation's insurers covered some acupuncture treatments in 1996. An acupuncturist may provide information about the number of treatments needed and how much each will cost. Generally, treatment may take place over a few days or several weeks. The cost per treatment typically ranges between $30 and $100, but it may be appreciably more. Physician acupuncturists may charge more than nonphysician practitioners.[13]

Check treatment procedures. To find out about the treatment procedures that will be used and their likelihood of success. You also should make certain that the practitioner uses a new set of disposable needles in a sealed package every time. The FDA requires the use of sterile, nontoxic needles that bear a labeling statement restricting their use to qualified practitioners. The practitioner also should swab the puncture site with alcohol or another disinfectant before inserting the needle. Some practitioners may use electroacupuncture; others may use moxibustion. These approaches are part of traditional Chinese medicine, and Western researchers are beginning to study whether they enhance acupuncture's effects.

During your first office visit, the practitioner may ask you at length about your health condition, lifestyle, and behavior. The practitioner will want to obtain a complete picture of your treatment needs and behaviors that may contribute to the condition. This holistic approach is typical of traditional Chinese medicine and many other alternative and complementary therapies.

Let the acupuncturist, or any doctor for that matter, know about all treatments or medications you are taking and whether you have a pacemaker, are pregnant, or have breast or other implants. Acupuncture may be risky to your health if you fail to tell the practitioner about any of these matters.

The Sensation of Acupuncture

Acupuncture needles are metallic, solid, and hair-thin, unlike the thicker, hollow hypodermic needles used in Western medicine to administer treatments or take blood samples. People experience acupuncture differently, but most feel minimal pain as the needles are inserted. Some people are energized by treatment, while others feel relaxed.[34] Some patients may fear acupuncture because they are afraid of needles. Improper needle placement, movement of the patient, or a defect in the needle can cause soreness and pain during treatment.[35] This is why it is so important to seek treatment from a qualified acupuncture practitioner.

As important research advances continue to be made on acupuncture worldwide, practitioners and doctors increasingly will work together to give you the best care available.

For More Information

For more information about acupuncture research sponsored by different parts of NIH, contact the respective Information Office or Clearinghouse. Call the NIH operator for assistance at 301-496-4000.

For more information about research on acupuncture, contact the NIH National Library of Medicine (NLM), which has published a bibliography of more than 2,000 citations to studies conducted on acupuncture. The bibliography is available on the Internet at http://www.nlm.nih.gov/pubs/cbm/acupuncture.html or by writing the NLM, 8600 Rockville Pike, Bethesda, MD 20894. The NLM also has a toll-free telephone number: 888-346-3656.

For a database of research on complementary and alternative medicine, including acupuncture, access the CAM Citation Index on the NCCAM Web site at http://nccam.nih.gov/nccam/resources/cam-ci/.

Glossary of Terms

Acupuncture: An ancient Chinese health practice that involves puncturing the skin with hair-thin needles at particular locations, called acupuncture points, on the patient's body. Acupuncture is believed to help reduce pain or change a body function. Sometimes the needles are twirled, given a slight electric charge (see electroacupuncture), or warmed (see moxibustion).

Attention deficit hyperactivity disorder: A syndrome primarily found in children and teenagers that is characterized by excessive physical movement, impulsiveness, and lack of attention.

Clinical studies: (Also clinical trials, clinical outcomes studies, controlled trials, case series, comparative trials, or practice audit evidence.) Tests of a treatment's effects in humans. Treatments undergo clinical studies only after they have shown promise in laboratory studies of animals. Clinical studies help researchers find out whether a promising treatment is safe and effective for people. They also tell scientists which treatments are more effective than others.

Electroacupuncture: A variation of traditional acupuncture treatment in which acupuncture or needle points are stimulated electronically.

Electromagnetic signals: The minute electrical impulses that transmit information through and between nerve cells. For example, electromagnetic signals convey information about pain and other sensations within the body's nervous system.

Fibromyalgia: A complex chronic condition having multiple symptoms, including muscle pain, weakness, and stiffness; fatigue; metabolic disorders; allergies; and headaches.

Holistic: Describes therapies based on facts about the "whole person," including spiritual and mental aspects, not only the specific part of the body being treated. Holistic practitioners may advise changes in diet, physical activity, and other lifestyle factors to help treat a patient's condition.

Meridians: A traditional Chinese medicine term for the 14 pathways throughout the body for the flow of qi, or vital energy, accessed through acupuncture points.

Moxibustion: The use of dried herbs in acupuncture. The herbs are placed on top of acupuncture needles and burned. This method is believed to be more effective at treating some health conditions than using acupuncture needles alone.

Neurohormones: Chemical substances made by tissue in the body's nervous system that can change the structure or function or direct the activity of an organ or organs.

Neurological: A term referring to the body's nervous system, which starts, oversees, and controls all body functions.

Neurotransmitters: Biochemical substances that stimulate or inhibit nerve impulses in the brain that relay information about external stimuli and sensations, such as pain.

Opioids: Synthetic or naturally occurring chemicals in the brain that may reduce pain and induce sleep.

Placebo: An inactive substance given to a participant in a research study as part of a test of the effects of another substance or treatment. Scientists often compare the effects of active and inactive substances to learn more about how the active substance affects participants.

Preclinical studies: Tests performed after a treatment has been shown in laboratory studies to have a desirable effect. Preclinical studies provide information about a treatment's harmful side effects and safety at different doses in animals.

Qi: (Pronounced "chee.") The Chinese term for vital energy or life force.

Randomized controlled clinical trials: A type of clinical study that is designed to provide information about whether a treatment is safe and effective in humans. These trials generally use two groups of people; one group receives the treatment and the other does not. The participants being studied do not know which group receives the actual treatment.

Traditional Chinese medicine: An ancient system of medicine and health care that is based on the concept of balanced qi, or vital energy, that flows throughout the body. Components of traditional Chinese medicine include herbal and nutritional therapy, restorative physical exercises, meditation, acupuncture, acupressure, and remedial massage.

Yang: The Chinese concept of positive energy and forces in the universe and human body. Acupuncture is believed to remove yang imbalances and bring the body into balance.

Yin: The Chinese concept of negative energy and forces in the universe and human body. Acupuncture is believed to remove yin imbalances and bring the body into balance.

References

1. Lytle, C.D. *An Overview of Acupuncture.* 1993. Washington, DC: United States Department of Health and Human Services, Health Sciences Branch, Division of Life Sciences, Office of Science and Technology, Center for Devices and Radiological Health, Food and Drug Administration.

2. Culliton, P.D. *"Current Utilization of Acupuncture by United States Patients."* National Institutes of Health Consensus Development Conference on Acupuncture, Program & Abstracts (Bethesda, MD, November 3-5, 1997). Sponsors: Office of Alternative Medicine and Office of Medical Applications Research. Bethesda, MD: National Institutes of Health, 1997.

3. Beinfield, H. and Korngold, E.L. *Between Heaven and Earth: A Guide to Chinese Medicine.* New York, NY: Ballantine Books, 1991.

4. Brown, D. "Three Generations of Alternative Medicine: Behavioral Medicine, Integrated Medicine, and Energy Medicine." *Boston University School of Medicine Alumni Report.* Fall 1996.

5. Senior, K. "Acupuncture: Can It Take the Pain Away? " *Molecular Medicine Today.* 1996. 2(4):150-3.

6. Raso, J. *Alternative Health Care: A Comprehensive Guide.* Buffalo, NY: Prometheus Books, 1994.

7. Eskinazi, D.P. "National Institutes of Health Technology Assessment Workshop on Alternative Medicine: Acupuncture." *Journal of Alternative and Complementary Medicine.* 1996. 2(1):1-253.

8. Tang, N.M., Dong, H.W., Wang, X.M., Tsui, Z.C., and Han, J.S. "Cholecystokinin Antisense RNA Increases the Analgesic Effect Induced by Electroacupuncture or Low Dose Morphine: Conversion of Low Responder Rats into High Responders." *Pain.* 1997. 71(1):71-80.

9. Cheng, X.D., Wu, G.C., He, Q.Z., and Cao, X.D. "Effect of Electroacupuncture on the Activities of Tyrosine Protein Kinase in Subcellular Fractions of Activated T Lymphocytes from the Traumatized Rats." *Acupuncture and Electro-Therapeutics Research.* 1998. 23(3-4):161-170.

10. Chen, L.B. and Li, S.X. "The Effects of Electrical Acupuncture of Neiguan on the PO2 of the Border Zone Between Ischemic and Non-Ischemic Myocardium in Dogs." *Journal of Traditional Chinese Medicine.* 1983. 3(2):83-8.

11. Lee, H.S. and Kim, J.Y. "Effects of Acupuncture on Blood Pressure and Plasma Renin Activity in Two-Kidney One Clip Goldblatt Hypertensive Rats." *American Journal of Chinese Medicine.* 1994. 22(3-4):215-9.

12. Okada, K., Oshima, M., and Kawakita, K. "Examination of the Afferent Fiber Responsible for the Suppression of Jaw-Opening Reflex in Heat, Cold and Manual Acupuncture Stimulation in Anesthetized Rats." *Brain Research.* 1996. 740(1-2):201-7.

13. National Institutes of Health. "Frequently Asked Questions About Acupuncture." Bethesda, MD: National Institutes of Health, 1997.

14. Dale, R.A. "Demythologizing Acupuncture. Part 1. The Scientific Mechanisms and the Clinical Uses." *Alternative & Complementary Therapies Journal.* April 1997. 3(2):125-31.

15. Takeshige, C. "Mechanism of Acupuncture Analgesia Based on Animal Experiments." *Scientific Bases of Acupuncture.* Berlin, Germany: Springer-Verlag, 1989.

16. Han, J. S. "Acupuncture Activates Endogenous Systems of Analgesia." *National Institutes of Health Consensus Conference on Acupuncture, Program & Abstracts* (Bethesda, MD, November 3-5, 1997). Sponsors: Office of Alternative Medicine and Office of Medical Applications of Research. Bethesda, MD: National Institutes of Health, 1997.

17. Wu, B., Zhou, R.X., and Zhou, M.S. "Effect of Acupuncture on Interleukin-2 Level and NK Cell Immunoactivity of Peripheral Blood of Malignant Tumor Patients." *Chung Kuo Chung Hsi I Chieh Ho Tsa Chich.* 1994. 14(9):537-9.

18. Wu, B. "Effect of Acupuncture on the Regulation of Cell-Mediated Immunity in Patients With Malignant Tumors." *Chen Tzu Yen Chiu.* 1995. 20(3):67-71.

19. National Institutes of Health Consensus Panel. Acupuncture. National Institutes of Health Consensus Development Statement (Bethesda, MD, November 3-5, 1997). Sponsors: Office of Alternative Medicine and Office of Medical Applications of Research. Bethesda, MD: National Institutes of Health, 1997.

20. Lao, L., Bergman, S., Langenberg, P., Wong, R., and Berman, B. "Efficacy of Chinese Acupuncture on Postoperative Oral Surgery Pain." *Oral Surgery, Oral Medicine, Oral Pathology.* 1995. 79(4):423-8.

21. Lewith, G.T. and Vincent, C. "On the Evaluation of the Clinical Effects of Acupuncture: A Problem Reassessed and a Framework for Future Research." *Journal of Alternative and Complementary Medicine.* 1996. 2(1):79-90.

22. Tsibuliak, V.N., Alisov, A.P., and Shatrova, V.P. "Acupuncture Analgesia and Analgesic Transcutaneous Electroneurostimulation in the Early Postoperative Period." *Anesthesiology and Reanimatology.* 1995. 2:93-8.

23. World Health Organization. *Viewpoint on Acupuncture.* Geneva, Switzerland: World Health Organization, 1979.

24. Bullock, M.L., Pheley, A.M., Kiresuk, T.J., Lenz, S.K., and Culliton, P.D. "Characteristics and Complaints of Patients Seeking Therapy at a Hospital-Based Alternative Medicine Clinic." *Journal of Alternative and Complementary Medicine.* 1997. 3(1):31-7.

25. Diehl, D.L., Kaplan, G., Coulter, I., Glik, D., and Hurwitz, E.L. "Use of Acupuncture by American Physicians." *Journal of Alternative and Complementary Medicine*. 1997. 3(2):119-26.

26. Levine, J.D., Gormley, J., and Fields, H.L. "Observations on the Analgesic Effects of Needle Puncture (Acupuncture)." *Pain*. 1976. 2(2):149-59.

27. Ter Reit, G., Kleijnen, J., and Knipschild, P. "Acupuncture and Chronic Pain: A Criteria-Based Meta-Analysis." *Clinical Epidemiology*. 1990. 43:1191-9.

28. U.S. Food and Drug Administration. "Acupuncture Needles No Longer Investigational." *FDA Consumer Magazine*. June 1996. 30(5).

29. Berman, B., Lao, L., Bergman, S., Langenberg, P., Wong, R., Loangenberg, P., and Hochberg, M. "Efficacy of Traditional Chinese Acupuncture in the Treatment of Osteoarthritis: A Pilot Study." *Osteoarthritis and Cartilage*. 1995. (3):139-42.

30. Allen, John J.B. "An Acupuncture Treatment Study for Unipolar Depression." *Psychological Science*. 1998. 9:397-401.

31. Sonenklar, N. "Acupuncture and Attention Deficit Hyperactivity Disorder." National Institutes of Health, Office of Alternative Medicine Research Grant #R21 RR09463. 1993.

32. Milligan, R. Breech Version by Acumoxa. National Institutes of Health, Office of Alternative Medicine Research Grant #R21 RR09527. 1993.

33. Cardini, F. and Weixin, H. "Moxibustion for Correction of Breech Presentation: A Randomized Controlled Trial." *Journal of the American Medical Association*. 1998. 280:1580-4.

34. American Academy of Medical Acupuncture. "Doctor, What's This Acupuncture All About? A Brief Explanation for Patients." Los Angeles, CA: American Academy of Medical Acupuncture, 1996.

35. Lao, L. "Safety Issues in Acupuncture." *Journal of Alternative and Complementary Medicine*. 1996. 2(1):27-9.

Organizations

American Academy of Medical Acupuncture
Medical Acupuncture Research Organization
5820 Wilshire Boulevard
Suite 500
Los Angeles, CA 90036
Toll Free: 800-521-2262
Tel: 323-937-5514
Fax: 323-937-0959
Internet: http://www.medicalacupuncture.org

A professional association of medical doctors who practice acupuncture. The academy provides a referral list of doctors who practice acupuncture. It also provides general information about acupuncture, legislative representation, publications, meetings, and proficiency examinations.

American Association of Oriental Medicine
433 Front Street
Catasauqua, PA 18032
Tel: 610-266-1433
Fax: 610-264-2768
Internet: http://www.aaom.org
E-Mail: aaom1@aol.com

A nonprofit professional organization of acupuncturists and practitioners of Oriental medicine. The association determines standards of practice and education through the National Certification Commission for Acupuncture and Oriental Medicine. It also funds research and provides a list of acupuncturists and Oriental medicine practitioners by geographic area. The association provides articles and fact sheets, membership and licensing information, a list of acupuncture schools, and a list of state acupuncture associations.

British Medical Acupuncture Society
Newton House, Newton Lane
Whitley, Warrington, Cheshire WA4 4JA
England UK
Tel: 01144 1925 730727
Fax: 01144 1925 730492
Internet: http://www.medical-acupuncture.co.uk
E-Mail: bmasadmin@aol.com

A group of doctors who practice acupuncture with more conventional treatments. The Society produces the journal Acupuncture in Medicine, published twice per year, covering original research and reviews.

Foundation for Traditional Chinese Medicine
122A Acomb Road
York YO2 4EY
England UK
Tel: 01144 1904 785120
Fax: 01144 1904 784828
Internet: http://www.demon.co.uk/acupuncture/index.html

The Foundation funds the Acupuncture Research Resource Center and provides information about acupuncture research listed by condition, including migraine and lower back pain.

International Council of Medical Acupuncture and Related Techniques
Rue de l'Amazone 62
1060 Brussels
Belgium
Tel: 011 3225 393900
Fax: 011 3225 393692
Internet: http://users.med.auth.gr/~karanik/english/icmart/intro.html

A nonprofit organization created in 1983 of more than 40 national acupuncture-related associations of medical doctors practicing acupuncture and/or related techniques.

National Acupuncture and Oriental Medicine Alliance
14637 Starr Road SE
Olalla, WA 98359
Tel: 253-851-6896
Fax: 253-851-6883
Internet: http://www.acuall.org

A professional society of state-licensed, registered, or certified acupuncturists, with membership open to consumers, schools, organizations, corporate sponsors, and health care providers. The Alliance lists thousands of acupuncturists across the country on its Web site and provides information about them to callers to their information and referral line. The Alliance requires documentation of state license or national board certification from all acupuncturists it lists.

National Acupuncture Detoxification Association
P.O. Box 1927
Vancouver, WA 98668-1927
Toll Free: 888-765-6232
Fax: 805-969-6051

A nonprofit organization that provides training and consultation for more than 500 drug and alcohol acupuncture treatment programs run by local agencies. The organization's clearinghouse provides a library of audiotapes, videotapes, and literature on using acupuncture to treat addiction and mental disorders.

National Acupuncture Foundation
P.O. Box 2271
Gig Harbor, WA 98335-4271
Tel: 253-851-6538
Fax: 253-851-6538

The Foundation publishes books, including the Acupuncture and Oriental Medicine Law Book and the Clean Needle Technique Manual. The Foundation filed the U.S. Food and Drug Administration needle reclassification petition of 1996.

Society for Acupuncture Research
6900 Wisconsin Avenue, Suite 700
Bethesda, MD 20815
Tel: 301-571-0624
Fax: 301-961-5340

A nonprofit organization that facilitates the scientific evaluation of acupuncture.

Training and Credentialing Organizations
Accreditation Commission for Acupuncture and Oriental Medicine
1010 Wayne Avenue, Suite 1270
Silver Spring, MD 20910
Tel: 301-608-9680
Fax: 301-608-9576
E-Mail: 73352.2467@compuserve.com

The Commission, established in 1982, evaluates professional master's degree and first professional master's-level certificate and diploma programs in acupuncture and Oriental medicine, with concentrations in both acupuncture and herbal therapy.

Council of Colleges of Acupuncture and Oriental Medicine

1010 Wayne Avenue, Suite 1270
Silver Spring, MD 20910
Tel: 301-608-9175
Fax: 301-608-9576
Internet: http://www.ccaom.org

This Council was formed in 1982 and has developed academic and clinical guidelines and core curriculum requirements for master's and doctoral programs in acupuncture as well as acupuncture and Oriental medicine.

NAFTA Acupuncture Commission Standards Management, Inc.

14637 Starr Road SE
Olalla, WA 98359
Tel: 253-851-6896
Fax: 253-851-6883

This group of educators, acupuncturists, medical doctors, and naturopathic doctors meet to exchange information and discuss training standards of competence for the practice of acupuncture and Oriental medicine in North America, including Mexico and Canada.

National Certification Commission for Acupuncture and Oriental Medicine

11 Canal Center Plaza, Suite 300
Alexandria, VA 22314
Tel: 703-548-9004
Fax: 703-548-9079
Internet: http://www.nccaom.org
E-Mail: info@nccaom.org

This Commission was established in 1982 to implement nationally recognized standards of competence for the practice of acupuncture and Oriental medicine. It provides information and programs on certification standards for acupuncturists.

Online Resources

The Internet is one of the fastest ways to access health information, but much of this information is not controlled or reviewed by qualified health professionals. Approach information from the

Internet with caution, as it may be misleading, incorrect, or even dangerous.

Acuall.org
Internet: http://www.acuall.org

A site sponsored by the National Acupuncture and Oriental Medicine Alliance with general information on acupuncture and Oriental medicine, referrals to practitioners, legislative status, national issues, conferences and workshops, publications, and information for potential students.

Healingpeople.com
Internet: http://www.healingpeople.com

Describes and summarizes acupuncture procedures, areas of research, and other pertinent information from multiple sources.

Health Info Library: Acupuncture
Internet: http://www.americanwholehealth.com/library/acupuncture/tcm.htm

A site by the health care company American WholeHealth that provides acupuncture articles and research.

Medical Matrix
Internet: http://www.medmatrix.org

A gateway to clinical medical resources, including numerous medical journals.

National Library of Medicine. Current Bibliographies in Medicine & Acupuncture
Internet: http://www.nlm.nih.gov/pubs/cbm/acupuncture.html

Bibliographies to 2,302 scientific papers collected between January 1970 and October 1997.

Summary of Controlled Clinical Studies Demonstrating the Effectiveness of Acupuncture Treatment for Various Conditions
Internet: http://www.halcyon.com/dember/studies.html

Summarizes studies on dental pain, migraine and headache, lower back pain, cervical pain, tennis elbow, dysmenorrhea (menstrual disorders), addiction, respiratory conditions, cardiovascular fitness, stroke, nausea, and sleep disorders.

Chapter 19

Biofeedback, Deep Relaxation, and Massage Therapy in Headache Management

Though the causes of headaches can be varied, with many medications touted for relief, there are also several effective non-drug options available for the management of the occasional or chronic headache pain. These non-drug options allow the patient to take control of headache pain.

Biofeedback

The word "biofeedback" was coined in the late 1960s to describe a training technique first developed in laboratory tests started in the 1940s. With this technique, research subjects were taught to improve their health, perfect their performance, and/or reduce pain by eliciting specific signals from their own bodies. It was one of the first of the mind-over-body practices. Its success opened the doors to other non-traditional pain management practices.

In biofeedback, various electronic instruments or mechanical devices are used to "feed back" information on how well a person is controlling bodily sensations. For example, one biofeedback device picks up electrical signals from muscles and translates the signals into a flashing color or beeping sound. One, or both, of these, are activated every time muscles become tense. To learn to relax tense muscles, a person must learn to slow down the flashing or beeping. In this way, people learn to associate sensations from the muscle with tension levels.

"Biofeedback, Deep Relaxation, and Massage Therapy in Headache Management," by Margareta-Erminia Cassani, © 2001 Omnigraphics, Inc.

After biofeedback training is completed, people are then able to re-create this tension-control response at will without being attached to the sensors of the device.

Benefits of Biofeedback

People have reported numerous benefits of biofeedback in the management of their headache pain, with the highest degree of success in migraine or tension type headache sufferers. The most important ones include:

- Patient gained a sense of calm during headaches.
- Reduction in intensity of headache.
- Ability to cut back on medication.
- Reduction in amount of time that headache lasted.
- Complete stoppage of headache in certain instances.

Types of Biofeedback

There are three types of biofeedback used in headache management-muscular, thermal and brain wave. In each, sensors are placed on a person's skin so that the biofeedback device can convert internal bodily responses to a signal that is either heard or seen. Common signals include a bell, buzzer, flashing light, colors, etc. which the person then learns to control.

Muscular—an electromyograph (EMG) measures the amount of electrical signal generated by muscles in the forehead. The muscular method of biofeedback would be used if your headaches are tension and/or muscle contraction-based in origin. Therapists also use EMGs to relieve muscle stiffness, treat incontinence, and recondition injured muscles.

Thermal / Skin Temperature—gauges, such as finger thermometers measure blood flow through the fingertips which are highly sensitive to stress and relaxation, indicated by blood vessel constriction and dilation. This method is used for migraine headaches which are vascular in nature. Biofeedback has been proven to be effective in migraine headache sufferers by enabling the ability to reduce the intensity or duration of the headaches with at least a 50% improvement. Galvanic skin response sensors (GSRs) monitor the amount of sweat produced to measure how well the skin conducts responses.

These thermal devices are often used to reduce anxiety which can contribute to triggering migraine headaches.

Brain wave—an electroencephalogram, or EEG, is used to monitor brain waves. This type of biofeedback is done best in a therapist's office setting as it is difficult for a patient to both monitor the energy output from brain waves and practice the necessary biofeedback techniques needed to control the brain energy responses.

How to Find a Biofeedback Therapist

- The Biofeedback Certification Institute of America (BCIA) is the certifying board for biofeedback therapists. Information about finding a practitioner can be obtained on the BCIA website at www.bcia.org.

- Consult the yellow pages of your local telephone directory under Biofeedback, Psychologists, or Physiologists.

- Call the Association for Applied Psychophysiology and Biofeedback at 800-477-8892. They direct you to your state's society for information on biofeedback therapists.

- Consult BiofeedbackZone.com which lists resources for many states as well as devices for at home use.

Deep Relaxation

Because many headaches are caused or worsened by stress and tension, the degree that you can learn to relax in general, especially during a headache, can influence the amount and severity of headaches you experience. Specific deep relaxation techniques can help you lessen the pain of a headache or completely prevent one from coming on.

Aerobic Exercise

Overall stress reduction is greatly helped by regular physical exercise, preferably in fresh air and sunshine. Even as little as a 20 minute walk outside on a nice day can reduce stress and tension levels considerably and brighten your mood by releasing the brain's natural pain-killing, "feel good" chemicals-endorphins. If you are unable to exercise outside, regular aerobic exercise (walking, stationary bicycling, swimming, running, tennis, etc.) done indoors, at the gym, or in classes at your local community college or high school can go a long way in helping you reduce the onset of headaches that are caused and/or aggravated by stress and tension. Aerobic exercise helps release tension in the face, neck, and shoulders, which can be the cause of painful tension headaches and migraines. Aerobic exercise done for a half an hour a day, three to four days a week can help lessen tension and stress associated with headaches.

There are other specific deep relaxation techniques you can practice either in tandem with taking a pain reliever or on their own to assist in relaxing you and reducing the pain of—or completely banishing—a headache once it has begun. These techniques can be done anywhere but work best if you can remove yourself from the stressful situation, preferably to an empty, dimly lit room where you can sit quietly without interruption and with open a window where you can take in a few deep breaths of fresh air.

Deep Breathing

If possible, open a window and take in several, slow deep breathes of fresh air. Breathe slowly and deeply through your nose. This serves to oxygenate your blood quickly and increases oxygen flow to your brain. By itself, this can alleviate a headache brought on by lack of oxygen in indoor air. Low oxygen levels in homes or office buildings occur more frequently in winter when furnaces are pumping out lots of warm, but stale, air into your living or working environment.

If you can't take a quick walk around the block, standing next to an open window and taking several deep breaths can rejuvenate and relax you. If you can't open a window, just taking in a few deep, slow breaths can help. In stressful situations where tensions are running high, taking deep breaths causes your autonomic nervous system to slow down your pulse rate and relax your muscles. When the pulse quickens, we tend to breathe in short, shallow spurts. This action can result in a lack of oxygen in the blood, thereby bringing on a headache. This deep breathing relaxation technique helps significantly in a crisis situation where you don't have a lot of time to "work" with an ensuing headache. However, if you have extra time to de-stress and de-tense, the following deep relaxation techniques can also help you. These techniques are best done in a quiet, darkened room where you will not be interrupted, and where you can stay for at least an hour to complete the exercises and get the most benefit.

Progressive Muscle Relaxation

This technique focuses on tensing and releasing each muscle group of the entire body, working on the premise that you can consciously "tell" your muscles to let-go. You may not realize how tense you are until you start practicing progressive muscle relaxation. This exercise is sometimes easier done with a helper—someone who will tell you what muscles to flex and relax. The sound of another person's voice as they quietly direct you can also help to calm and de-stress you. It can also be easier to focus on someone else's verbal instructions rather than your own thoughts if stress and/or bad headache pain makes it difficult to concentrate. The purpose of this exercise is to train you in how a relaxed muscle feels. Once you put this information into your brain bank, you can call on it to get yourself to that relaxed state faster. Here's how to perform progressive muscle relaxation:

- Sit in a comfortable chair (like a recliner) where you can put your feet up, or lie on a bed or on a blanket on the floor. If its practical and you want, you may even put on some very peaceful, "dreamy" type music at low volume to assist you in relaxing.

- Starting with your toes, flex, or tighten, your toe/foot muscles for about 10 seconds. Then let them go. Repeat twice, or three times, until your toe/foot muscles feel completely relaxed.

- Next, move to your leg muscles and, again, flex and release your leg muscles 2-3 times, for about 10 seconds each, until that muscle group feels completely relaxed.

- Repeat this flexing/releasing of all muscle groups until you have gone through each muscle group of your entire body. At the end of this exercise, you should feel very relaxed and your headache pain greatly alleviated if not completely gone.

The next three deep relaxation techniques take a little longer to perform and require more mental concentration from you. Therefore, they may be more helpful as "maintenance" type techniques to keep you relaxed and de-stressed thereby minimizing painful headache occurrences.

Creative or Guided Imagery

This method of deep relaxation uses visualization techniques to help you feel the same satisfying sensations you feel when you experience a pleasant situation, for example, lying in the sun or floating on a raft.

You can even combine deep breathing and progressive relaxation with the imagery technique. Here's how:

- Sit in a comfortable chair or lie on a comfortable surface and begin with deep breathing.

- Next, try to relax all your muscles as you would doing progressive muscle relaxation techniques.

- Focus your mind on some pleasant place such, as lying on a warm, sunny beach, feeling the sun on your skin, hearing the sound of the ocean rhythmically rolling in and out on the shore, a comfortable, light breeze kissing your skin now and then. Try to actually "project" your mind into that created scene.

- Then imagine all your tension and stress leaving just as it would if you were actually in that scene. You can talk to yourself during this technique saying things like, "Everything's fine. I don't have a care in the world. My body and mind are free from tension. All my stress and worry are melting away. The warm sun is relaxing my neck, my face, and all my muscles. My headache is drifting away out to sea."

Deep Relaxation Training Resources

- Your local high school, community college, YMCA, or nearest state university may offer specific classes in some aspect of deep relaxation technique training.

- Videos and books are available. Check your local library or bookstore.

- Sports medicine clinics or physical therapists may offer specific programs geared at deep relaxation techniques. You will find them in your yellow pages directory under Physicians, Sports Medicine and/or Physical Therapy.

- The Mind-Body Medical Institute (617-632-9525) can refer you to health and wellness centers in your area that offer relaxation-training classes.

Massage Therapy

The hands-on rubbing of sore spots is the most innate and perhaps oldest form of treatment/healing. When we bump ourselves, we immediately, instinctively rub the area as a way to alleviate pain. When we get a headache, many of us unconsciously rub our forehead, the bridge of our nose, the top of our head, or our temple areas.

Scientists believe this has to do with the fact that human physical touch, like exercise, stimulates the brain to produce the "feel good" chemicals (endorphins) that function as natural pain killers and mood elevators. Massage also works by increasing blood flow to muscles helping them to relax. When muscles are tight, the blood vessels supplying oxygen and other chemical micronutrients to them become constricted, cutting off the flow of oxygen and nutrients. This causes the muscle to operate in a "starvation" state, and it starts hurting as a result.

What's Massage Therapy Like?

Professional massage therapy is an enjoyable, relaxing experience. You may choose to go to a massage therapy clinic or to have a massage therapist visit your home. Most "traveling" massage therapists own their own portable massage tables and can work right in your living room if you so desire. The cost of a professional massage therapist varies, but generally they are in the $40-60/hour range. With a little preliminary instruction and practice, however, your spouse, children, or friend can learn to do an effective massage that can help alleviate your headache pain.

If you have neck or head injuries, get clearance from your doctor before trying massage therapy. They may refer you to a clinical massage therapist who can work with your doctor for your specific injuries. Massage therapy, especially if neck or head injuries are involved, must be deep in pressure. Initially there may be some discomfort associated with pressing on certain pressure points. In time, this should lessen or completely disappear.

To be relaxing and most effective, massage should be done in a darkened, comfortable- temperature room. Most professional massage therapists opt to use candles and soft, relaxing music. The degree your entire body is relaxed contributes to relieving the severity and/or duration of a headache. To that end, most professional massage therapists ask you to remove all of your clothing (except underwear) to improve skin-to-skin contact, transference of body heat, and aid in the application of oil, gel, or lotion to loosen overly tightened muscles. A sheet and/or blanket will be placed over you for your privacy, and the massage therapist will help you discreetly turn either in order to target the specific problem muscle groups. For the headache sufferer, these muscles will be the large and small muscles of the upper back, neck, head, and face. However, a general body massage done first will help you relax.

If you (or someone you designate) are doing your massage at home, you may want to create this same relaxing atmosphere. Choose a quiet place and time of day where you won't be interrupted and can turn the phone off.

Healing a Headache With Massage

Most tension headaches originate in the muscles surrounding the face and neck. Migraine headaches can also be brought on and/or worsened by tension in these muscles. Although a headache may have varied causes, the actual pain of the headache itself usually comes from specific pressure, or trigger, points located in certain muscles of the head and neck. Consequently, if these trigger points can be released through direct pressure, or massage, the headache pain can also be released.

If you cannot afford the time or expense of a professional massage therapist, and would like to try relieving your headache pain with self-massage or have your spouse, friend, or child perform the massage for you, these basic head, face and neck massage steps can help.

- First apply warmed almond or olive oil to clean, dry skin. Gently massage into the neck and upper shoulders. Go over these areas at least 3 times to help relax the muscles.

- If the neck muscles are stiff and sore, let your head drop forward until your chin nearly reaches your chest. Place the palms of the hands on the back of the head, apply gentle pressure so that the neck stretches but does not strain. Using creative imagery and "self-talk" to make your muscle smooth, loose, and stress-free. If the muscles are hard and/or knotted, spend extra time gently applying pressure and/or an "ironing" action with the palms of the hands to try and un-knot these muscles.

- Always keeping contact with the skin, gently slide the thumb and fingers down the back of the neck, all the way from the skull to the shoulders.

- When the neck muscles begin to relax, glide your fingers up to the temples area, front of ears, and then back down to the neck.

- Press the balls of each thumb gently into the base of the skull on either side, holding for a moment. This directs pressure to one of the trigger points that cause headache pain. Rotate the pads of the thumbs against the scalp in small circles.

- Slide the palms of your hands against the sides of your head, using slightly more pressure at the soft temples area. Don't press in though, rather slide the palms up toward the top of the head. This helps to unkink the band of muscles surrounding the head that can tighten during stress and tension causing a headache.

- Next work the facial muscles by placing three or four fingers of each hand on the cheeks and smoothing the face outward/upward over the cheekbones toward the temples and area in front of the ears.

- Next work the forehead muscles by placing a hand flat on the forehead at the bridge of the nose area. If someone else is doing this maneuver for you, have them place one hand behind your head to hold it steady. Adding gentle pressure, slide the palm of the hand upwards on the forehead toward the hairline in an ironing manner, allowing the hand to slide off the hair.

- Repeat each massage movement 3 times.

- If your headache seems to intensify with these maneuvers, try to work gently through it as many headaches reach a pain peak and then go away. However, if you experience sudden, sharp pain, stop the massage immediately. Do not press hard on temple areas because this can compress blood flow in the temporal artery. Also, do not bend the neck sharply backwards because this can compress nerve outlets in the upper cervical (neck) spine.

Resources for Massage Therapy

- Consult your physician first if you have any head or neck injuries. He or she can clear you for massage therapy and refer you to a licensed massage therapist.

- Call the American Massage Therapy Association at 847-864-0123 for a referral.

- Your yellow pages lists massage therapists under Massage or Massage Therapy.

- A chiropractor may employ a massage therapist or perform the massage.

157

Some massage therapists use a soft, gentle touch and others use a more invigorating, aggressive touch. It's a good idea to experiment with different massage therapists to find one who has the right touch for you. Go with what feels comfortable. Massage therapy is meant to relax you and relieve pain-it shouldn't cause pain.

For Additional Information

American Massage Therapy Association
820 Davis Street, Suite 100
Evanston, IL 60201-4444
Tel: 847-864-0123
Fax: 847-864-1178
Internet: http://
www.amtamassage.org

Association for Applied Psychophysiology and Biofeedback
10200 W. 44th Avenue, Suite 304
Wheat Ridge, CO 80033-2840
Toll Free: 800-477-8892
Tel: 303-422-8436
Fax: 303-422-8894
Internet: http://www.aapb.org
E-Mail: aapb@resourcenter.com

Biofeedback Certification Institute of America (BCIA)
10200 W. 44th Avenue, Suite 310
Wheat Ridge, CO 80030
Tel: 303-420-2902
Fax: 303-422-8894
www.bcia.org
E-Mail: bcia@resourcenter.com

The BiofeedbackZone
13200 Summit Square Center
Route 413 and
Doublewoods Road
Langhorne, PA 19047
Tel: 215-968-2186
Fax: 801-459-8096
Internet:
www.biofeedbackzone.com
E-Mail: bio@webideas.com

Excedrin Library Article 15-1097, Biofeedback, Deep Relaxation and Massage.
Internet: http://
www.excedrin.com/6_library/articles/01_adverse.html

Mind-Body Medical Institute
75 Mt. Auburn Street
Cambridge, MA 02138
Tel: 617-632-9525
Fax: 617-496-1135
Internet: http://
www.mindbody.harvard.edu

—by Margareta-Erminia Cassani

M.E. Cassani is a freelance health/medicine writer from Livonia, Michigan.

Chapter 20

Oxygen Therapy

Oxygen treatment of headaches was first mentioned in literature in 1939. Mr. Charles E. Rhein, Linde Air Products Co., reported to Dr. Alvarez at the Mayo Clinic in Rochester, MN the successful treatment of severe "migraine" attacks by breathing pure oxygen. Subsequently, Dr. Alvarez noted that the treatment with 100 percent oxygen at a flow of six to eight liters a minute would often produce relief. Sometimes, patients would not be able to obtain relief with this treatment, whereas, at other times they would. In 1940, Dr. Alvarez reported the treatment of over 100 persons suffering from headache attacks. They were treated with oxygen with a nasal type of mask and a flow of six to eight liters a minute. He found that 80 percent of "migrainous" headaches were completely or significantly relieved. Dr. Alvarez also found that patients with other types of headaches were often helped through the use of oxygen inhalation and that the prompt institution of therapy had a better chance of resulting in relief than if it was delayed. This work was much less rigorous than that done recently.

The first significant work done on oxygen inhalation was that of Dr. Kudrow who investigated patients with cluster headaches. Fifty-two out-patients were treated with 100 percent oxygen at a flow of seven liters per minute. 75 percent of these patients had "complete or almost complete cessation of head pain within 15 minutes: for at least seven of 10 attacks." Dr. Kudrow found that there is greater effect of oxygen inhalation in patients with episodic cluster. Patients younger than 50 years of age appeared to have a better response than those above age 50. However, this was not considered statistically significant. Also of interest, 62 percent of those responding to oxygen had their attacks relieved within seven minutes of starting therapy. Dr. Kudrow did a second trial in a crossover fashion, comparing sublingual ergotamine tartrate and oxygen inhalation in the abortive treatment of cluster headache. Fifty patients selected at random used either 100 percent oxygen or the ergotamine to treat their headaches. After 10 cluster headaches were treated with one modality the patient then used the other treatment for 10 headaches. Eighty-two percent of the subjects found at least seven out of 10 cluster headaches were successfully relieved by the oxygen, while 70 percent treated their headaches successfully with ergotamine. These results were not considered statistically different.

Dr. Fogan studied 19 patients with cluster headache in the most rigorous fashion possible through a double-blind crossover study comparing oxygen versus air inhalation. He found there was a significant difference in the relief obtained in those patients inhaling oxygen versus air. By making this comparison Dr. Fogan was able to be sure that the oxygen was the significant factor in successfully treating the cluster headaches. He eliminated the other associated factors involved with the inhalation of a gas, such as the gas tank and the oxygen mask.

The way in which oxygen inhalation reduces headache pain is unknown. Researchers have shown that there is an increased blood flow in the brain in both cluster and migraine headaches, although both headaches do not have the same degree of increased flow. It has been shown that oxygen causes a marked decrease in cerebral blood flow that is coincident with the reduced degree of pain in cluster headache.

While it is clear that oxygen is a very useful therapy in cluster headaches, its utility in migraine headaches is less well documented. It is unlikely that the literature of the 1930s and 1940s was able to distinguish between migraine and cluster headaches. Thus, any belief ascribed to migraine headaches in that era could have confused patients with cluster headaches with those of migraine headaches. Some investigators have found it useful, however, to use oxygen therapy in patients with migraine headaches. I have found approximately 50 percent of my patients with migraine headaches will be able to achieve some relief with oxygen therapy. They use 100 percent oxygen for eight to nine liters a minute for up to 30 minutes. If no effect has been achieved by that time, it is unlikely that one will occur.

The side effects of oxygen inhalation are rare. Cluster headache patients are very often smokers and if one should happen to light up while an oxygen tank is open, the result can be explosive. Another side effect of oxygen use was found by Dr. Kudrow who noticed that 25 percent of his study patients had rebound cluster headaches after oxygen inhalation therapy. No other side effects have been found and therefore, oxygen therapy is safe. Oxygen could be preferred to ergotamine's use since ergotamine often causes nausea and vomiting as well as a sense of unreality and leg cramps. Ergotamine cannot be used in patients with hypertension, peripheral vascular disease or infections when oxygen obviously can be. It has been suggested that oxygen therapy when used together with ergotamine will give greater relief than the sum of the effect found by using either one alone.

Oxygen therapy is not a well-known modality for headache patients. Many physicians are unaware of the benefits of oxygen therapy, as are third-party payers who hesitate to reimburse for its use. Sometimes this can be overcome by a letter from the treating physician. Since approximately 50 percent of patients respond to oxygen therapy, it is worth trying it before going to the expense and effort of having an oxygen tank installed in one's home.

Chapter 21

Alternative Medicine

What Is Complementary and Alternative Medicine?

Complementary and alternative medicine (CAM) covers a broad range of healing philosophies, approaches, and therapies. Generally, it is defined as those treatments and healthcare practices not taught widely in medical schools, not generally used in hospitals, and not usually reimbursed by medical insurance companies.

Many therapies are termed "holistic," which generally means that the healthcare practitioner considers the whole person, including physical, mental, emotional, and spiritual aspects. Many therapies are also known as "preventive," which means that the practitioner educates and treats the person to prevent health problems from arising, rather than treating symptoms after problems have occurred.

People use these treatments and therapies in a variety of ways. Therapies are used alone (often referred to as alternative), in combination with other alternative therapies, or in addition to conventional therapies (sometimes referred to as complementary).

Some approaches are consistent with physiological principles of Western medicine, while others constitute healing systems with a different origin. While some therapies are far outside the realm of accepted Western medical theory and practice, others are becoming established in mainstream medicine.

From a fact sheet produced by the National Center for Complementary and Alternative Medicine (NCCAM), February 2001.

How Can I Find More Information about Complementary and Alternative Medical Practices?

Ask your healthcare provider about complementary and alternative medical treatments and practices in general, and about those particular practices used for your specific health problems.

Increasingly, healthcare providers are becoming familiar with alternative treatments or are able to refer you to someone who is. For scientific information about the safety and effectiveness of a particular treatment, ask your healthcare provider to obtain valid information for you.

If your healthcare provider cannot provide information, medical libraries, public libraries, and popular bookstores are good places to find information about particular complementary and alternative medical practices.

Other resources for information are the 25 Institutes and Centers (ICs) at the NIH. For information on a wide range of specific diseases or medical conditions, call 301-496-4000 and ask the operator to direct you to the appropriate NIH office.

Also, you may want to ask practitioners of complementary and alternative healthcare about their practices. Many practitioners belong to a growing number of professional associations, educational organizations, and research institutions that provide information about complementary and alternative medical practices. Many organizations are developing Internet Web sites. Most internet browser programs will have a mechanism for searching the World Wide Web by keyword or concept.

Remember that these organizations may advocate a specific therapy or treatment and may be unable to provide complete and objective health information.

CAM on PubMed

If you have access to a computer with an Internet connection, you may be able to search medical libraries and databases for specific conditions and alternative treatments. CAM on PubMed, developed jointly by the National Library of Medicine and the National Center for Complementary and Alternative Medicine, contains bibliographic citations (1966-present) related to complementary and alternative medicine. These citations are a subset of the National Library of Medicine's PubMed system that contains over 11 million journal citations from the MEDLINE database and additional life science journals important to health researchers, practitioners and consumers. CAM on PubMed also displays links to publisher web sites offering full text of articles.

How Can I Find a Practitioner in My Area?

To find a qualified complementary and alternative medical healthcare practitioner, you may want to contact medical regulatory and licensing agencies in your state. These agencies may be able to provide information about a specific practitioner's credentials and background. Many states license practitioners who provide alternative therapies such as acupuncture, chiropractic services, naturopathy, herbal medicine, homeopathy, and massage therapy.

You may also locate practitioners by asking your healthcare provider, or by contacting a professional association or organization. These organizations can provide names of local practitioners, and provide information about how to determine the quality of a specific practitioner's services. Contact the NCCAM Clearinghouse to obtain the fact sheet, "Considering Complementary and Alternative Therapies," which provides helpful hints and questions to consider when choosing an alternative healthcare practitioner.

Also, you may find complementary and alternative healthcare practitioners by asking people you trust, like friends and family members, who may have experience with practitioners of complementary and alternative medicine.

Can I Receive an Alternative Treatment at the National Center for Complementary and Alternative Medicine (NCCAM)?

The NCCAM is not a treatment facility and cannot answer specific medical questions. The NCCAM cannot make referrals to individual practitioners or recommend particular therapies for patients.

Will My Experience Help in the Evaluation of Complementary and Alternative Medical Therapies?

Many people write to the NCCAM with their own testimony about a successful treatment or a particular healer or healthcare practitioner. To have this information reviewed, people may ask their practitioners whether he/she is collecting information on the success of their treatments. A practitioner can collect and organize the information and present it to the NCCAM once there is sufficient data to make a case for the effectiveness of a particular treatment.

Will the NCCAM Evaluate My Own Invention or Treatment?

Many people contact the NCCAM with ideas for alternative medical cures. To have a method or cure tested, one must formulate a research protocol. This entails collaborating with individuals who have expertise in research and evaluation, if one does not possess this expertise.

The NCCAM supports rigorous research into a range of alternative medical treatments either by awarding grants or by setting up studies. For further information, please contact the NCCAM Clearinghouse to obtain the "Research Information Package."

Can Complementary and Alternative Medicine Be Investigated Using the Same Methods Used in Conventional Medicine?

People sometimes ask whether the NCCAM uses the same standard of science as conventional medicine. Complementary and alternative medicine needs to be investigated using the same scientific methods used in conventional medicine. The NCCAM encourages valid information about complementary and alternative medicine, applying at least as rigorous, and, in some cases, even more rigorous research methods than the current standard in conventional medicine. This is because the research often involves novel concepts and claims, and uses complex systems of practice that need systematic, explicit, and comprehensive knowledge and skills to investigate.

Chapter 22

Experimental Treatments

The scalpel has failed. The IV tubing stands abandoned on the side of the room. Friends and nurses visit less often. The doctors say the limits of medical knowledge have been reached and there is nothing left for you to do but go home and put your affairs in order.

This is a crushing moment. It's even more frightening than the day the doctors announced that you had a serious and life-threatening disease, such as AIDS, cancer or Alzheimer's disease. For many people, however, the limitations of medical knowledge do not define the limits of human hope. As long as life lingers, many patients will fight on, refusing to give up even when biology is against them. So, they set out on a search for treatment options.

And many alternatives exist. In today's medical bazaar, options range from alternative and complementary therapies like acupuncture and homeopathic and naturopathic medicine to nutritional supplements and macrobiotic diets, home-brewed remedies, and even outright frauds like laetrile. But greater promise resides in the drug development pipeline where tomorrow's therapeutics await proof that they work. Unlike alternative therapies, billions of dollars and decades of scientific study often have been invested in the research that leads to promising new therapies. Might there be, somewhere in that high-priced gauntlet, just the right molecule that cures a patient who is running out of time?

"Experimental Treatments? Unapproved But Not Always Unavailable," by Larry Thompson *FDA Consumer Magazine*, U.S. Food and Drug Administration (FDA), January-February 2000.

The answer is possibly, but finding it isn't easy. Short of randomly hearing about a promising study through the media, most people know relatively little about what drugs are in development. Even if experimental drugs existed in a database, "it is hard to know which drugs are truly promising," says David Banks of the Food and Drug Administration's Office of Special Health Issues. But on average, about 80 percent of the drugs in testing will ultimately be approved.

Getting your hands on a novel medicine can be even more difficult. Usually, only the company has any supply of the new medicine, which is extremely limited to begin with, and most of what is made will be used in clinical studies.

As if these hurdles are not enough, there is the long-held, but incorrect, public perception that FDA erects regulatory barriers that block patients from getting investigational new drugs (INDs). These are drugs that pharmaceutical companies have in clinical trials to demonstrate their safety and effectiveness, but which have yet to be approved by FDA for marketing. For those with a serious illness, the agency rarely blocks access to unproven medications. But FDA does strive to protect all patients, even those who may be dying, from undue risks associated with investigational new drugs. At the same time, FDA believes that the best way to benefit all patients is to speed promising new therapies through the development and approval process so safety, effectiveness and proper use can be established.

"FDA has worked diligently to balance two compelling, and sometimes competing, factors," says FDA Commissioner Jane E. Henney, M.D. "On one hand, there is the need for the disciplined, systematic, scientifically controlled studies necessary to identify treatments that may improve patient health and that lead to the approval of new drugs. At the same time, there is the desire of seriously ill persons, with no effective options available, to have the earliest access to unapproved products that could be the best therapy for them."

Over the last decade, FDA's institutional philosophy has evolved to be more supportive of thoughtful risk-taking by patients who have run out of options. As a result, the agency has put in place a number of regulatory mechanisms and worked with manufacturers to ensure that seriously ill patients can get access to promising, but not fully evaluated, products. At the same time, FDA has protected the critical scientific studies that must be carried out so that patients, physicians and the agency can determine which drugs are truly safe and effective, and how they can best be used. "We believe that the best means of providing access to useful medical treatments for all Americans is to continue to shorten the review times," Henney says, "and to continue to work with the industry to shorten development times for drugs, biologics and medical devices."

Before the 1980s, a more paternalistic medical community argued that it was the government's job to protect patients from possible harm by withholding experimental drugs until there is proof that they work and are safe.

AIDS helped alter that view. Not only did that lethal disease spread with terrifying speed, but it struck a patient population capable of mounting a political response that grabbed the nation's attention and galvanized public health policymakers to reconsider long-held beliefs.

Experimental treatments should be available, The Washington Post quoted one activist at the time, "so people would be able to choose for themselves, working with their doctors, whether they want to risk taking a drug because of the possible benefits." Critics accused FDA of denying dying patients access to possibly lifesaving drugs. To drive home the point, in October 1988, more than 1,000 gay activists staged a protest outside FDA's Rockville, Md., headquarters, trapping the agency's staff inside.

"FDA is the nexus between the government, the private sector and the consumer," the spokeswoman for one of the protest organizers told the Post. "That's why we're targeting [the agency]."

The protest had an effect. The agency, already focused on the issue by the urgency of AIDS, accelerated its reexamination of the way people with serious and life-threatening diseases could gain access to unproven remedies. Although the treatment IND regulations were finalized in 1987, FDA put in place additional mechanisms to make experimental drugs available to seriously ill patients earlier in the drug development process.

With the activism around AIDS and the demands of people with other serious illnesses for access to unproven treatments, the medical community, including FDA, began to appreciate that the traditional risk/benefit models may have been inappropriate for people with serious and life-threatening diseases. Dying patients were willing to take bigger risks for even the slenderest hope of benefit.

"The hope part of it is that it might work and keep them alive a little longer," says Theresa Toigo, associate commissioner for the Office of Special Health Issues. "Even if it is only two months, by then there might be a cure. It is a wonderful survival instinct."

Getting Access

For patients in search of a cutting edge treatment, the possibilities have improved dramatically. First of all, there are more clinical studies under way than ever before. FDA has on file more than 13,000 active drug and biologic studies. These range from a few dozen patients to as many as 50,000 participating in a single investigational new drug trial. More than 100,000 patients are enrolled each year in National Institutes of Health-sponsored studies conducted all over the United States.

Studies with investigational new drugs can be conducted by the federal government, primarily through the National Institutes of Health; by research universities, usually with federal funding, though also through private foundations or drug companies; and by private, for-profit companies on behalf of pharmaceutical manufacturers.

Clinical trials are essential to the development and approval of new drugs. In these studies, a group of human volunteers receiving the investigational therapy are compared with another group that receives either the standard treatment or a placebo. Placebos, sometimes called sugar pills, are any fake treatment that has no therapeutic benefit. This allows the researchers to compare the effect of the treatment to no treatment in otherwise similar patients. When the control group is given the standard treatment, researchers are able to determine whether the experimental treatment provides a better outcome than what is already available.

The clinical trial setting helps ensure that risks are minimized because the research protocol, the set of rules by which the clinical trial is conducted, have been scrutinized by FDA and a local ethics committee called an institutional review board.

"We want to encourage people to participate in the clinical trial process because that is where information is best developed about the drug product," says David Lepay, M.D., director of the division of scientific investigation in FDA's Center for Drug Evaluation and Research.

The downside of being in a clinical trial, indeed the downside of using any unproved medication, is that the new drug may not work. It may even be dangerous and, sometimes, deadly. Not everyone who wants to participate in a clinical trial can do so. Limits on the number of participants and specific eligibility criteria keep some people out. In addition, it is often inconvenient for the patient to travel to the research center. When individuals are unable to participate in a clinical study, FDA provides alternative mechanisms for patients and their doctors to get their hands on a promising new drug.

Beyond Clinical Trials

In 1987, FDA created a regulatory mechanism (first proposed in 1982) to permit expanded access to investigational drugs outside of controlled clinical trials. The "treatment IND" allows people with serious and life-threatening illnesses to take investigational drugs while the products are being tested in a clinical trial. Typically, however, drugs allowed under treatment INDs already have shown promise and proven safety. In addition to the benefit to individual patients, treatment INDs generate useful information about how the drug affects larger segments of the patient population than might otherwise receive it in a clinical study.

For example, the AIDS drug Videx (ddI) was made available to people with AIDS outside the clinical trial at a time when the choices for AIDS therapy were few and many people had already exhausted the then available options. Although patients seeking treatment with ddI were told that it was still under study and that there were risks, more than 20,000 decided to take ddI anyway. This not only gave them a better chance to survive but also gave researchers more information about the drug's safety than would have been possible from the some 4,000 patients involved in the clinical studies.

Since the final treatment IND rule was published more than a decade ago, FDA has made more than 40 drug or biologic investigational products available to patients early and has approved 36. Of these, nearly a dozen were for cancer and another dozen for AIDS or AIDS-related conditions.

Single-Patient INDs

As with a clinical trial, there may not be an appropriate treatment IND for an individual patient's condition, but there may be a new drug still working its way through development. If enough is known about the drug's safety, and there is some clinical evidence of effectiveness, FDA may allow a patient to become his or her own study. This so-called single-patient IND, or compassionate use IND, virtually ensures that any patient can get access to any investigational new drug.

Although FDA's requirements for a single-patient IND are relatively simple, setting up this kind of access for an individual patient is not. First of all, the company must be willing to provide the new drug to the patient. This can be expensive and time consuming for the company since, in addition to providing the drug, the company needs to track shipments of the drug, create special instructions for its use, and create a way of collecting safety data and a mechanism for tracking outcomes for each patient. Second, the patient must give informed consent, understanding that the drug is not approved and may cause side effects from mild to fatal. Third, the patient's physician must be willing to take responsibility for treating the patient and agree to collect information about the effects of the drug.

Companies sometimes say that they cannot make the drug available to a patient because FDA won't allow it, but that is rarely true. FDA only denies access when there is evidence that the risk of using the experimental drug clearly outweighs any potential benefit to the patient.

If a drug is frequently used in single-patient INDs, FDA streamlines the process for obtaining permission. One example is thalidomide, a drug initially associated with birth defects in the 1950s but now being used experimentally to treat cancer. (FDA approved thalidomide in 1998 to treat leprosy.) FDA has similar rules that give patients access to investigational new medical devices.

A Difficult Decision

All things being equal, is it worth it for a patient to get access to an experimental medication? For society the additional safety information about the new drug may prove useful. And sometimes it does make a difference for individual patients. For example, people with AIDS who participated in the clinical trials for a category of drugs called protease inhibitors probably benefited because this class of drugs proved so dramatically effective. But for many other INDs, the success rates are much less impressive, such as tacrine (Cognex) for the treatment of Alzheimer's disease.

Even if access does not change long-term survival, it may provide for the patient and the family a sense that they are doing something and are not simply victims of some serious disease. Biomedical research advances rapidly and breakthroughs come from unexpected places, all feeding the hope that the next experimental drug will be the one that cures our ills.

Finding Information About Investigational New Drugs

While finding and getting into an appropriate clinical trial for your individual disease is something like a scavenger hunt, the Internet has made it much easier to track down these studies. The following is a listing of major Internet sites where you can search for a clinical trial that may benefit you.

Information Program on Clinical Trials, (www.lhncbc.nlm.nih.gov/clin/) mandated by the FDA Modernization Act of 1997, is a joint FDA/National Institutes of Health resource. While initially containing only NIH studies, it will eventually include all federally and privately financed clinical studies.

CancerNet (http://cancernet.nci.nih.gov) is run by NIH's National Cancer Institute (NCI). It provides information on clinical trials. Information is also available through NCI's Cancer Information Service at 1-800-4-CANCER.

ACTIS (www.actis.org), the AIDS Clinical Trials Information Service, provides a wide range of information on current AIDS research, including drug trials, vaccine trials, and other educational material. Sponsored by the U.S. Public Health Service, including FDA, NIAID, Centers for Disease Control and Prevention, and the National Library of Medicine, ACTIS also can be reached at 1-800-TRIALS-A.

Information regarding clinical trials for rare disease can be found at http://rarediseases.info.nih.gov/ord/research-ct.html, a database compiled by NIH's Office of Rare Diseases.

CenterWatch Clinical Trials Listing Service (www.centerwatch.com) is published on the Internet by CenterWatch Inc., a multimedia publishing company in Boston, Mass. It provides information on more than 5,000 active clinical trials as well as other information.

When a clinical trial is not an option, FDA facilitates access to an investigational new drug or an investigational medical device through other programs. For information on programs for, or access to, an unapproved investigational new drug, call FDA's Office of Special Health Initiatives at 301-827-4460.

Is the Risk Worth It?

No matter how promising a clinical trial or investigational new drug seems, there is no way to know about all the risks before the study begins. While the hope is that the study will produce a cure, it's important to recognize that risks can prove significant. For example, in 1992, tests for a promising hepatitis B drug severely damaged the liver in 10 patients. Some died and others required liver transplants.

Because of these inherent uncertainties the health-care professionals conducting the study must ensure that the patient understands the risks as well as the benefits beforehand and is willing to proceed.

Here are some questions patients might want to ask to make sure they understand the consequences of entering a study or using an investigational new drug:

1.   What are the potential benefits from the treatment being studied? What have the animal or other human studies shown about the effectiveness of the drug?

2.   What are the potential dangers from using this drug? Again, what do other animal and human studies show about the side effects?

3.   In what phase is this clinical trial?

     Clinical trials are generally performed in three phases. A phase 1 trial is primarily designed to assess the safety profile in a small number of patients. Phase 2 tests the effectiveness of the treatment in a relatively small number of patients. Many drugs never progress beyond phase 2 because they are not effective. In phase 3, a large number of patients receive the drug to substantiate that the effectiveness seen in phase 2 is real and to work out the details of its use. Individual patients are most likely to benefit from drugs in the later phases of development.

4.   Will there be a control group?

     For a clinical trial to produce useful information, the group of patients receiving the new treatment needs to be compared with patients who receive something—or nothing—else. Often, patients in the control group receive whatever is the current standard therapy for the disease. Sometimes, the control group patients will receive a placebo—so-called sugar pills that produce no therapeutic benefit. In a clinical study, patients are randomly assigned to either the group treated with the experimental drug or to a group receiving the standard therapy or placebo.

5.   How do I know if I am eligible to be in the study?

     Every trial has a set of criteria to select the people that will be included in the study. These criteria generally relate to general health, stage of disease, and prior treatments and are designed to produce useful scientific information.

6.   Do I have to pay to be in a clinical study?

     Generally, studies funded by the federal government are free for the patient. Many studies funded by drug companies also do not cost anything. Some costs, however, may be paid by a patient's health insurance or managed-care plan.

7. So I'm just a guinea pig, right?

    By the time most studies reach the stage where the new drug is being tested in people, a great deal is known about how it affects the body. While there is always the chance that something could go wrong, the safety of most drugs being studied is well understood. It is true, however, that researchers do not know if a treatment being studied works better than current therapies or not.

What FDA Does Not Do

Although FDA is responsible for overseeing the field of drug development, there are a number of services the agency cannot provide to individual patients. For one thing, it cannot give out the name of drugs in development, a common request from patients who call the agency. Unless the company publicly releases information about the experimental treatment, FDA is currently forbidden to even acknowledge that it knows about the drug.

Along the same lines, FDA cannot make the drug available to individual patients or physicians. The agency simply does not have the product; only the company that is developing the drug has a supply. And FDA has no authority to require that the company make its drug available outside of the clinical trial.

FDA, itself, does not conduct any clinical trials or drug studies. The agency carries out its drug review and approval responsibilities by examining clinical and other data generated by the drug company.

And lastly, FDA does not give advice. While staff from the Office of Special Health Issues and the Center for Drug Evaluation and Research's drug information branch will often provide detailed information and explain the process for getting access to an experimental medication, the agency does not steer patients in one direction or the other. Information is provided so patients, in consultation with their physicians, can make their own informed decisions.

Chapter 23

The Truth about Choosing Medical Treatments

Choosing Treatments to Get Better

When you're sick it isn't always easy to get well again. There are lots of medicines and other ways to treat health problems. You may hear about some from a friend. Or you may see an ad on TV or in the paper. Or your doctor may recommend a treatment. It's FDA's job to make sure the medicines and other treatments people buy are safe and really work. Most treatments you can buy have FDA's OK. But some don't.

An FDA-approved medicine may help you get better. Some are phony and are a waste of your money. Some can even make you sicker. Just because a product is advertised doesn't mean it can really do what the ad says it can. A phony medicine may make you sicker.

Unproven Treatments

Sometimes there are no treatments with FDA's OK that will help you. This is mainly true for very bad sicknesses like some cancers and AIDS, or with sicknesses that last a long time like arthritis. Then you might hear about a treatment that's still being tested.

There are many unproven treatments. Some you may have heard of are:

- imagery (With imagery, you learn to imagine yourself in a certain way. For example, you might be guided to think of yourself

U. S. Food and Drug Administration (FDA), FDA Pub. No. 00-1248, 2000.

as very strong and healthy and think of your sickness as weak and easy to destroy.)

- hypnosis

- biofeedback (You try to make yourself better by learning to control body functions like your heart rate, temperature, and muscles.)

There are many unproven treatments. They may work or they may not work. If you want to try an unproven treatment, do these things first:

- Talk to people who have tried the treatment. Ask them about everything that happened during and after the treatment—both good and bad.

- Ask the person who is giving the treatment what kind of training they've had and how long they have been doing the treatment.

- Ask how much it will cost. Health insurance may not pay for unproven treatments.

- Tell your doctor you're thinking about trying a new treatment.

The best way to try an unproven treatment is to get into a clinical trial. A clinical trial is an experiment to see if the treatment is safe and really works. Clinical trials must follow exact steps to protect patients. Your doctor may be able to help you find a clinical trial. Before you try an unproven treatment talk to someone who knows about it.

Watch Out for Phony Treatments

How can you tell if a medicine or other treatment is phony? One way to tell is to look for certain tricks. People who sell phony health products often use tricks to gain your trust and get your money.
Watch out for ads that talk about:

- secret formulas (Real scientists share what they know.)

- amazing breakthroughs or miracle cures (Real breakthroughs don't happen very often. When they do, real scientists don't call them amazing or miracles.)

178

- easy weight loss (For most people, the only way to lose weight is to eat less and exercise more.)

- quick, painless, or guaranteed cures.

Remember

- Phony medicines or other treatments cheat you out of your money. Some phony treatments might not hurt you but they won't make you any better either.

- Some phony treatments might make you even sicker. The best advice: If it sounds too good to be true, it probably isn't true.

- Ask your doctor or the pharmacist at the drug store about treatments that may help you.

Questions?

Do you have questions about any kind of medical treatment? FDA may have an office near you. Look for their number in the blue pages of the phone book.

You can also contact FDA through its toll-free number, 1-888-INFO-FDA (1-888-463-6332). Or, on the World Wide Web at http://www.fda.gov.

Do you have questions about experimental medicine or clinical trials? Ask your doctor or write a letter to:

National Institutes of Health
National Center for Complementary and
Alternative Medicine Clearinghouse
P. O. Box 8218
Silver Spring, MD 20907-8218
Toll-Free: 888-644-6226
Internet: http://nccam.nih.gov

Chapter 24

Tips for Dealing with Chronic Pain

Introduction

What was the worst pain you can remember? Was it the time you scratched the cornea of your eye? Was it a kidney stone? Childbirth? Rare is the person who has not experienced some beyond-belief episode of pain and misery. Mercifully, relief finally came. Your eye healed, the stone was passed, the baby born. In each of those cases pain flared up in response to a known cause. With treatment, or with the body's healing powers alone, you got better and the pain went away. Doctors call that kind of pain acute pain. It is a normal sensation triggered in the nervous system to alert you to possible injury and the need to take care of yourself.

Chronic pain is different. Chronic pain persists. Fiendishly, uselessly, pain signals keep firing in the nervous system for weeks, months, even years. There may have been an initial mishap—a sprained back, a serious infection-from which you've long since recovered. There may be an ongoing cause of pain—arthritis, cancer, ear infection, or headache. But some people suffer chronic pain in the absence of any past injury or evidence of body damage.

Pain's "Terrible Triad"

Pain of such proportions overwhelms all other symptoms and becomes the problem. People so afflicted often cannot work. Their appetite falls

From "Chronic Pain: Hope Through Research," National Institute of Neurological Disorders and Stroke (NINDS), NIH Pub. No. 98-2406, September 1998.

off. Physical activity of any kind is exhausting and may aggravate the pain. Soon the person becomes the victim of a vicious circle in which total preoccupation with pain leads to irritability and depression. The sufferer can't sleep at night and the next day's weariness compounds the problem—leading to more irritability, depression, and pain. Specialists call that unhappy state the "terrible triad" of suffering, sleeplessness, and sadness, a calamity that is as hard on the family as it is on the victim. The urge to do something—anything—to stop the pain makes some patients drug dependent and drives others to undergo repeated operations or resort to questionable practitioners who promise quick and permanent "cures."

Many chronic pain conditions affect older adults. Arthritis, cancer, angina—the chest-binding, breath-catching spasms of pain associated with coronary artery disease—commonly take their greatest toll among the middle-aged and elderly. Trigeminal neuralgia (tic douloureux) is a recurrent, stabbing facial pain that is rare among young adults. But ask anyone living in a community for retired persons if there are any trigeminal neuralgia sufferers around and you are sure to hear of cases. So the fact that Americans are living longer contributes to a widespread and growing concern about pain.

Neuroscientists share that concern. At a time when people are living longer and painful conditions abound, the scientists who study the brain have made landmark discoveries that are leading to a better understanding of pain and more effective treatments.

In the forefront of pain research are scientists supported by the National Institute of Neurological Disorders and Stroke (NINDS), a component of the National Institutes of Health (NIH). Other institutes at NIH that support pain research include the National Institute of Dental Research (NIDR), the National Cancer Institute (NCI), the National Institute of Nursing Research (NINR), the National Institute on Drug Abuse (NIDA), and the National Institute of Mental Health (NIMH).

Theories of Pain

In the past several decades, important discoveries about pain-suppressing chemicals came about because scientists were curious about how morphine and other opium-derived painkillers, or analgesics, work. For some time neuroscientists had known that chemicals were important in conducting nerve signals (small bursts of electric current) from cell to cell. In order for the signal from one cell to reach the next in line, the first cell secretes a chemical, called a "neurotransmitter," from the tip of a long fiber that extends from the cell body. The transmitter molecules cross the gap separating the two cells and attach to special receptor sites on the neighboring cell surface. Some neurotransmitters excite the second cell—allowing it to generate an electrical signal. Others inhibit the second cell—preventing it from generating a signal.

When investigators injected morphine into experimental animals, they found that the morphine molecules fit snugly into receptors on certain brain and spinal cord neurons. Why, the scientists wondered, should the human brain—the product of millions of years of evolution—come equipped with receptors for a man-made drug? Perhaps there were naturally occurring brain chemicals that behaved exactly like morphine.

Numerous studies around the world led to the discovery of not just one pain-suppressing chemical in the brain, but a whole family of such proteins. The smaller members of the family were named enkephalins (meaning "in the head"). In time, the larger proteins were isolated and called endorphins, meaning the "morphine within." The term endorphins is now often used to describe the group as a whole.

The discovery of the endorphins lent weight to an overarching theory of pain: endorphins released from brain nerve cells might inhibit spinal cord pain cells through pathways descending from the brain to the spinal cord. Laboratory experiments subsequently confirmed that painful stimulation led to the release of endorphins from nerve cells. Some of these chemicals then turned up in cerebrospinal fluid, the liquid that circulates in the spinal cord and brain. Laced with endorphins, the fluid could bring a soothing balm to quiet nerve cells.

A New Look at Pain Treatments

Further evidence that endorphins figure importantly in pain control came from studies of some of the oldest and newest pain treatments. These studies involved the use of a drug called naloxone that prevents endorphins and morphine from working. Injections of naloxone resulted in a return of pain which had been relieved by morphine and certain other treatments. But, interestingly, some pain treatments are not affected by naloxone: their success in controlling pain apparently does not depend on endorphins. Thus nature has provided us with more than one means of achieving pain relief.

Acupuncture

Probably no therapy for pain has stirred more controversy in recent years than acupuncture, the 2,000-year-old Chinese technique of inserting fine needles under the skin at selected points in the body. The needles are manipulated by the practitioner to produce pain relief which some individuals report lasts for hours, or even days. Does acupuncture really work? Opinion is divided. Many specialists agree that patients report benefit when the needles are placed near the site of the pain, not at the body points indicated on traditional Chinese acupuncture charts.

The case for acupuncture has been made by investigators who argue that local needling of the skin excites endorphin systems of pain control. Wiring the needles to stimulate nerve endings electrically (electroacupuncture) also activates endorphin systems, they believe. Further, some experiments have shown that there are higher levels of endorphins in cerebrospinal fluid following acupuncture.

Those same investigators note that naloxone injections can block pain relief produced by acupuncture. Others have not been able to repeat those findings. Skeptics also cite long-term studies of chronic pain patients that showed no lasting benefit from acupuncture treatments. Current opinion is that more controlled trials are needed to define which pain conditions might be helped by acupuncture and which patients are most likely to benefit.

Local Electrical Stimulation

Applying brief pulses of electricity to nerve endings under the skin, a procedure called transcutaneous electrical nerve stimulation (TENS), yields excellent pain relief in some chronic pain patients. The stimulation works best when applied to the skin near where the pain is felt and where other sensibilities like touch or pressure have not been damaged. Both the frequency and voltage of the electrical stimulation are important in obtaining pain relief.

Brain Stimulation

Another electrical method for controlling pain, especially the widespread and severe pain of advanced cancer, is through surgically implanted electrodes in the brain. The patient determines when and how much stimulation is needed by operating an external transmitter that beams electronic signals to a receiver under the skin that is connected to the electrodes. Stimulation-produced analgesia is a costly procedure that involves the risk of brain surgery. However, patients who have used this technique report that their pain "seems to melt away." The pain relief is also remarkably specific: the other senses remain intact, and there is no mental confusion or cloudiness as with opiate drugs.

Placebo Effects

For years doctors have known that a harmless sugar pill or an injection of salt water can make many patients feel better—even after major surgery. The placebo effect, as it is called, has been thought to be due to suggestion, distraction, the patient's optimism that something is being done, or the desire to please the doctor (placebo means "I will please" in Latin).

Later experiments suggested that the placebo effect may be neurochemical, and that people who respond to a placebo for pain relief—a remarkably consistent 35 percent in any experiment using placebos—are able to tap into their brains' endorphin systems. To evaluate it, investigators designed an ingenious experiment. They asked adults scheduled for wisdom teeth removal to volunteer in a pain experiment. Following surgery, some patients were given morphine, some naloxone, and some a placebo. As expected, about a third of those given the placebo reported pain relief. The investigators then gave these people naloxone. All reported a return of pain.

How people who benefit from placebos gain access to pain control systems in the brain is not known. Scientists cannot even predict whether someone who responds to a placebo in one situation will respond in another. Some investigators suspect that stress may be a factor. Patients who are very anxious or under stress are more likely to react to a placebo for pain than those who are more calm, cool, and collected. But dental surgery itself may be sufficiently stressful to trigger the release of endorphins—with or without the effects of placebo. For that reason, many specialists believe further studies are indicated to analyze the placebo effect.

As research continues to reveal the role of endorphins in the brain, neuroscientists have been able to draw more detailed brain maps of the areas and pathways important in pain perception and control and have found other members of the endorphin family. At the same time, clinical investigators have tested chronic pain patients and found that they often have lower-than-normal levels of endorphins in their spinal fluid. If we could just boost their stores with man-made endorphins, perhaps the problems of chronic pain patients could be solved.

Some endorphins are quickly broken down after release from nerve cells. Other endorphins are longer lasting, but there are problems in manufacturing the compounds in quantity and getting them into the right places in the brain or spinal cord. In a few promising studies, clinical investigators have injected an endorphin called beta—endorphin under the membranes surrounding the spinal cord. Patients reported excellent pain relief lasting for many hours. Morphine compounds injected in the same area are similarly effective in producing long-lasting pain relief.

But spinal cord injections or other techniques designed to raise the level of endorphins circulating in the brain require surgery and hospitalization. And even if less drastic means of getting endorphins into the nervous system could be found, they are probably not the ideal answer to chronic pain. Endorphins are also involved in other nervous system activities such as controlling blood flow. Increasing the amount of endorphins might have undesirable effects on these other body activities. Endorphins also appear to share with morphine a potential for addiction or tolerance.

Meanwhile, chemists are synthesizing new analgesics and discovering painkilling virtues in drugs not normally prescribed for pain. Much of the drug research is aimed at developing nonnarcotic painkillers. The motivation for the research is not only to avoid introducing potentially addictive drugs on the market, but is based on the observation that narcotic drugs are simply not effective in treating a variety of chronic pain conditions. Developments in nondrug treatments are also progressing, ranging from new surgical techniques to therapies like exercise, hypnosis, and biofeedback.

New and Old Drugs for Pain

When you complain of headache or low back pain and the doctor says take two aspirins every 4 hours and stay in bed, you may think your pain is being dismissed lightly. Not at all. Aspirin, one of the most universally used medications is an excellent painkiller. Scientists still cannot explain all the ways aspirin works, but they do know that it interferes with pain signals where they usually originate, at the nerve endings outside the brain and spinal cord: peripheral nerves. Aspirin also inhibits the production of chemicals called prostaglandins that are manufactured in the blood to promote blood clotting and wound healing.

Unfortunately, prostaglandins, released from cells at the site of injury, are pain-causing substances. They actually sensitize nerve endings, making them-and you-feel more pain. Along with increasing the blood supply to the area, these chemicals contribute to inflammation—the pain, heat, redness, and swelling of tissue damage.

Some investigators now think that the continued release of pain-causing substances in chronic pain conditions may lead to long-term nervous system changes in some patients, making them hypersensitive to pain. People suffering such hyperalgesia can cry out in pain at the gentlest touch, or even when a soft breeze blows over the affected area. In addition to the prostaglandins, blister fluid and certain insect and snake venoms also contain pain-causing substances. Presumably these chemicals alert you to the need for care—a fine reaction in an emergency, but not in chronic pain.

There are several prescription drugs that usually can provide stronger pain relief than aspirin. These include the opiate-related compounds codeine, propoxyphene, morphine, and meperidine. All these drugs have some potential for abuse, and may have unpleasant and even harmful side effects. In combination with other medications or alcohol, some can be dangerous. Used wisely, however, they are important recruits in the chemical fight against pain.

In the search for effective analgesics, physicians have discovered pain-relieving benefits from drugs not normally prescribed for pain. Certain antidepressants are used to treat several particularly severe pain conditions, notably the riveting pain of facial neuralgias like trigeminal neuralgia and the excruciating pain that can follow an attack of shingles.

Interestingly, pain patients who benefit from antidepressants report pain relief before any uplift in mood. Pain specialists think that the antidepressant works because it increases the supply of a naturally produced neurotransmitter, serotonin. (Doctors have long associated decreased amounts of serotonin with severe depression.) But now scientists have evidence that cells using serotonin are also an integral part of a pain-controlling pathway that starts with endorphin-rich nerve cells high up in the brain and ends with inhibition of pain-conducting nerve cells lower in the brain or spinal cord.

Antiepileptic drugs have also been used successfully in treating trigeminal neuralgia. The rationale for the use of antiepileptic drugs (principally carbamazepine) is based on the theory that a healthy nervous system depends on a proper balance of incoming and outgoing nerve signals.

Trigeminal neuralgia and other facial pains or neuralgias are thought to result from damage to facial nerves. That means that the normal flow of messages to and from the brain is disturbed. The nervous system may react by becoming hypersensitive: it may create its own powerful discharge of nerve signals, as though screaming to the outside world "Why aren't you contacting me?" Antiepileptic drugs—

187

used to quiet the excessive brain discharges associated with epileptic seizures—quiet the distress signals and in that way may relieve pain.

Nondrug Treatments

Treatment for pain can include counseling, relaxation training, meditation, hypnosis, biofeedback, or behavior modification. The philosophy common to all of these approaches is the belief that patients can do something on their own to manage their pain. That something may mean changing attitudes, feelings, or behaviors associated with pain.

Psychotherapy

Some patients may benefit from individual or group counseling. Trained professionals can help the chronic pain sufferer learn valuable coping skills. They also provide the patient with much needed support—both psychological and emotional—for dealing with pain.

Relaxation and Meditation Therapies

These methods enable people to relax tense muscles, reduce anxiety, and alter mental states. Both physical and mental tension can make pain worse, and in conditions such as headache or back pain, tension may be at the root of the problem. Meditation, which aims at producing a state of relaxed but alert awareness, is sometimes combined with therapies that encourage people to think of pain as something remote and apart from them. The methods promote a sense of detachment so that the patient thinks of the pain as confined to a particular body part over which he or she has control. The approach may be particularly helpful when pain is associated with fear, as in cancer.

Hypnosis

No longer considered magic, hypnosis is a technique in which an individual's susceptibility to suggestion is heightened. Normal volunteers who prove to be excellent subjects for hypnosis often report a marked reduction or obliteration of experimentally induced pain, such as that produced by a mild electric shock. The hypnotic state does not lower the volunteer's heart rate, respiration, or other autonomic responses. These physical reactions show the expected increases normally associated with painful stimulation.

The role of hypnosis in treating chronic pain patients is uncertain. Some studies have shown that 15 to 20 percent of hypnotizable patients with moderate to severe pain can achieve total relief with hypnosis. Other studies report that hypnosis reduces anxiety and depression. By lowering the burden of emotional suffering, pain may become more bearable.

Biofeedback

Some individuals can learn voluntary control over certain body activities if they are provided with information about how the system is working—how fast their heart is beating, how tense their head or neck muscles are, how cold their hands are. The information is usually supplied through visual or auditory cues that code the body activity in some obvious way—a louder sound meaning an increase in muscle tension, for example. How people use this biofeedback to learn control is not understood, but some practitioners of the art report that imagery helps: they may think of a warm tropical beach, for example, when they want to raise the temperature of their hands. Biofeedback may be a logical approach in pain conditions that involve tense muscles, like tension headache or low back pain. But results are mixed.

Behavior Modification

This psychological technique (sometimes called operant conditioning) is aimed at changing habits, behaviors, and attitudes that can develop in chronic pain patients. Some patients become dependent, anxious, and homebound—if not bedridden. For some, too, chronic pain may be a welcome friend, relieving them of the boredom of a dull job or the burden of family responsibilities. These psychological rewards—sometimes combined with financial gains from compensation payments or insurance—work against improvements in the patient's condition, and can encourage increased drug dependency, repeated surgery, and multiple doctor and clinic visits.

There is no question that the patient feels pain. The hope of behavior modification is that pain relief can be obtained from a program aimed at changing the individual's lifestyle. The program begins with a complete assessment of the painful condition and a thorough explanation of how the program works. It is essential to enlist the full cooperation of both the patient and family members. The treatment is aimed at reducing pain medication and increasing mobility and independence through a graduated program of exercise, diet, and other activities. The patient is rewarded for positive efforts with praise and attention. Rewards are withheld when the patient retreats into negative attitudes or demanding and dependent behavior.

How effective are any of these treatment methods? Are some superior to others? Who is most likely to benefit? Do the benefits last? The answers are not yet in hand. Patient selection and patient cooperation are all-important. Analysis of individuals who have improved dramatically with one or another of these approaches is helping to pinpoint what factors are likely to lead to successful treatment.

Surgery to Relieve Pain

Surgery is often considered the court of last resort for pain: when all else fails, cut the nerve endings. Surgery can bring about instant, almost magical release from pain. But surgery may also destroy other sensations as well, or, inadvertently, become the source of new pain. Further, relief is not necessarily permanent. After 6 months or a year, pain may return.

For all those reasons, the decision for surgery must always involve a careful weighing of the patient's condition and the outlook for the future. If surgery can mean the difference between a pain-wracked existence ending in death, versus a pain-free time in which to compose one's life and see friends and family, then surgery is clearly a humane and compassionate choice.

There are a variety of operations to relieve pain. The most common is cordotomy: severing the nerve fibers on one or both sides of the spinal cord that travel the express routes to the brain. Cordotomy affects the sense of temperature as well as pain, since the fibers travel together in the express route.

Besides cordotomy, surgery within the brain or spinal cord to relieve pain includes severing connections at major junctions in pain pathways, such as at the places where pain fibers cross from one side of the cord to the other, or destroying parts of important relay stations in the brain like the thalamus, an egg-shaped cluster of nerve cells near the center of the brain. In addition, surgeons sometimes can relieve pain by destroying nerve fibers or their parent cell bodies outside the brain or spinal cord.

A case in point is the destruction of sympathetic nerves (a part of the autonomic nervous system) to relieve the severe pain that sometimes follows a penetrating wound from a sharp instrument or bullet.

When pain affects the upper extremities, or is widespread, the surgeon has fewer options and surgery may not be as effective. Still, skilled neurosurgeons have achieved excellent results with upper spinal cord or brain surgery to treat severe intractable pain. These procedures may employ chemicals or use heat or freezing treatments to destroy tissue, as well as the more traditional use of the scalpel.

Some surgeons have reported success with a brain operation called cingulotomy to relieve intractable pain in patients with severe psychiatric problems. The nerve fibers destroyed are part of a pathway important in emotions and motivation. The surgery appears to eliminate the discomfort and suffering the patient feels, but does not interfere with other mental faculties such as thinking and memory.

Prior to operating, physicians can often test the effectiveness of surgery by using anesthetic drugs to block nerves temporarily. In some chronic pain conditions—like the pain from a penetrating wound—these temporary blocks can in themselves be beneficial, promoting repair of nerve damage.

How do these current treatments apply to the more common chronic pain conditions? What follows is a brief survey of major pain disorders and the treatments most in use today.

The Major Pains

Headache

Tension headache, involving continued contractions of head and neck muscles, is one of the most common forms of headache. The other common variety is the vascular headache, involving changes in the pressure of blood vessels serving the head. Migraine headaches are of the vascular type, associated with throbbing pain on one side of the head. Genetic factors play a role in determining who will have migraines, but many other factors are important as well. A major difficulty in treating migraine headache is that changes occur throughout the course of the headache.

Blood vessels may first constrict and then dilate. Changing levels of neurotransmitters have also been noted. While a number of drugs can relieve migraine pain, their usefulness often depends on when they are taken. Some are only effective if taken at the onset. Several drugs for the prevention of migraine have been developed in recent years, including serotonin agonists which mimic the action of this key brain chemical. Prompt administration of these drugs is important.

Drugs are also the most common treatment for tension headache, although attempts to use biofeedback to control muscle tension have

191

had some success. Physical methods such as heat or cold applications often provide additional, if only temporary, relief.

Low Back Pain

The combination of pain-killers and modest amounts of a muscle relaxant are usually prescribed for the first-time low back pain patient. At the initial examination, the physician will also note if the patient is overweight or works under conditions (such as driving a truck or sitting at a desk for long hours) that offer little opportunity for exercise. Some authorities believe that low back pain is particularly prevalent in Western society because of the combination of overweight, bad posture (made worse if there is added weight up front), and infrequent exercise.

Although bed rest may be necessary for severe back problems, exercise is now considered to be an important addition to treatment and can help speed recovery for many patients with low back pain. Exercise helps reduce stress on the lower back by increasing flexibility and strength. To avoid injury, however, carefully follow the exercise routine prescribed by your doctor. In some cases, a full neurological examination may be necessary, including tests to determine if there may be a ruptured disc or other source of pressure on the cord or nerve roots.

Sometimes x-rays will show a disc problem that can be helped by surgery. Milder analgesics (aspirin, acetaminophen, or stronger non-narcotic medications) and electrical stimulation—using TENS or implanted brain electrodes—can be very effective for low back pain. What is not effective is long-term use of muscle-relaxant tranquilizers. Many specialists are convinced that chronic use of these drugs is detrimental to the back pain patient, adding to depression and increasing pain. Massage and manipulative therapy are used by some clinicians but, except for individual patient reports, their usefulness is still undocumented.

Cancer Pain

The pain of cancer can result from the pressure of a growing tumor or the infiltration of tumor cells into other organs. Or the pain can come about as the result of radiation or chemotherapy. These treatments can cause fluid accumulation and swelling (edema), irritate or destroy healthy tissue causing pain and inflammation, and possibly sensitize nerve endings. Ideally, the treatment for cancer pain is to remove the cancerous tissue. When that is not possible, pain can be treated by any or all of the currently available therapies: electrical stimulation, psychological methods, surgery, and strong pain-killers.

Arthritis Pain

Arthritis is a general descriptive term meaning a disorder of the joints. The two most common forms are osteoarthritis that typically affects the fingers and may spread to important weight-bearing joints in the spine or hips, and rheumatoid arthritis, an inflammatory joint disease associated with swelling, congestion, and thickening of the soft tissue around joints. Current treatments for arthritis include aspirin, acetaminophen, and nonsteroidal anti-inflammatory drugs like indomethacin and ibuprofen. Steroid drugs—important anti-inflammatory agents modeled after the body's own chemicals produced in the adrenal glands—were introduced and hailed as lifesavers in the 1950's. But the long-term use of steroids has serious consequences, among them the lowering of resistance to infection, hemorrhaging, and facial puffiness—producing the so-called moonface.

TENS and acupuncture have been tried with mixed results. In cases where tissue has been destroyed, surgery to replace a diseased joint with an artificial part has been very successful. The total hip replacement operation is an example.

Arthritis is best treated early, say the experts. A modest program of drugs combined with exercise can do much to restore full function and forestall long-term degenerative changes. Exercise in warm water is especially good since the water is both relaxing and provides buoyancy that makes exercises easier to perform. Physical treatments with warm or cold compresses are helpful sources of temporary pain relief.

Neurogenic Pain

The most difficult pains to treat are those that result from damage to the peripheral nerves or to the central nervous system itself. Mentioned earlier in this brochure as examples of extraordinarily searing pain were trigeminal neuralgia and shingles, along with several drugs that can help in these conditions. In addition, trigeminal neuralgia sufferers can benefit from surgery to destroy the nerve cells that supply pain-sensation fibers to the face. An advantage to using a treatment called "thermocoagulation"—which uses heat supplied by an electrical current to destroy nerve cells—is that pain fibers are more sensitive to the treatment resulting in less destruction of other sensations (such as touch and temperature).

Sometimes specialists treating trigeminal neuralgia find that certain blood vessels in the brain lie near the group of nerve cells supplying sensory fibers to the face, exerting pressure that causes pain. The surgical insertion of a small sponge between the blood vessels and the nerve cells can relieve the pressure and eliminate pain.

Among other notoriously painful neurogenic disorders is pain from an amputated or paralyzed limb—so called "phantom" pain—that affects a significant number of amputees and paraplegia patients. Various combinations of antidepressants and weak narcotics like propoxyphene are sometimes effective. Surgery, too, is occasionally successful. Many experts now think that the electrical stimulating techniques hold the greatest promise for relieving these pains.

Psychogenic Pain

Some cases of pain are not due to past disease or injury, nor is there any detectable sign of damage inside or outside the nervous system. Such pain may benefit from any of the psychological pain therapies listed earlier. It is also possible that some new methods used to diagnose pain may be useful. One method gaining in popularity is thermography, which measures the temperature of surface tissue as a reflection of blood flow. A color-coded "thermogram" of a person with a headache or other painful condition often shows an altered blood supply to the painful area, appearing as a darker or lighter shade than the surrounding areas or the corresponding part on the other side of the body.

Thus an abnormal thermogram in a patient who complains of pain in the absence of any other evidence may provide a valuable clue that can lead to a diagnosis and treatment.

Where to Go for Help

People with chronic pain have usually seen a family doctor and several other specialists as well. Eventually they are referred to neurologists, orthopedists, or neurosurgeons. The patient/doctor relationship is extremely important in dealing with chronic pain. Both patients and family members should seek out knowledgeable specialists who neither dismiss nor indulge the patient, physicians who understand full well how pain has come to dominate the patient's life and the lives of everyone else in the family.

Contrary to what many people think, pain patients are not malingerers or hypochondriacs. They are men and women of all ages, education, and social background, suffering a wide variety of painful conditions.

People with pain problems may feel isolated, helpless, or hopeless. But many of those who suffer with a pain problem can be helped if they—and their families—understand all the causes of pain, and the many and varied steps that can now be taken to undo what chronic pain has done. As a result of the strides neuroscience has made in tracking down pain in the brain—and in the mind—we can expect more and better treatments in the years to come. The days when patients were told "I'm sorry, but you'll have to learn to live with the pain" will be gone forever.

Part Four

Headaches, Hormones, and Other Co-Existing Conditions

Chapter 25

Women and Headaches: An Overview

History of Headache and Migraine

People suffered from headache as far back as 7000 BC. During this time, a large hole (trepanation) was placed in the scull possibly thought to relieve the "evil spirits or demons" inside the head that caused such pain. During the next several thousand years, continued descriptions and treatments for headaches are seen scattered throughout art, literature and medicine.

Aretaeus of Cappodocia (2nd century AD) often is considered as being "the discover" of migraine because of his classic descriptions of the condition. Some of the causes of such headaches also were recognized during this era when Celsus (215-300 AD) clearly described what is currently define as some common migraine triggers: "drinking wine, or crudity (dyspepsia), or cold, or heat of fire, or the sun."

During this era, most of these artistic, literary, and medical descriptions of migraine or headache used males as the sufferers, despite the likely higher prevalence in females than males. By the 12th century, Abbess Hildegarde of Bingen clearly described her own migraine aura. "I saw a great star, most splendid and beautiful, and with

Text in this chapter is from the following documents: "History of Women's Health," American Council for Headache Education (ACHE) © 2000. Reprinted from the web site of the American Council for Headache Education (www.achenet.org); reprinted with permission. And, "Women and Headaches," American Headache Society (AHS), © 2000, available online at http://www.ahsnet.org; reprinted with permission.

it an exceeding multitude of falling sparks with which the star followed southward... and suddenly they were all annihilated, being turned into black coals... and cast into the abyss so that I could see them no more."

Despite the long history of headache and migraine, the prevalence of migraine in women was not clearly documented in epidemiological studies until this century.

Women's Health in the United States

Prior to the 20th century, there was a general low state of health specifically for women. Most medicines were created for men that predominantly affected illnesses for men. Medicines were tested predominantly in men. Women assumed a role of "self care" with patent medicines like Lydia Pinkham's Vegetable Compound. Because life expectancy was short, other health concerns specific to women were nonexistent such as breast and uterine cancers, or menopause.

Health care in the 20th century expanded and included more women's health concerns, however, the standard of care was still inferior to men. Part of the reason for this was environmental, but also, many of the biological differences between men and women were not well understood. Differences in the physiology between men and women were unexplored until recently. For example, onset of heart disease occurs at an earlier age in men than in women.

Also, in the 20th century, the role of women in the field of medicine has dramatically changed compared to previous centuries. Specifically, the majority of all health care workers are now female. Women in general carry a tremendous responsibility for health care in the United States and in many other countries worldwide. Beside the increasing number of women physicians in this country, women often:

- Fulfill the doctors' orders,

- Deliver treatments,

- Teach patients about health,

- Provide the majority of nursing care,

- Identify, describe and report signs and symptoms of illness, and

- Are the first to be told when someone in the family does not feel well.

Despite their important role in the health care system during the last 100 years, women have only become proactive in demanding high quality health care during the last 20 years. Many women feel that there is a "stigma" regarding women within the field of medicine, so many are discouraged from seeking help that is now readily available. This comes, in part, from a history of women not being taken seriously by "male doctors" or other family members. Women's health concerns that historically have not been taken seriously and often have been considered attributable to the "hysterical" women include:

- Biological changes resulting from PMS (hormone changes causing fatigue, irritability, aching, swelling, among others)
- Menopause (hot flashes, fatigue, among others), and even
- Headaches (considered psychological in origin)

Clearly, medical advances show that these conditions are not psychological or "hysterical" in nature, but are caused by real biological factors. The higher prevalence of headaches in women, like the increased incidence of certain cancers, are specific to women and require individualized treatment that has been clinically tested specifically in women. Likewise, other medical conditions can be researched and tested specifically in men given their gender-specific origins, such as prostate cancer or high blood pressure, among others.

Myths about Headache in Women

One of the reasons that specific treatments for migraine in women have not been well studied are the myths and stigmas that women and headache have assumed over time. Many believed that headaches were an "excuse" and not a true medical condition. The pathophysiology of migraine is evident, and myths about migraine and headache need to be corrected.

Myth 1: "Not Tonight Dear, I Have a Headache"

Some believe that women use "migraine" or "headache" as an excuse to avoid sex. However, sex and many other forms of physical activity can make a migraine worse. Avoiding sex often is not an attempt to avoid intimacy with a spouse or partner, rather, an attempt to avoid making the headache worse. Migraine is usually associated with disability including disability within the family and social life. Women with migraine need to remember that their husbands need to be reassured that a migraine attack is not a feeble attempt to avoid intimacy. One way couples can cope with a mild or moderate migraine might be to spend a quite evening, with the lights low, relaxing, and trying some relaxation or massage therapy.

Myth 2: Migraines Are "All In Your Head"

For years, health care providers and family members believed that many women complaining of headache had psychological problems. Interestingly, history documents the reality of the pain and the disability associated with migraine, but this was not transferred to women with migraine. Most migraine patients experience mood changes, irritability and even depression prior to the onset of an attack. This may be one of the reasons doctors and family members were led to believe that these patients had a mood or psychological disorder. Recent advances have shown that mood changes, irritability and even depression result from biochemical changes in the brain. Indeed, migraine is a biological condition, and the pathophysiology of its origin is biologically based.

Myth 3: Women Get Migraine and It Is Just Part of Their "PMS"

The relation of migraine to menstruation occurs in only a fraction of women. Most women experience migraine attacks throughout the month, only of which a portion of these attacks are associated with their menstrual cycle. Indeed migraine is more prevalent in women than men, but several million men in the United States suffer from migraine too. (The hardest part of this myth is that there are thousands of men who are afraid to admit they have migraine headaches because they do not want to think they have psychological problems or are "weak in character" [part of another myth that migraine is "all in your head"]).

Women and Headache Facts

- In 1992, women made 10,000,000 visits to their primary care physicians for evaluation of headache.

- In the United States, 8,700,000 women suffer from migraine each year, and 3,400,000 (just less than half of the women) have more than one migraine attack per month.

- The highest prevalence for migraine occurs in women between the ages of 35 and 45—a period when many women are at the height of their professional career, family responsibilities, and social life.

- An average, 16 out of every 100 women (or 16%) suffer from migraine headaches.

- In women migraine sufferers, 60% of them experience migraine during menses as well as during other times of the month; 14% of women only have migraine during their menstrual period.

- Changes in hormones, such as decrease in estrogen levels, are likely to be a trigger for migraine in some women.

- Aura occurs in about 15% of all migraine attacks.

- In the first century, Arateus of Cappadocia (Asia) was the first physician to accurately document the symptoms of migraine.

- Headache is one of the most common causes for absenteeism from work. On average headache sufferers lose an average of 1.1 days of work every three months (or over 4 workdays per year).

Women and Headaches

Menstrual Migraine

About 15% of women who have migraines will only get them two or three days before or after the start of their menstrual period. Over 60% will describe consistent worsening migraines at this time, although they have some migraines that occur at other times as well. Yet other women will report that they have a predictable headache at some part of their cycle, perhaps at ovulation. It's easy to see, then, that the hormones of the menstrual cycle account for a significant part of the increased risk for headache in women.

If you suspect that your headaches vary with your periods, note on your calendar when your periods and your headaches occur. After a few months, you and your doctor will then be able to tell just how strong the link is, and that may help your doctor choose among treatment options.

The vast majority of women with menstrual migraine do not have abnormalities of their hormones. Rather, they have a biological predisposition to migraine, and the normal changes in hormones over the cycle serve as headache triggers that increase their vulnerability to headache.

Current thinking is that a drop in estrogen following several days of high levels serves as the hormonal trigger for most women. This is the natural pattern just before the period starts, and accounts for the strong link between menstruation and migraine. The first step in controlling menstrual migraine is usually to treat it like any other migraine. Any of the medications currently available for migraine can be used to stop an attack of menstrual migraine, provided there is no significant chance of pregnancy. Many women find the newer "triptan" medications most effective, although virtually all of the currently available medications have helped some women. If migraines are exclusively menstrual, occurring only once a month, there is little danger of developing a pattern of medication overuse that can result in daily "drug rebound" headache.

Some women like to try to prevent the migraine from starting in the first place. For exclusively menstrual migraines, a regular prescription dose of an anti-inflammatory medication such as ibuprofen or naproxen started about two days before the expected migraine can be helpful. When the headache-prone period is over, the drug is stopped until the next month. Other medications that have been used in migraine prevention can also be used in this fashion.

For women with migraines at other times of the month as well, or whose periods are irregular, using a regular migraine preventive throughout the month may be most effective. Choice of a preventive will depend on your particular headache pattern and type, as well as your medical history. Sometimes a small boost in dosage of the preventive just before the menstrual migraine can help prevent that particular headache type. Hormonal manipulation for menstrual migraine can be tried, but the results are not always predictable. Adding a little estrogen in the form of either a pill or a patch, beginning a few days before the period, has been useful to some women. Stronger hormonal manipulations, such as drugs to eliminate menstrual periods or counteract estrogens, are also possible for more severe problems. Finally, many women ask about hysterectomy. In general, this is not a recommended treatment for menstrual migraine. For the most part it is a drastic step that just doesn't work.

Oral Contraceptives

Because of the relationship of estrogen levels to migraine, oral contraceptives (OCs) may have significant impact on women's migraines. Some women have reported improvement of migraine on OCs, but it's more common for women to report worsening migraine with OCs. This effect usually occurs right away but may only become apparent after longer-term use. OCs have been known to bring on migraines in women who may have a biological tendency to migraine but never had headaches previously, and discontinuation of OCs may not result in improvement for many months. Even non-estrogen hormonal methods of birth control such as Depo-Provera injection seem to aggravate headaches in some women.

Women who have problems with migraine and suspect their OCs as a trigger are probably best advised to use non-hormonal methods of birth control, at least until the headaches are under control or it is relatively certain that the OCs are not at fault. There are some very personal issues involved with decisions about birth control, though, and it is important to also consider the physical, social, and psychological risks of an unwanted pregnancy.

Yet another issue relating to oral contraceptives involves the risk of stroke in migraine patients. In women who have migraines with auras, there appears to be a small increase in the risk of stroke if they also take OCs. To put this into perspective, the risk of stroke in young women is very small, and even doubling that risk still leaves stroke as a very unlikely occurrence. However, that risk increases again if the woman is older, and particularly if she smokes as well. Many physicians feel that the migraine patient who smokes should not use OCs, but again it must be acknowledged that there are many personal issues involved in these choices.

Pregnancy and Breastfeeding

The peak occurrence of migraine for women is the child-bearing years. Pre-existing migraine can become worse during the first trimester of pregnancy and then disappear for the last two. However, about 25% of women with migraine will go through their pregnancy with their headache pattern unchanged. Migraine can also appear for the first time during pregnancy or soon after giving birth.

Many women with migraine may see an improvement in their headaches during pregnancy, probably due to the sustained high levels of estrogens. Women who have menstrual migraine tend to have a higher rate of disappearance or improvement.

Managing migraine during pregnancy and breastfeeding can be problematic, for now there are two patients to be considered. Generally non-drug treatment is preferred. Avoidance of triggers, especially dietary ones, is important. Exercise, biofeedback and other relaxation techniques are other good options.

Medical treatment is advisable when headache is disabling and associated symptoms such as severe nausea, vomiting and dehydration are potentially harmful to the fetus as well. One must weigh the potential risk of the medication against the risk to the mother and fetus if left untreated. For the isolated attack, the best treatment is rest, reassurance and ice packs.

Although the absolute safety of specific drugs during pregnancy has not been established, there are some that are felt to be relatively safe. These include acetaminophen, codeine, caffeine and aspirin. Aspirin should be avoided in late pregnancy, since it may inhibit uterine contractions and cause increased bleeding in mother and newborn. Nonsteroidal anti-inflammatory drugs (NSAIDs) such as ibuprofen and indomethacin (Indocin) can be used, but their use should be limited to 48 hours since they can inhibit labor and prolong pregnancy. Promethazine (Phenergan) is useful for nausea and vomiting as well as headache control. This and other common anti-nausea treatments are thought to be safe if used occasionally in low doses. Women should be assured that the presence of migraine, whether mild or disabling, does not result in more miscarriages, birth defects or other complications than occur among women without migraine.

The same principles hold true for breastfeeding. The baby is now receiving whatever the mother is taking, so avoiding medication use whenever possible is the safest approach. If medication is needed, the mother can use a short-acting drug such as ibuprofen or sumatriptan, then pump and dump the breast milk a few hours later, feeding the baby formula or stored breast milk in the meantime. Women should consult their obstetrician and their neurologist or primary care doctor for guidance regarding the relative risks and benefits of treatment.

Menopause

Headaches may reappear at menopause after years of absence, or become more severe or more frequent. In general, most women experience an overall lessening of their headaches, and they often change in nature. Women who have had migraine with aura may continue to have the aura but without the subsequent headache. They will often state that they no longer have "killer" headaches marked by vomiting, diarrhea and inability to function, but rather headaches they "can live with." Following natural menopause, there is a reported 60% decrease in headache. With surgical menopause (hysterectomy) this number decreases to about 30%. Those who have had primarily menstrual migraine earlier in life seem to benefit most from menopause.

Somewhere between 50% to 80% of women have disagreeable symptoms related to menopause or serious health concerns such as higher risk of osteoporosis or heart disease. These can be treated by hormone replacement therapy (HRT). Although still a controversial issue, in most of these cases the benefits of HRT outweigh the risks, which include a slightly increased risk of uterine cancer and possibly of breast cancer and blood clotting abnormalities. The decision to start HRT should be made by the woman and her doctor based on her individual needs and requirements for optimal health and well-being.

For women with migraine, it is difficult to predict how their headaches will respond to HRT. Some improve while others find their headaches are worse. To reduce the risk of uterine cancer, progesterone is often given along with estrogen to those women who still have a uterus. Women with migraine seem to do better when they receive a daily dose of progesterone days 1-25 rather than just days 16-25, probably because their hormone levels remain more stable throughout the month.

If the headaches get worse with HRT, changing the way the estrogen dose is delivered (oral, transdermal patch or topical) may help. The topical form gives a more limited dose and is not protective against osteoporosis or cardiovascular disease. Currently, little information is available regarding how headache is affected by natural plant hormones or by the newer selective estrogen agent raloxifene (Evista).

Headache Triggers

Headache triggers do not "cause" headache. Instead, triggers are events that activate or bring on a headache in a headache-prone person. Recognizing and modifying events that trigger headaches can be very helpful in reducing headache frequency and the need for medication.

Stress. Stress is by far the most common headache trigger. Most women and men report that they are more likely to have headaches during or after periods of stress. The fact that stress can trigger headache attacks does not mean the headaches are a psychological problem. As you may know, stress can also trigger heart attacks in someone who has pre-existing heart disease, such as coronary artery disease. The illness is biological but its severity is influenced by environment, lifestyle and other non-biological factors.

We know that major life events, such as a death in the family or a move across country cause stress, but it is actually the day-to-day stress or daily hassles that are most likely to trigger headaches. Women are likely to have multiple role stress due to juggling many different roles and responsibilities. Roles often include being a mother, wife, professional working woman, and caretaker of the home. Often these important roles come into conflict with one another, and women are forced to make tough choices between competing demands. Often women overextend themselves trying to do it all. Either situation equals stress.

Women are also prone to caregiver stress, charged with providing most of the attention needed by their small children, aging parents, or ill family members. This can be a physically and emotionally taxing responsibility. Most jobs are 40 hours per week, but caregiving often requires one to be on-call 24 hours a day, 7 days a week. Ironically, for some women a bad migraine attack may be the only time they have to themselves, even though it's the last way they'd like to spend it. Whatever your responsibilities, it's important for you to make time for yourself. If you are always putting other people first, try making a weekly appointment to do something you want to do, or to do nothing at all, whatever helps you to "de-stress." If others ask you to do something at that scheduled time, just say, "Sorry, I have an appointment."

Environmental and Behavioral Triggers. Natural events in the environment are known to trigger headache for some people. Weather patterns like heat, humidity, and sudden changes in barometric pressure can act as headache triggers. Dust, smoke, glare and strong odors may also be triggers.

Our own lifestyles and behaviors can increase headache. For example, eye strain, physical exertion, and chronically clenching the jaw or tensing muscles can trigger headache. Altering sleep patterns tends to provoke headache. Irregular sleep schedules, shift-work, and oversleeping are known headache triggers. Women are particularly prone to insomnia and headache brought on by insufficient sleep. Notably, sleeping can help reduce a headache episode once it is underway.

Diet and Dietary Habits. Alcohol, aged cheeses, nuts, dairy products, shellfish, and chocolate are triggers for some but not all migraine sufferers. Some are sensitive to food additives and preservatives, such as MSG, the artificial sweetener aspartame, and nitrates used as preservatives. How we eat can be just as important as what we eat. Often because of time pressures or in an attempt to lose weight, women skip meals, making them more vulnerable to a headache.

The relationship between headache and diet can be complex. For example, it may be the withdrawal of caffeine after regular use, rather than the caffeine itself, that triggers a headache. Sometimes diet interacts with a second factor to trigger headache. For some people, alcohol alone will not trigger headache, but drinking alcohol when sleep-deprived will lead to a severe headache. Keeping a food and headache diary can help you identify any dietary headache triggers.

Depression. The link between headache and depression works both ways. Having a chronic illness like headache increases the risk for depression. As headaches become more frequent and more severe, the likelihood for depression also increases. Individuals with daily headache are at the highest risk for developing depression.

In turn, depression can make pain more intense and difficult to treat. Depression also tends to decrease energy, disturb sleep, and influence appetite and eating habits. These sleep and dietary changes can then contribute to the headache problem. Although most women with headaches are not depressed, it is important to identify even mild levels of depression. The usual drug and non-drug treatments for headache are not as effective when the headache sufferer is also troubled by depression.

Getting Support and Treatment

Women with headache may be taken less seriously by the medical profession when they do seek care for their headaches. There is evidence that men with headache are more likely to receive intensive medical scrutiny for underlying causes of headache, whereas women with similar headache complaints are more likely to be diagnosed with depression or viewed as having a psychologically based illness. Women themselves may not take their problems seriously and be reluctant to "bother" their doctor about a headache that "only" comes once a month.

The more you understand about headache as a biological disorder, the better able you will be to seek and find effective treatment. A little education and support can go a long way into making treatment more available. The American Council for Headache Education (ACHE) produces a variety of headache education materials and sponsors over 50 active support groups nationwide. Many resources are available to these support groups. Online sites on CompuServe, AOL, Prodigy and the World Wide Web (http://www.achenet.org) include information and chat rooms. A variety of headache specialists contribute to

ACHE's quarterly newsletter. Features include topics of interest to women and an "Ask the Doctor" column. If you are in search of a headache specialist in your region, ACHE can help. Call 1-800-255-ACHE for lists of support groups and headache specialists in your region.

Chapter 26

Oral Contraceptives and Headaches

Why Is Headache Associated with Oral Contraceptive Use?

To begin with, OCs contain hormones (usually a small amount of estrogen and progesterone, although there are "progesterone only" pills available as well). These hormones fool the body and the master gland in the brain (the pituitary gland) that controls the release of eggs from the ovaries into not releasing an egg monthly (ovulation). No ovulation usually means no pregnancy. Used correctly (without skipping or missing pills) OCs are 99% effective in preventing pregnancy.

Women experiencing migraine or headache while on combination OCs (varying doses and proportions of synthetic estrogen and progesterone) tend to have attacks during the week that hormone levels are withdrawn (also know as the "placebo" week). This suggests that estrogen withdrawal can trigger migraine. How OCs influence migraine is still unknown.

Will Using Oral Contraceptives Make My Headaches Worse?

Many women with migraine who take OCs experience no difference in their migraine pattern. One third of women may actually experience

Text in this chapter is from the American Council for Headache Education (ACHE) © 2000. Reprinted from the web site of the American Council for Headache Education (www.achenet.org); reprinted with permission.

fewer attacks or they may be less severe (and about one third have more severe headaches). However, significantly more women start having migraine when starting OCs than when not using OCs, suggesting a causal relationship. A family history of migraine may increase the risk for some women when they start taking OCs.

What about women who do notice a connection between hormone fluctuations and headaches? Will their headaches worsen on OCs? Based on studies done in the 1960s by Dr. Brian Somerville, it is thought that the drop in estrogen levels that occurs a few days before a normal menstrual period increases susceptibility to headache in some (but not all) women with migraine. Specifically, is has been suggested that the decrease in estrogen levels primes cranial vessels for certain chemicals such as serotonin. These women are more likely to have headaches during the week when they are off OCs, when estrogen levels fall.

Some women notice no change in their headaches when they are on OCs, and other women notice an improvement in their headaches when on OCs. Switching to a pill with a different dose or type of estrogen can also change headaches (make them better or worse). If headaches are a problem only during the week off OCs, it is possible to take the OC continuously, skipping the placebo pill or pill-free week. Doing this will cause women to have unpredictable light spotting for a few months, usually followed by minimal bleeding. Most gynecologists are familiar with using OCs this way to treat endometriosis, and are comfortable doing it for women with headache problems as well. The drawback to continuous use is that women will not have monthly withdrawal bleeding, which many women find reassuring as evidence that they are not pregnant.

Treatments for Migraine Associated with Oral Contraceptive Use

Treatment of migraine in women using OCs is similar to migraine treatment in women with menstrual migraine who are not on the OCs. Preventive therapy beginning several days before an anticipated migraine attack may be more effective under these circumstances because OCs improve the regularity of the menstrual cycle. If conventional anti-migraine therapies are not effective or not well tolerated, OCs should be discontinued and alternative means of contraception considered.

Migraines may stop immediately after OCs are stopped or relief may be delayed for as long as six months to a year. If migraine frequency does increase when taking OCs and preventive therapies do not help, discontinuation of the OCs should be considered. Women may find that headaches may persist for up to three months after discontinuing OC therapy because it takes a while for menstrual cycles to normalize. After that time, headache frequency may return to previous baselines levels as noted before starting OCs.

Oral Contraceptives and Stroke

"Stroke" is a medical term commonly used to mean damage to part of the brain caused by a lack of blood flow. Blood flow may be reduced by a blood clot, an embolus (a clot forming in one place and moving to another place), or a ruptured artery that delivers blood to that part of the brain.

"Risk factors" increase the chance that someone will have a stroke. Some of the most common risk factors for stroke include high blood pressure, diabetes, high blood cholesterol, and smoking. In patients with migraine without aura, taking OCs seems to slightly increase the risk of stroke, particularly in women during their childbearing years. OCs containing low doses of estrogen (less than 50 micrograms) do not appear to substantially increase the rate of stroke in women without traditional stroke risk factors. Low-dose OCs also may carry less risk of life-threatening events than can occur with pregnancy. There is, however, a greater risk of stroke with OC use in older women (over 35 years of age) and in those who smoke, have hypertension or diabetes, or have a history of stroke or transient ischemic attack (also known as "TIA").

Recent data suggests that combined OC pills, including those with low estrogen levels, increase the risk of stroke in women with migraine even if no other risk factors for stroke exist. The absolute risk of stroke in this population, however, is small. Therefore, it is difficult to make any definitive recommendations.

Women who have migraine with aura (especially prolonged or complicated auras involving numbness, weakness or loss of vision) may have an increased risk of a stroke. How high is that risk? Unfortunately, no one knows for sure; some estimates put it at around 14 times the risk of someone in the general population. In the United Kingdom, OCs are not traditionally prescribed for women who have migraine with aura. In contrast, some clinicians think that aspirin and migraine-preventing medications may give some protection against stroke for migraine sufferers. Women with migraine who take OCs and develop aura for the first time, who have more severe aura symptoms, or whose headaches worsen significantly should discontinue using OCs and contact their doctor immediately.

If the decision is made to use OCs, using a lower dose of estrogen and taking it continuously (skipping the placebo pill or pill-free week) may be the most effective way to avoid worsening headaches. Many experts also recommend choosing an OC that has stable levels of hormones rather than changing doses throughout the month. This is based on the theory that increases and decreases in circulating levels of estrogen may not be well tolerated by women with headaches influenced by hormones.

The question remains whether putting these two things together (migraine and using OCs) increases the risk of a stroke to unacceptable levels. Some experts agree that women who have migraine without aura can probably safely take OCs. The risks of unintended pregnancy for those women may outweigh the small increase in risk of stroke. In light of this uncertainty, using OCs in patients with migraine is a decision that needs to be made on an individual basis.

Chapter 27

Migraine during Pregnancy

Planning Pregnancy while Managing Migraine

Many women with headaches worry about what will happen to their headaches once they are pregnant. Actually, the "periconceptional" period—when someone is trying to get pregnant but is not sure if they are or are not pregnant—can be a challenging time. Most women do not realize that they are pregnant until a week or so after they have missed a period. Urine pregnancy tests, although good and getting better, may not be positive that early. A migraine patient is concerned that medications taken early in pregnancy to treat headache could be harmful to the developing fetus.

Many commonly used headache medications have unknown effects during pregnancy. However, to minimize potential problems, many headache experts recommend that women with headache pay special attention when planning their pregnancies. For example, it helps to minimize the number of months where patients have to wonder whether or not they are pregnant. Making an effort to conceive quickly can do this. Couples may use an ovulation predictor kit sold in drugstores to monitor ovulation and concentrate intercourse to that period. Doctors disagree on how often patients should have intercourse when trying to become pregnant, but some suggest once a day is optimal.

Many headache experts recommend tapering off daily preventive medications if planning to get pregnant. Generally patients do not

Text in this chapter is from the American Council for Headache Education (ACHE) © 2000. Reprinted from the web site of the American Council for Headache Education (www.achenet.org); reprinted with permission.

need to avoid their preventive medications for several months before attempting to conceive; but about a week or so is fine (check with your doctor to determine specific treatment strategy changes). Some women with very severe headache problems are not able to taper off their daily medications. In that case, discuss the potential risks of these medications with the doctor before becoming pregnant. While some commonly used preventive therapies (beta-blockers and tricyclics) have a reassuring track record when used in pregnancy, others (especially sodium valproate or Depakote®) are known to cause birth defects. Many birth defects occur early in pregnancy, often during the first three months, when major organ systems are forming. Therefore, waiting until after conceiving to make decisions about preventive medication for migraine is not recommended. For a review of medications and their use in pregnancy and menstrual migraine, see Table 27.1.

Drug Labeling in Pregnancy

If a headache sufferer becomes pregnant (approximately 44% of all pregnancies resulting in live births are unintended) 12 and has been taking medication, they should not panic! Although it is difficult to say with certainty, it is unlikely that commonly used headache medications will cause major problems. There are many sources of information about the risks of medications when taken during pregnancy. Manufacturers include information in the package insert, and many agencies have telephone hot lines, and other information is available in the published literature.

General "headache hygiene" is crucial for women who have headaches and are trying to get pregnant. Many physicians recommend that women continue their current therapy or even start nonpharmacological headache treatments for headache. Other nonpharmacological ways to improve headache management include:

1. exercise regularly,

2. maintain a normal sleep schedule,

3. avoid headache triggers including alcohol and tobacco,

4. do not skip meals, and

5. eat a healthy balanced diet that includes folic acid. Many multivitamins include folic acid as an ingredient. Women in their childbearing years often do not get adequate amounts of folic acid. Supplemental folic acid during pregnancy can decrease the risk of certain birth defects.

Table 27.1. Medications and Their Use in Pregnancy (continued on pages 218–220)

	Fetal Risk	*Breast Feeding[1]*
Analgesics		
Simple Analgesics		
Aspirin	C*	Caution
Acetaminophen	B*	Compatible
Caffeine	B	Compatible

* D if used during 3rd trimester

	Fetal Risk	*Breast Feeding*
Narcotics		
Butorphanol	B**	Compatible
Codeine	C**	Compatible
Hydromorphone	B**	Compatible
Meperidine	C**	Compatible
Methadone	B**	Compatible
Morphine	B**	Compatible
Propoxyphene	C**	Compatible

** D if prolonged or at term

Nonsteroidal Anti-inflammatory Drugs (NSAIDs)

	Fetal Risk	*Breast Feeding*
NSAIDs		
Fenoprofen	B*	Compatible
Ibuprofen	B*	Compatible
Indomethacine	B*	Compatible
Meclofenamate	B*	Compatible
Naproxen	B*	Compatible
Sulindac	B*	Compatible
Tolmetin	B*	Compatible

* D if used during 3rd trimester

Sedatives/Hypnotics

	Fetal Risk	*Breast Feeding*
Barbituates		
Butalbital	C	Caution (sedation)
Phenobarbital	D	Caution (sedation)
Benzodiazepams		
Chlordiazepoxide	D	Concern***
Diazepam	D	Concern
Lorazepam	D	Concern
Clonazepam	C	Concern

*** effects unknown

Table 27.1. Medications and Their Use in Pregnancy (continued from page 217; continues on pages 219–220).

	Fetal Risk	*Breast Feeding*[1]
Neuroleptics/Antiemetics		
Antihistamines		
Cyclizine (Marezine)	B	NA
Cyproheptadine	B	Contraindicated
Dimenhydrinate (Dramamine)	B	NA
Meclizine (Antivert)	B	NA
Other		
Emetrol	B	Compatible
Doxylamine succinate		
and Vitamin B6 (Bendectin)	B	NA
Trimethobenzamide (Tigan)	C	NA
Neuroleptics		
Phenothiazines	C	Concern
Chlorpromazine (Thorazine)	C	Concern
Prochlorperazine (Compazine)	C	Compatible
Promazine (Sparine)	C	NA
Haloperidol (Haldol)	C	Concern
Thiothixene (Navane)	C	NA
Metoclopramide (Reglan)	C	Concern
Ergots and Serotonin Agents		
Ergots and Serotonin Agonists		
Ergotamine	X	Contraindicated***
Dihydroergotamine	X	Contraindicated
Methylergonovine maleate	C	Caution
Methysergide	D	Caution
Naratriptan	C	Caution
Rizatriptan	C	Caution
Sumatriptan	C	Caution
Zolmitriptan	C	Caution

*** Vomiting, diarrhea, convulsions

Antihypertensives		
Beta-blockers		
Atenolol	C	Compatible
Metoprolol	B	Compatible
Nadolol	C	Compatible
Propranolol	C	Compatible
Timolol	C	Compatible

Table 27.1. Medications and Their Use in Pregnancy (continued from pages 217–218; continues on page 220).

	Fetal Risk	Breast Feeding[1]
Antihypertensives, continued		
Adrenergic Blocker		
Clonidine	C	Compatible
Calcium Channel Blocker		
Diltiazem	C	Compatible
Nifedipine	C	Compatible
Verapamil	C	Compatible
Antidepressants		
Amitriptyline	D	Concern
Amoxapine	C	Concern
Bupropion	B	Concern
Desipramine	C	Concern
Doxepin	C	Concern
Fluoxetine	B	Concern
Imipramine	D	Concern
Nefazodone	C	Concern
Nortriptypline	D	Concern
Sertraline	C	Concern
Paroxetine	C	Concern
Phenelzine	C	Concern
Protriptyline	C	Concern
Venlafaxine	C	Concern
Other Drugs		
Anticonvulsants		
Carbamazapine	C	Compatible
Gabapentin	C	?
Lamotrigine	C	?
Phenobarbital	D	Compatible
Phenytoin	D	Compatible
Topiramate	D	?
Valproic acid	D	Compatible
Corticosteroids		
Cortisone	D	Compatible
Dexamethasone	C	Compatible
Prednisone	B	Compatible

Table 27.1. Medications and Their Use in Pregnancy (continued from pages 217–219)

	Fetal Risk	Breast Feeding[1]
Other Drugs, continued		
Other		
Bromocriptine	C	Contraindicated*
Diphenoxylate	C	Compatible
Lidocaine	C	NA
Lithium	C	Contraindicated**
Paregoric	B***	Compatible

* Suppresses lactation
** 1/3 to 1/2 therapeutic blood levels in infants
*** D if prolonged use of 3rd trimester
A,B,C,D,X, see Table 27.2.

[1]*Editor's note*: Other sources sometimes indicate different levels of breast feeding concern. Breast feeding women should check with their physicians for further information.

Table 27.2. The Food and Drug Administration lists five categories of fetal risk in labeling for drug use in pregnancy.

Category A: Controlled studies show no risk.Adequate, well-controlled studies in pregnant women fail to demonstrate a risk to the fetus.

Category B: No evidence of risk in humans.Either animal-reproduction studies have not demonstrated a fetal risk but there are no controlled studies in pregnant women, or animal-reproduction studies have shown an adverse effect (other than a decrease in fertility) that was not confirmed in controlled studies in women.

Category C: Risk cannot be ruled out.Either studies in animals have revealed adverse effects on the fetus (teratogenic or embryocidal or other) and there are no controlled studies in woman, or studies in women and animals are not available. Drugs should be given only if the potential benefit justifies the potential risk to the fetus.

Category D: Positive evidence of risk.There is positive evidence of human fetal risk, but the benefits from use in pregnant women may be acceptable despite the risk.

Category X: Contraindicated in pregnancy.Studies in animals or human beings have demonstrated fetal abnormalities, or there is evidence of fetal risk based on human experience, or both, and the risk of the use of the drug in pregnant women clearly outweighs any possible benefit.

Treatment of Migraine During Pregnancy

Most women are highly motivated to avoid using unnecessary medications during pregnancy. If at all possible, it is best to minimize medication during the important first trimester of pregnancy, when many organ systems are developing in the fetus. Drugs or environmental factors that cause birth defects or problems usually cause that particular problem only if they are present during the stage at which the organ system is developing. If the fetus is exposed to these factors before or after the development of the organ system they affect, there is generally no effect. Since so much development takes place during the first trimester, it is best to be off medication at that time, if at all possible.

Growth and development of the fetus continues throughout the second and third trimesters. Many things can still negatively affect the central nervous system (brain and spinal cord) during this time. For this reason, most women and their doctors try hard to minimize medication use throughout pregnancy. There are times, however, where the benefits of medication treatment might outweigh the potential risks. For example, if a woman is so ill from headaches that she is vomiting frequently, dehydrated, losing weight and unable to function, most people would accept that headache treatment might be necessary despite potential risks, since the pregnancy itself can be threatened.

As a general rule, use of medications should be restricted during pregnancy to avoid harming the fetus. Some medications may be associated with birth defects, embryo toxicity, delayed fetal growth, interference with uterine contractions during labor, or direct effects on the newborn baby. For this reason, nonpharmacological therapies are often recommended during pregnancy.

Pharmacological (Medication) Treatments

Acute Treatments

Proving which drugs are "safe" during pregnancy is not an easy matter. For one thing, since most pregnant women avoid using medication, it can take a long time to collect information about the effects of drugs in pregnancy. Furthermore, no drug manufacturer will study use of a drug in pregnant women because it is ethically impossible to justify doing randomized, controlled clinical research on pregnant women. Another problem is figuring out if reported adverse events were actually attributed to the medication or might they have happened anyway. Studies show that 1% to 2% of babies will have some type of malformation or congenital problem at birth, even when they are not exposed to drugs or other problem-causing substances.

Long-term experience with some types of medications causes us to believe that they are relatively safe for use during pregnancy. Even these drugs, though, need to be used in moderation and under careful medical supervision. Headache medications that most physicians feel can be used in pregnancy include:

- acetaminophen (Tylenol®),
- narcotics (like Percocet® or Vicodin®), and
- some of the preventive headache medications such as beta-blockers or antidepressants.

The Food and Drug Administration (FDA) classify triptans as medications that should be used during pregnancy "only if the potential benefit to the mother outweighs the potential risk to the fetus." This means that, as with any medication women consider using during pregnancy, a careful discussion with the doctor is necessary to weigh the pros and cons for the mother and the baby.

Triptans, Ergotamine, and Dihydroergotamine

The long-term effect of migraine medications that cause blood vessel constriction (narrowing) is not clearly established. These drugs (e.g., triptans, ergotamine, dihydroergotamine) should be monitored closely or even avoided during pregnancy. However, many companies that make these medications support pregnancy registries. Women who take medications such as triptans can enroll in these registries and provide valuable information regarding the safety of these medications for use during pregnancy.

NSAIDS and Combination Analgesics

For pregnant patients that need medication for their migraine attack, acetaminophen is considered safe and is the drug of choice for mild-to-moderate headache. Codeine occasionally may be added to increase the efficacy of acetaminophen when treating more severe migraine attacks. Caffeine may help in the acute treatment of migraine, either alone or in combination with other measures. Moderate (less than 300 mg per day 14) caffeine use is not considered harmful to the fetus.

Aspirin and NSAIDs may increase the risk of bleeding in the mother and fetus, and when used late in pregnancy these agents may interfere with labor. For these reasons, their use is generally restricted during pregnancy.

Narcotics

Selected narcotic medications are considered relatively safe for use during pregnancy (caution should be taken to avoid overuse and address dependency concerns).

Treatment of Nausea and Vomiting

Medications to help with nausea and vomiting may also be needed. Emetrol® which acts on the wall of the gastrointestinal tract, and trimethobenzamide (Tigan®) are felt to be safe agents for treatment of nausea and vomiting. If headache or nausea and vomiting are severe and do not respond to conservative management, patients may require hospitalization in order to receive intravenous fluids and treatment with narcotics.

Preventive Therapy

Preventative medications that have been used safely during pregnancy include selected beta-blockers, tricyclic antidepressants, and calcium channel blockers, although these should be used only when absolutely necessary. Patients should always discuss the use of all medications with their obstetrician, especially if there is a different physician for treatment of migraine or for headache management in general.

Non-Pharmacological Techniques

Nonpharmacological techniques can help for almost every headache patient, and their use should be particularly stressed during pregnancy. Some nonpharmacological measures can be started at home and require no formal treatment plan. These include:

- avoidance of identified triggers (e.g., diet, sleep, stress)
- moderate exercise, and
- ice packs.

Formal nonpharmacological techniques include biofeedback, relaxation training, massage therapy, postural training, hypnosis and acupuncture. Local anesthetic also may be injected into trigger points of the head and neck region, if indicated. Dr. Dawn Marcus has studied the use of biofeedback training to treat headaches during pregnancy and shown that this is very helpful for many women. If headaches continue to be especially troublesome, consider reducing work hours or other responsibilities. Many physicians would rather write a letter to a patient's employer asking for reduced work hours than prescribe medication for headache control.

Postpartum Migraine

Frequency and Cause of Postpartum Migraine

Headache within the first week after delivering (first postpartum week) occurs in over one third of all women, but in nearly two thirds of women with migraine. The postpartum headache is often less severe than one's typical migraine headache.

During the final trimester of pregnancy, estrogen levels increase to 100 times what they were prior to pregnancy. After delivery of the baby, estrogen levels fall quickly. This rapid change in estrogen levels may trigger an attack in patients with a predisposition to migraine. Although estrogen levels are higher during pregnancy, the rapid decline in estrogen at the time of birth resembles the withdrawal of estrogen that occurs monthly before the menstrual period.

Treatment of Postpartum Migraine

Safe treatment of migraine after pregnancy depends on whether a woman is breastfeeding the infant. Medications that should be avoided include bromocriptine, ergotamine, cyproheptadine, and lithium. There is very little data regarding the use of triptans while breastfeeding. Benzodiazepam (e.g, Ativan®, Valium®), barbiturates (e.g., Fioricet®, Fiorinal®, Esgic®), antidepressants (e.g., Elavil®, Pamelor®) and neuroleptics (drugs that work on the dopamine system of the brain, e.g., Risperdal®, Seroquel®) should be used cautiously. Acetaminophen is preferred over aspirin.

Managing Migraine when Breastfeeding

Breastfeeding has many advantages for the baby (and some for the mother, as well) compared with formula feeding. It would be a shame if concerns over headaches prevented women from breastfeeding.

Several issues need to be considered when deciding to breastfeed while managing headaches. Importantly, there are several "tricks" that women can do that will allow them to make decisions about medication while breastfeeding.

Delaying Return of the Menstrual Cycle

If women are breastfeeding exclusively, with little or no formula supplementation, the return of the menstrual cycle probably will be delayed. For women who experience migraine with their menstrual cycle, this is a positive feature of continued breastfeeding. However, this is not true for everyone. Sleep deprivation for the mother is not uncommon after she has a new baby, and the stresses of being a new parent can cause an increase in headaches for some women. Once the baby starts eating solid food, or if the mother decreases the frequency of breastfeeding (such as if they return to work), the menstrual cycle may come back. For many women, headaches will likely return to their pre-pregnancy pattern.

Medications Excreted in Breast Milk

Unfortunately, many medications that the mother might take to help manage headache are released (excreted) into the breast milk and can be passed on to the baby. For example, sedative or narcotic medications can make the breastfeeding infant sleepy and may not be advisable. Many commonly used acute headache medications have short half-lives, which means they do not stay in the mother's system for very long. Among the triptans, for example, sumatriptan, rizatriptan, and zolmitriptan have half-lives of about 2-3 hours and should be essentially gone from the mother's system in 8 to12 hours. Some headache experts feel that pumping and discarding milk during the 8 to12 hours after using these drugs is a way to continue breastfeeding and still be able to treat headaches when they occur. However, very little is known about excretion into breast milk of most headache medications, and little is known about the dangers of exposing babies to these drugs while breastfeeding.

Pediatricians and obstetricians are aware of the concerns regarding medications that can be excreted into breast milk. Check with the pediatrician or obstetrician for specific information about using headache medication (or any medication) while breastfeeding.

Chapter 28

Migraine during Menopause

Changes in Headache during Menopause and Aging

For women whose headaches have been closely linked with their menstrual periods, the elimination of that headache trigger with menopause can result in real improvement in headaches, although it is rare for them to disappear entirely. Getting older also usually is associated with headaches becoming less severe. Many women, for example, notice that nausea, vomiting and even headache pain are much less severe as time goes by. So it may not be only menopause, but also aging, which produces headache improvement in many cases.

In women experiencing spontaneous menopause, migraine headache improved in 67%, was unchanged in 24% and worsened in 9%. Surgical ovariectomy (removal of the ovaries) on the other hand, led to improvement in 33% and worsening in 67%.

Unfortunately, not all women find menopause improves their headaches. For some women, the worsening of migraine (and occasionally even the onset of migraine) is seen just prior to the onset of menopause, and sometimes may be associated with estrogen replacement therapy that is frequently prescribed during menopause.

Text in this chapter is from "Causes of Migraine during Menopause," American Council for Headache Education (ACHE) © 2000. Reprinted from the web site of the American Council for Headache Education (www.achenet.org); reprinted with permission.

Causes of Migraine during Menopause

The worsening of migraine just prior to menopause in some women may be related to hormone fluctuations. As menopause progresses, the plasma levels of sex steroids decline and migraine headaches frequently abate. Researchers feel that, at least in part, these changing levels of hormones cause headache for some women. However, in the general population over the age of 55 to 60, the incidence of migraine in females is still higher than males (2:1). This suggests that some factors other than sex hormones contributes to the predominance of migraine in women, and reasons for this are not well understood.

Estrogen Replacement Therapy

Estrogen replacement therapy (ERT) is prescribed to combat hot flashes and other uncomfortable symptoms (e.g., fatigue, dizziness, insomnia, and decreased concentration and libido). Given alone, estrogen stimulates growth of the uterine lining; if this continues unchecked, it can lead to cancer of the uterine lining. For this reason, unless the uterus was removed, estrogen is given in conjunction with another hormone called progesterone, which prevents proliferation of the uterine lining. Estrogen can also be stopped for a few days to allow bleeding and shedding of the uterine lining. This interrupted method of giving ERT is referred to as "intermittent ERT" or "cyclical ERT." ERT given daily is called "continuous ERT" or "non-cyclical ERT." For women who have headaches during their menstrual period or the "week off" of the oral contraceptive, continuous use of ERT is less likely to cause headaches. This is because they will avoid the sudden drop in estrogen levels that seems especially likely to provoke headache in susceptible women.

Taking ERT is not the only way to obtain estrogen. Many foods, particularly soy-based products and yams, contain plant-based estrogens. Unfortunately, reliable information is lacking on how much of these foods women need to eat, and there are no studies that demonstrate dietary (natural) estrogens and progesterone can actually prevent osteoporosis (thinning and weakening of the bones that occurs in everyone with age but which is accelerated after menopause).

As with most things in life, there are pros and cons to be considered when deciding on ERT. Some of these include:

- Headache
- Hot flashes and other symptoms

- Osteoporosis
- Coronary artery disease
- Blood clotting, and
- Breast cancer

Taking ERT is a personal decision that women should make in conjunction with their doctor. The doctor can be either their primary care physician or obstetrician-gynecologist.

Headaches

The effect of ERT on headaches is not predictable. Some women find that they are very sensitive to estrogen, and feel it worsens their headache (although, it may not be the estrogen itself but the way it is administered that causes the problem). Still other women find that ERT has no effect on their headaches. Some women feel that stable estrogen levels obtained on ERT actually improve headaches. Faced with such differences in response among different women, the presence or absence of other medical issues (hot flashes, osteoporosis, risk of blood clotting, among others) may play a role in the decision making process. When starting any medication, patients should keep track of headaches before starting ERT and then after beginning ERT. This will help clarify if headaches are improving or deteriorating with ERT. If headaches worsen, it is not always necessary to stop ERT. Such things as lowering the dose, switching from natural estrogen (such as Premarin®, which is derived from the urine of pregnant female horses) to a synthetic estrogen, or trying the patch instead of pills, might help.

Hot Flashes and Other Symptoms

Many, but not all, women experience such things as hot flashes, vaginal dryness or mood changes with declining estrogen levels during menopause. For some women, these symptoms are mild and get better over time without specific treatment. Other women find these problems to be disabling and do not experience improvement with time. ERT reduces or eliminates these complaints, and for many women the major reason to use ERT is to improve their comfort level.

Osteoporosis

ERT has clearly been shown to reduce the risk and progression of osteoporosis (thinning and weakening of the bones that occurs in everyone with age but which is accelerated after menopause). Estrogen stimulates formation of new bone and decreases the breakdown of bone that is already present. Women who smoke, who are thin, who take medications such as steroids for other medical problems or who have a family history of osteoporosis are at highest risk for this problem.

Although osteoporosis itself is not life-threatening, it can cause severe pain from fractures in the spine and put women at risk for hip fractures, which causes serious disability and even death (from complications).

Treatment of osteoporosis, once the problem has occurred, is not very successful. For this reason, efforts to prevent bone loss are very important. Estrogen is the most powerful method of replenishing bone loss; weight-bearing exercise and calcium intake are less effective but can help prevent osteoporosis. Newer drugs called selective estrogen receptor modulators (SERMs) such as raloxifene (Evista®) have the same effect estrogen does on bone, but do not affect the uterus or breast. These drugs do not prevent hot flashes, and while they do help preserve bone, it is not yet clear whether they work as well as estrogen does. Their use right now is reserved for women who can not take estrogen for specific reasons, but who need protection against bone loss. As we learn more about them, it is possible that they will be recommended for other situations. There is some early evidence that they may actually be helpful for women with headaches, but it is too early to encourage their use for that reason.

Coronary Artery Disease

Many studies suggest that estrogen may help prevent the onset of heart attack or other cardiac problems. Higher estrogen levels may explain why women as a group tend to develop heart problems 10 to 15 years later than men. Estrogen improves levels of "good" cholesterol and may have beneficial effects on blood vessels as well. The benefits of estrogen on heart problems are not as clear as the benefits of estrogen on osteoporosis. Some scientists suggest that women who take estrogen tend to be better educated, less likely to smoke, and more likely to exercise. In other words, this group of women are less likely to get heart disease because of other lifestyle factors. These confounding factors might make it look like estrogen helps prevent heart problems, when in fact it, it might be the lifestyle of this group of women who happen to also take estrogen.

Additional studies are needed to better understand the effect of estrogen and these other factors on coronary artery disease in post-menopausal women.

Blood Clotting

Estrogen increases the amount of certain clotting factors that are in the blood. Women who are on ERT or on oral contraceptives have a greater tendency to have blood clots. Development of these blood clots can be life-threatening depending on where they occur and how quickly they are recognized and treated. Fortunately, problems like this are rare. For women who do not have underlying clotting problems to begin with, this drawback is probably not common enough to make someone avoid ERT. Women with a history of blood clots, or who have been told that their blood clots more easily than it should, ERT may not be recommended.

Breast Cancer

Most scientists feel that estrogen does not cause breast cancer, but once breast cancer is present it may act like "fertilizer" by making it easier for the cancer to grow and spread. In fact, treatment for some kinds of breast cancer includes the use of drugs like tamoxifen that oppose (inhibit) the action of estrogen. In some cases of premenopausal breast cancer, the ovaries may be removed or drugs given to stop estrogen production, as a way of retarding cancer growth.

Many large-scale studies have been done to see if women who take ERT are at higher risk of developing or dying from breast cancer. Unfortunately, even these large studies do not provide clear evidence one way or the other. In some, there was no increased risk of breast cancer apparent in women who took ERT. In others, there appeared to be a small increased risk of breast cancer. Many doctors believe it is unlikely that ERT greatly increases the risk of breast cancer, and many women decide that the benefits of ERT outweigh the risk of breast cancer. However, this is a decision that patients need to make on an individual level.

Treatment for Headaches Associated with ERT

When migraine headaches are associated with hormone replacement therapy, a number of different options are available that may help reduce frequency and severity of headaches. These involve altering the dose of hormone therapy. Any changes in hormone therapy should be discussed with the physician first before modifying dose or delivery techniques. Some options include:

- using synthetic estrogen instead of natural extracts,
- using an estrogen patch instead of pill,
- switching to daily estrogen instead of cycling,
- reducing the dosage of estrogen,
- eliminating progesterone, and
- adding testosterone

The first three options may work by decreasing the fluctuations in estrogen which are thought to trigger migraine. Importantly, any change in hormone therapy should be discussed with the physician before hand.

For many patients, good control of migraines may not be achieved with the first treatment, and it may take several different attempts over several months before success is achieved. Also, there are a variety of different estrogen preparations available for oral, parenteral, and transdermal use, although conjugated equine estrogen tablets (e.g., Premarin®, Estratab®) are most commonly used. Specific decisions about which preparation is right for each individual patient should be made through discussions with the doctor.

Chapter 29

Migraine and Co-Existing Conditions

"Clinical depression? My doctor had to be kidding me!"

"I have severe migraines and for a while, I often felt hopeless and immobile. There were times when everything seemed dark like I was in a pit of molasses. I blamed myself for these times; I told myself I just wasn't trying hard enough."

"These were not common symptoms of migraine, and it took me a while to accept that I had another invisible illness to live with — clinical depression."

"I am thankful, however, that both the migraine and clinical depression can be treated with medications. it also helped me to be told that both these illnesses were genetically based and were not my fault..."

—M.L.

What Is Migraine?

Migraine is one of the more common types of headache. Approximately 17 to 18% of all women and 6% of all men suffer from migraine headaches. This type of headache is partly due to expansion (dilation) and inflammation of brain blood vessels, causing pain messages to

Text in this chapter is from the American Council for Headache Education (ACHE) © 2000. Reprinted from the web site of the American Council for Headache Education (www.achenet.org); reprinted with permission.

travel to the brain. Although these affected blood vessels are located in the scalp, skull, and surface of the brain, the pain feels like it is coming from inside the head. The pain associated with a migraine attack usually lasts 4 to 72 hours.

Migraine headaches are often localized to one side of the head, and the pain can be pounding or throbbing in nature. Some people feel nauseated, and others actually vomit. Noises and light can make the headache worse. Up to 25% of migraine sufferers have an "aura" prior to the onset of pain. An aura is recognized by seeing flashing lights or curved lines, arm or leg numbness or tingling, or rarely, one-sided weakness.

Source: Stewart, WF, Lipton RB, Celentano DD, Reed ML. Prevalence of migraine headache in the United States. Relation to age, income, race and other sociodemographic factors. *JAMA.* 1992; 267 (1):64–69.

What are Co-Existing Conditions?

Co-existing medical conditions are multiple illnesses or health conditions that can occur at the same time. For example, some children with seizures also may have headaches. Headache sufferers may have co-existing health conditions or illnesses, such as depression, anxiety, high blood pressure, or a sleep disorder. Nearly half of the patients with chronic tension-type headache also suffer from mood or anxiety disorders. Sometimes these co-existing conditions are related biologically to each other, and sometimes they are independent from each other. One person with migraine may suffer from depression, while another migraine sufferer may have asthma. Both asthma and depression are co-existing conditions with migraine, but it is likely that only depression and migraine are related. Some researchers believe that changes in brain chemicals, such as serotonin, may be a common underlying factor related to specific co-existing conditions and migraine.

Why Diagnose Co-Existing Conditions?

Diagnosing and acknowledging the presence of migraine and co-existing conditions are steps to successful migraine management. For the migraine sufferer, it is important to:

• Recognize that there are two or more conditions.

• Accept the need for treatment of these conditions.

- Work with the physician to develop a treatment plan that fits with lifestyle issues.

- Understand that treating more than one condition at a time is complex, and requires added medical attention and long-term, follow-up care.

Can Co-Existing Conditions Make Migraine Worse?

There are at least two critical reasons to diagnose and appropriately manage migraine along with co-existing conditions.

Cause

Some health conditions may increase the frequency or severity of migraine attacks. By gaining control of the co-existing condition, the migraine attacks may become less frequent or less severe and, in some cases, completely go away.

Treatment

Some medications used to treat co-existing conditions can make migraines worse. Fortunately, other medications used to treat specific medical conditions also will treat migraine successfully.

Can Modification of Lifestyle Help?

Feeling good about "life" is an important part of successful migraine management and also may help with managing co-existing conditions. Some lifestyle changes are simple and easily incorporated into a daily routine, while others may require a little more effort. Here are a few ways migraine sufferers can gain control of their headaches—and their lives:

- *Diet*—avoid foods that may trigger migraine (red wine, food additives [MSG, nitrates], chocolate, caffeine, peanuts, aged cheeses). Remember that the best way to identify a food trigger is to keep a calendar/diary.

- *Exercise*—exercise regularly with moderation; too much or too little exercise may trigger migraine.

- *Meals*—eat regularly; fasting and hypoglycemia may trigger migraine.

- *Sleep*—engage in a normal sleeping routine; sleep deprivation and changes in sleeping patterns may cause migraine. This is often seen with long-distance travelers that suffer from "jet-lag."

- *Stress*—reduce work and personal stress. High stress may cause anxiety, depression, panic, and other emotional fluctuations that may trigger migraine.

- *Hormones* (women)—be aware of monthly biological changes. Fluctuations in hormones during menstruation, ovulation, and while using birth control pills may trigger migraine. Talk with a health care provider about how to incorporate lifestyle changes that may prevent or relieve both migraine AND other co-existing conditions.

Are Some Medical Conditions More Common?

For reasons that are not well understood, some medical conditions are more commonly associated with migraine. Some of these include:

- *Condition*—Description

- *Asthma*—Inflammation of the airways leading to breathing difficulty and shortness of breath

- *Fatigue (chronic fatigue syndrome)*—A combination of unexplained fatigue (lack of energy) with memory or concentration problems, sleep difficulty, muscle or joint pain, or headaches

- *Hypertension*—High blood pressure; long-term effects include kidney disease, vision loss, heart attack, and stroke

- *Raynaud's Phenomena*—Spasms in the arteries in the fingers leading to numbness or decreased blood flow to the fingers

- *Stroke*—Sudden neurological condition usually related to blocking of the blood supply to an area of the brain

While many of these conditions are associated with headache and are more common in individuals with migraine, most migraine is not caused by one of the above medical conditions. Individuals who think that they may have migraine along with at least one of these co-existing conditions should discuss this with the doctor.

What Psychological Conditions are Associated with Migraine?

Many conditions that affect behavior and mood are more frequent in migraine sufferers. This is likely due to changes in the brain chemical serotonin. Certain brain cells that use serotonin as a messenger are involved in controlling mood, attention, sleep, and pain. If serotonin levels suddenly drop, a migraine may develop. Chronic changes in serotonin levels may also lead to psychological conditions.

People with anxiety or panic disorder develop an overwhelming sense of fear or nervousness without any clear reason. This may be so severe that they are unable to function at work or at home. An actual attack can last for several days.

Depression is a change in a person's mood that lasts for an extended period of time. People with depression often feel sad, alone, or isolated. They also have decreased energy and do not enjoy activities that they would enjoy normally. Some people with depression have decreased appetite and lose weight; others will eat continuously even though they are not hungry. Sleep problems—including difficulty falling asleep, waking up during the night or early in the morning, and not feeling rested in the morning—are also part of depression.

Stress is the human body's response to outside factors that a person perceives as dangerous, damaging, painful, or which may have a negative impact on the person. Thousands of years ago, human stresses were mostly physical. Today, many stresses are directed toward a person's emotional and psychological well-being. These stresses can come from work and family responsibilities, changing relationships, and financial difficulties. Stress may be triggered by positive changes as well, such as taking on a new job, buying a house, getting married, or having a child. While everyone is exposed to daily stresses, the migraine sufferer's nervous system may respond in such a way that it causes greater negative effects on the body.

Talking to Your Doctor

Headache sufferers should make a specific appointment to talk to their doctor about headaches. This way both the doctor and the headache sufferer will plan enough time to discuss all aspects of the headaches and possible co-existing conditions. The doctor will want to discuss other symptoms that may not appear to be related directly to headaches. These symptoms may be a clue that one or more co-existing conditions are present. During the office visit, it is critical to establish

237

an open and honest dialogue with the doctor. Specific characteristics of migraine and co-existing conditions will influence the treatment plan. For example, issues to discuss honestly with a doctor might include:

- Ability to cope with stress
- Severity of pain
- Degree of disability
- Rate of pain onset
- Treatment preferences
- Lifestyle preferences

Here are steps that will help prepare headache sufferers for an office visit:

1. Keep track of headaches and associated symptoms (use a headache diary).

2. Make a list of questions to discuss with the doctor or nurse; during the course of the office visit, it can be difficult to remember all the questions or concerns that most migraine sufferers have.

3. Bring all the medicines taken daily or on a routine basis (including successful and unsuccessful headache medications, allergy medicines, vitamins, and others).

During the office visit, it is important that the doctor and migraine sufferer review each condition and its relationship to migraine. Understanding why each medicine is used will help ensure their appropriate use. Furthermore, it is critical to review lifestyle issues during the office visit. Sometimes simple modifications in lifestyle will dramatically improve the frequency and severity of migraines.

Treatment of Migraine with Co-Existing Conditions

Headache characteristics and the presence of co-existing conditions CLEARLY will affect the specific treatment plan designed for each migraine sufferer. For example, treatment of a co-existing condition alone may make migraine less frequent and less severe. And, treatment of migraine also could decrease the disability caused by co-existing conditions.

An individually designed headache treatment plan should:

- Alleviate the pain from migraine,

- Reduce the disability from migraine attack,

- Allow the sufferer to return to normal activities as quickly as possible, and

- Reduce the impact of co-existing conditions on activities.

Two general approaches are used to treat migraine:

- *Acute Treatment*—Everyone requires medication that is taken when the migraine begins or during the course of the headache. The goal of acute treatment is to allow the migraine sufferer to be pain-free and to return to normal functioning as quickly as possible.

- *Preventive Treatment*—Some migraine sufferers require medication to prevent migraine from developing. These medications are used by patients with relatively frequent or severely disabling migraines. Many of these medications also can be beneficial for treating co-existing conditions.

The doctor must screen carefully for co-existing conditions because some migraine medications may not be appropriate to use in the presence of such conditions as heart disease, high blood pressure, depression, asthma, pregnancy, seizure disorder, or risk of stroke.

Migraine sufferers may be able to decrease the impact of migraine as well as certain co-existing conditions by using nonpharmacologic (nondrug) approaches. Some patients may benefit from certain behavioral treatments and physical therapies.

Behavioral treatments may include biofeedback training, relaxation training, stress-management training, and even hypnosis. Physical therapies include massage, acupuncture, and cervical manipulation. These techniques have not been rigorously tested in clinical trials for migraine patients, but many patients have found them useful. The goals of nonpharmacological therapies are to:

- Improve the overall management of migraine and possible co-existing conditions,

- Reduce the need for multiple medications to treat migraine and co-existing conditions over a long period of time, and

- Provide the migraine sufferer with alternate tools to gain control of their migraine attacks.

It is important to make the doctor aware of nonpharmacological treatments or alternative therapy approaches used for managing migraine or other co-existing conditions.

Taking Control

The burden of dealing with migraine can be shared by the patient, family, loved ones, coworkers, and doctor. Health care providers and doctors will guide migraine sufferers through treatment regimens and lifestyle changes, but ONLY the sufferer can be fully responsible for gaining control of migraine. How can sufferers gain control of their migraines? Following are a few steps to begin with.

Step 1: Learn About Each Condition

Doctors and other health care providers are prepared to answer questions and explain what migraine is and why the various medications are needed.

Remember: The only silly question is the one not asked.

Step 2: Follow the Treatment Plan Established with the Doctor

- Be sure to understand what to do when the next migraine attack comes.

- Take medications EXACTLY as recommended by the doctor.

- Take only medications recommended by the doctor.

- Take acute medications as soon as it is clear that the headache is a migraine.

- Carry medications at all times.

- If preventive therapies are prescribed, follow the treatment plan EXACTLY as agreed upon. If the treatment plan is too hard to follow, contact the doctor.

- Do not increase or decrease the amount of medication without talking to the doctor FIRST.

Step 3: Monitor Headaches

One important part of migraine management is being able to accurately recognize improvement or deterioration in migraines. A headache calendar will help identify headache patterns, triggers, and responses to treatments.

Important tips:

- Acute medication may not work every time, therefore, rescue medication prescribed by the doctor may be necessary.

- Preventive medication may take a few weeks to show improvement.

- Call the doctor if side effects occur from medication.

- Record headache activity on a daily basis using a headache diary.

- Make and keep follow-up appointments with the doctor.

Migraine can be effectively managed. If a treatment plan is not as effective as expected, it might be possible to modify it. Establishment of a successful treatment plan may require several changes. Medications should be adjusted after considering co-existing conditions and lifestyle needs. Changes in the treatment plan must be discussed with the doctor.

Chapter 30

Sinusitis and Headaches

You're coughing and sneezing and tired and achy. You think that you might be getting a cold. Later, when the medicines you've been taking to relieve the symptoms of the common cold are not working and you've now got a terrible headache, you finally drag yourself to the doctor. After listening to your history of symptoms, examining your face and forehead, and perhaps doing a sinus X-ray, the doctor says you have sinusitis.

Sinusitis simply means inflammation of the sinuses, but this gives little indication of the misery and pain this condition can cause. Chronic sinusitis, sinusitis that persists for at least 3 weeks, affects an estimated 32 million people in the United States. Americans spend millions of dollars each year for medications that promise relief from their sinus symptoms.

Sinuses are hollow air spaces, of which there are many in the human body. When people say, "I'm having a sinus attack," they usually are referring to symptoms in one or more of four pairs of cavities, or spaces, known as paranasal sinuses. These cavities, located within the skull or bones of the head surrounding the nose, include the frontal sinuses over the eyes in the brow area; the maxillary sinuses inside each cheekbone; the ethmoids just behind the bridge of the nose and between the eyes; and behind them, the sphenoids in the upper region of the nose and behind the eyes.

"Sinusitis," National Institute of Allergy and Infectious Diseases (NIAID), April 2001.

Each sinus has an opening into the nose for the free exchange of air and mucus, and each is joined with the nasal passages by a continuous mucous membrane lining. Therefore, anything that causes a swelling in the nose—an infection or an allergic reaction—also can affect the sinuses. Air trapped within an obstructed sinus, along with pus or other secretions, may cause pressure on the sinus wall. The result is the sometimes intense pain of a sinus attack. Similarly, when air is prevented from entering a paranasal sinus by a swollen membrane at the opening, a vacuum can be created that also causes pain.

Symptoms

Sinusitis has its own localized pain signals, depending upon the particular sinus affected. Headache upon awakening in the morning is characteristic of sinus involvement. Pain when the forehead over the frontal sinuses is touched may indicate inflammation of the frontal sinuses. Infection in the maxillary sinuses can cause the upper jaw and teeth to ache and the cheeks to become tender to the touch. Since the ethmoid sinuses are near the tear ducts in the corner of the eyes, inflammation of these cavities often causes swelling of the eyelids and tissues around the eyes, and pain between the eyes. Ethmoid inflammation also can cause tenderness when the sides of the nose are touched, a loss of smell, and a stuffy nose. Although the sphenoid sinuses are less frequently affected, infection in this area can cause earaches, neck pain, and deep aching at the top of the head.

However, most patients with sinusitis have pain or tenderness in several locations, and symptoms usually do not clearly define which sinuses are inflamed.

Other symptoms of sinusitis can include fever, weakness, tiredness, a cough that may be more severe at night, and runny nose or nasal congestion. In addition, drainage of mucus from the sphenoids (or other sinuses) down the back of the throat (postnasal drip) can cause a sore throat and can irritate the membranes lining the larynx (upper windpipe). On rare occasions, acute sinusitis can result in brain infection and serious complications.

Causes

Most cases of acute sinusitis are preceded by virus-induced "colds." These viral "colds" do not cause symptoms of sinusitis, but they do cause inflammation of the sinuses. Both the "cold" and the sinus inflammation usually resolve without treatment in two weeks. However, the inflammation might explain why colds increase the likelihood of developing acute sinusitis. For example, the nose reacts to an invasion by viruses that cause infections such as the common cold, flu, or measles by producing mucus and sending white blood cells to the lining of the nose, which congest and swell the nasal passages. When this swelling involves the adjacent mucous membranes of the sinuses, air and mucus are trapped behind the narrowed openings of the sinuses. If the sinus openings become too narrow to permit drainage of the mucus, then bacteria, which normally are present in the respiratory tract, begin to multiply. Most healthy people harbor bacteria, such as Streptococcus pneumoniae and Haemophilus influenzae, in their upper respiratory tracts with no ill effects until the body's defenses are weakened or drainage from the sinuses is blocked by a cold or other viral infection. The bacteria that may have been living harmlessly in the nose or throat can multiply and cause an acute sinus infection.

Sometimes, fungal infections can cause acute sinusitis. Although these organisms are abundant in the environment, they usually are harmless to healthy people, indicating that the human body has a natural resistance to them. Fungi, such as Aspergillus, can cause serious illness in people whose immune systems are not functioning properly. Some people with fungal sinusitis have an allergic-type reaction to the fungi.

Chronic inflammation of the nasal passages (rhinitis) also can lead to sinusitis. Allergic rhinitis or hay fever may be complicated by episodes of acute sinusitis. Patients with allergic rhinitis also often have chronic sinusitis. Vasomotor rhinitis, caused by humidity, cold air, alcohol, perfumes, and other environmental conditions, also may be complicated by sinus infections.

Acute sinusitis is much more common in certain patients than in the general population. For example, sinusitis occurs more often in patients with reduced immune function (such as patients with immune deficiencies and HIV infection) and with abnormality of mucus secretion or mucus movement (such as cystic fibrosis and diseases of abnormal cilia [Kartagener's syndrome]).

Chronic Sinusitis

Chronic sinusitis refers to inflammation of the sinuses that continues for at least 3 weeks, but often continues for months or even years.

Allergies are frequently associated with chronic sinusitis. Patients with asthma have a particularly high frequency of chronic sinusitis.

Inhalation of airborne allergens (substances that provoke an allergic reaction), such as dust, mold, and pollen, often set off allergic reactions (allergic rhinitis) that, in turn, may contribute to sinusitis. People who are allergic to fungi can develop a condition called "allergic fungal sinusitis."

Damp weather, especially in northern temperate climates, or pollutants in the air and in buildings also can affect people subject to chronic sinusitis.

Like acute sinusitis, chronic sinusitis is more common in patients with immune deficiency or abnormalities of mucus secretion or movement (e.g., immune deficiency, HIV infection, cystic fibrosis, Kartagener's syndrome). In addition, some patients have severe asthma, nasal polyps, and severe asthmatic responses to aspirin and aspirin-like medications (so-called non-steroidal anti-inflammatory drugs, or NSAIDs). These latter patients have a high frequency of chronic sinusitis.

Diagnosis

Although a stuffy nose can occur in other conditions, like the common cold, many people confuse simple nasal congestion with sinusitis. A cold, however, usually lasts about 7 to 14 days and disappears without treatment. Acute sinusitis often lasts longer and typically causes more symptoms than just a cold. A doctor can diagnose sinusitis by medical history, physical examination, X-rays, and if necessary, MRIs or CT scans (magnetic resonance imaging and computed tomography).

Treatment

After diagnosing sinusitis and identifying a possible cause, a doctor can prescribe a course of treatment that will reduce the inflammation and relieve the symptoms. Acute sinusitis is treated by re-establishing drainage of the nasal passages, controlling or eliminating the source of the inflammation, and relieving the pain. Doctors generally recommend decongestants to reduce the congestion, antibiotics to control a bacterial infection, if present, and pain relievers to reduce the pain.

Over-the-counter and prescription decongestant nose drops and sprays, however, should not be used for more than a few days. When used for longer periods, these drugs can lead to even more congestion and swelling of the nasal passages.

Most patients with sinusitis that is caused by bacteria can be treated successfully with antibiotics used along with a nasal or oral decongestant. An antibiotic that fights the bacteria most commonly associated with sinusitis is the initial treatment recommended.

Many cases of acute sinusitis resolve without antibiotics. However, patients with underlying allergic disease, and infectious sinusitis, need to be treated to relieve their allergy symptoms. Patients with asthma and infectious sinusitis often have exacerbations of asthma which need to be treated. Many physicians feel that some patients with severe asthma have dramatic symptom improvement when their chronic sinusitis is treated with antibiotics. Doctors often prescribe steroid nasal sprays, along with other treatments, to reduce the congestion, swelling, and inflammation of sinusitis.

Chronic sinusitis is often difficult to treat successfully, as symptoms persist even after prolonged courses of antibiotics. In general, the treatment of chronic sinusitis, such as with antibiotics and decongestants, is similar to treatment of acute sinusitis. However, the role of bacterial infections, and hence the usefulness of antibiotics in treating chronic sinusitis, is debated.

Steroid nasal sprays are commonly used to reduce inflammation in chronic sinusitis. Although these nasal sprays are occasionally used for long-term treatment for patients with chronic sinusitis, the long-term safety of these medications, especially in children, is not fully understood, and the benefits and risks need to be balanced. For patients with severe chronic sinusitis, a doctor may prescribe oral steroids, such as prednisone. Because oral steroids can have significant side effects, they are prescribed only when other medications have not been effective.

Although sinus infection cannot be cured by home remedies, people can use them to lessen their discomfort. Inhaling steam from a vaporizer or a hot cup of water can soothe inflamed sinus cavities. Another treatment is saline nasal spray, which can be purchased in a pharmacy. A hot water bottle; hot, wet compresses; or an electric heating pad applied over the inflamed area also can be comforting.

When medical treatment fails, surgery may be the only alternative for treating chronic sinusitis. Studies suggest that the vast majority of patients who undergo surgery have fewer symptoms and better quality of life. In children, problems often are eliminated by removal of adenoids obstructing nasal-sinus passages. Adults who have had allergic and infectious conditions over the years sometimes develop nasal polyps that interfere with proper drainage. Removal of these polyps and/or repair of a deviated septum to ensure an open airway often provides considerable relief from sinus symptoms. The most common surgery done today is functional endoscopic sinus surgery, in which the natural openings from the sinuses are enlarged to allow drainage. This type of surgery is less invasive than conventional sinus surgery and serious complications are rare.

Prevention

Although people cannot prevent all sinus disorders—any more than they can avoid all colds or bacterial infections—they can take certain measures to reduce the number and severity of the attacks and possibly prevent sinusitis from becoming chronic.

Many people with sinusitis find partial relief from their symptoms when humidifiers are installed in their homes, particularly if room air is heated by a dry forced-air system. Air conditioners help to provide an even temperature, and electrostatic filters attached to heating and air conditioning equipment are helpful in removing allergens from the air.

A person susceptible to sinus disorders, particularly one who also is allergic, should avoid cigarette smoke and other air pollutants. Inflammation in the nose caused by allergies predisposes a patient to a strong reaction to all irritants. Drinking alcohol also causes the nasal-sinus membranes to swell.

Sinusitis-prone persons may be uncomfortable in swimming pools treated with chlorine, since it irritates the lining of the nose and sinuses. Divers often experience congestion with resulting infection when water is forced into the sinuses from the nasal passages.

Air travel, too, poses a problem for the individual suffering from acute or chronic sinusitis. A bubble of air trapped within the body expands as air pressure in a plane is reduced. This expansion causes pressure on surrounding tissues and can result in a blockage of the sinuses or the eustachian tubes in the ears. The result may be discomfort in the sinus or middle ear during the plane's ascent or descent. Doctors recommend using decongestant nose drops or inhalers before the flight to avoid this difficulty.

People who suspect that their sinus inflammation may be related to dust, mold, pollen, or food—or any of the hundreds of allergens that can trigger a respiratory reaction—should consult a doctor. Various tests can determine the cause of the allergy and also help the doctor recommend steps to reduce or limit allergy symptoms.

Chapter 31

Headaches and Stroke Risks

How Do You Recognize Stroke?

Symptoms of stroke appear suddenly. Watch for these symptoms and be prepared to act quickly for yourself or on behalf of someone you are with:

- Sudden numbness or weakness of the face, arm, or leg, especially on one side of the body.

- Sudden confusion, trouble talking, or understanding speech.

- Sudden trouble seeing in one or both eyes.

- Sudden trouble walking, dizziness, or loss of balance or coordination.

- Sudden severe headache with no known cause.

If you suspect you or someone you know is experiencing any of these symptoms indicative of a stroke, do not wait. Call 911 emergency immediately. There are now effective therapies for stroke that must be administered at a hospital, but they lose their effectiveness if not given within the first 3 hours after stroke symptoms appear. Every minute counts!

From "Stroke: Hope through Research," National Institute of Neurological Disorders and Stroke (NINDS), NIH Pub. No. 99-2222, May 1999; reviewed July 2001.

How Is the Cause of Stroke Determined?

Physicians have several diagnostic techniques and imaging tools to help diagnose the cause of stroke quickly and accurately. The first step in diagnosis is a short neurological examination. When a possible stroke patient arrives at a hospital, a health care professional, usually a doctor or nurse, will ask the patient or a companion what happened and when the symptoms began. Blood tests, an electrocardiogram, and CT scans will often be done. One test that helps doctors judge the severity of a stroke is the standardized NIH Stroke Scale, developed by the NINDS. Health care professionals use the NIH Stroke Scale to measure a patient's neurological deficits by asking the patient to answer questions and to perform several physical and mental tests. Other scales include the Glasgow Coma Scale, the Hunt and Hess Scale, the Modified Rankin Scale, and the Barthel Index.

More than 2,400 years ago the father of medicine, Hippocrates, recognized and described stroke—the sudden onset of paralysis. Until recently, modern medicine has had very little power over this disease, but the world of stroke medicine is changing and new and better therapies are being developed every day. Today, some people who have a stroke can walk away from the attack with no or few disabilities if they are treated promptly. Doctors can finally offer stroke patients and their families the one thing that until now has been so hard to give: hope.

In ancient times stroke was called apoplexy, a general term that physicians applied to anyone suddenly struck down with paralysis. Because many conditions can lead to sudden paralysis, the term apoplexy did not indicate a specific diagnosis or cause. Physicians knew very little about the cause of stroke and the only established therapy was to feed and care for the patient until the attack ran its course.

The first person to investigate the pathological signs of apoplexy was Johann Jacob Wepfer. Born in Schaffhausen, Switzerland, in 1620, Wepfer studied medicine and was the first to identify postmortem signs of bleeding in the brains of patients who died of apoplexy. From autopsy studies he gained knowledge of the carotid and vertebral arteries that supply the brain with blood. He also was the first person to suggest that apoplexy, in addition to being caused by bleeding in the brain, could be caused by a blockage of one of the main arteries supplying blood to the brain; thus stroke became known as a cerebrovascular disease ("cerebro" refers to a part of the brain; "vascular" refers to the blood vessels and arteries).

Medical science would eventually confirm Wepfer's hypotheses, but until very recently doctors could offer little in the area of therapy. Over the last two decades basic and clinical investigators, many of them sponsored and funded in part by the National Institute of Neurological Disorders and Stroke (NINDS), have learned a great deal about stroke. They have identified major risk factors for the disease and have developed surgical techniques and drug treatments for the prevention of stroke. But perhaps the most exciting new development in the field of stroke research is the recent approval of a drug treatment that can reverse the course of stroke if given during the first few hours after the onset of symptoms.

Studies with animals have shown that brain injury occurs within minutes of a stroke and can become irreversible within as little as an hour. In humans, brain damage begins from the moment the stroke starts and often continues for days afterward. Scientists now know that there is a very short window of opportunity for treatment of the most common form of stroke. Because of these and other advances in the field of cerebrovascular disease stroke patients now have a chance for survival and recovery.

What Is Stroke?

A stroke occurs when the blood supply to part of the brain is suddenly interrupted or when a blood vessel in the brain bursts, spilling blood into the spaces surrounding brain cells. In the same way that a person suffering a loss of blood flow to the heart is said to be having a heart attack, a person with a loss of blood flow to the brain or sudden bleeding in the brain can be said to be having a "brain attack."

Brain cells die when they no longer receive oxygen and nutrients from the blood or when they are damaged by sudden bleeding into or around the brain. Ischemia is the term used to describe the loss of oxygen and nutrients for brain cells when there is inadequate blood flow. Ischemia ultimately leads to infarction, the death of brain cells which are eventually replaced by a fluid-filled cavity (or infarct) in the injured brain.

When blood flow to the brain is interrupted, some brain cells die immediately, while others remain at risk for death. These damaged cells make up the ischemic penumbra and can linger in a compromised state for several hours. With timely treatment these cells can be saved.

Even though a stroke occurs in the unseen reaches of the brain, the symptoms of a stroke are easy to spot. They include sudden numbness or weakness, especially on one side of the body; sudden confusion

251

or trouble speaking or understanding speech; sudden trouble seeing in one or both eyes; sudden trouble walking, dizziness, or loss of balance or coordination; or sudden severe headache with no known cause. All of the symptoms of stroke appear suddenly, and often there is more than one symptom at the same time. Therefore stroke can usually be distinguished from other causes of dizziness or headache. These symptoms may indicate that a stroke has occurred and that medical attention is needed immediately.

There are two forms of stroke: ischemic—blockage of a blood vessel supplying the brain, and hemorrhagic—bleeding into or around the brain.

Ischemic Stroke

An ischemic stroke occurs when an artery supplying the brain with blood becomes blocked, suddenly decreasing or stopping blood flow and ultimately causing a brain infarction. This type of stroke accounts for approximately 80 percent of all strokes. Blood clots are the most common cause of artery blockage and brain infarction. The process of clotting is necessary and beneficial throughout the body because it stops bleeding and allows repair of damaged areas of arteries or veins. However, when blood clots develop in the wrong place within an artery they can cause devastating injury by interfering with the normal flow of blood. Problems with clotting become more frequent as people age.

Blood clots can cause ischemia and infarction in two ways. A clot that forms in a part of the body other than the brain can travel through blood vessels and become wedged in a brain artery. This free-roaming clot is called an embolus and often forms in the heart. A stroke caused by an embolus is called an embolic stroke. The second kind of ischemic stroke, called a thrombotic stroke, is caused by thrombosis, the formation of a blood clot in one of the cerebral arteries that stays attached to the artery wall until it grows large enough to block blood flow.

Ischemic strokes can also be caused by stenosis, or a narrowing of the artery due to the buildup of plaque (a mixture of fatty substances, including cholesterol and other lipids) and blood clots along the artery wall. Stenosis can occur in large arteries and small arteries and is therefore called large vessel disease or small vessel disease, respectively. When a stroke occurs due to small vessel disease, a very small infarction results, sometimes called a lacunar infarction, from the French word "lacune" meaning "gap" or "cavity."

The most common blood vessel disease that causes stenosis is atherosclerosis. In atherosclerosis, deposits of plaque build up along the inner walls of large and medium-sized arteries, causing thickening, hardening, and loss of elasticity of artery walls and decreased blood flow.

Hemorrhagic Stroke

In a healthy, functioning brain, neurons do not come into direct contact with blood. The vital oxygen and nutrients the neurons need from the blood come to the neurons across the thin walls of the cerebral capillaries. The glia (nervous system cells that support and protect neurons) form a blood-brain barrier, an elaborate meshwork that surrounds blood vessels and capillaries and regulates which elements of the blood can pass through to the neurons.

When an artery in the brain bursts, blood spews out into the surrounding tissue and upsets not only the blood supply but the delicate chemical balance neurons require to function. This is called a hemorrhagic stroke. Such strokes account for approximately 20 percent of all strokes.

Hemorrhage can occur in several ways. One common cause is a bleeding aneurysm, a weak or thin spot on an artery wall. Over time, these weak spots stretch or balloon out under high arterial pressure. The thin walls of these ballooning aneurysms can rupture and spill blood into the space surrounding brain cells.

Hemorrhage also occurs when arterial walls break open. Plaque-encrusted artery walls eventually lose their elasticity and become brittle and thin, prone to cracking. Hypertension, or high blood pressure, increases the risk that a brittle artery wall will give way and release blood into the surrounding brain tissue.

A person with an arteriovenous malformation (AVM) also has an increased risk of hemorrhagic stroke. AVMs are a tangle of defective blood vessels and capillaries within the brain that have thin walls and can therefore rupture.

Bleeding from ruptured brain arteries can either go into the substance of the brain or into the various spaces surrounding the brain. Intracerebral hemorrhage occurs when a vessel within the brain leaks blood into the brain itself. Subarachnoid hemorrhage is bleeding under the meninges, or outer membranes, of the brain into the thin fluid-filled space that surrounds the brain.

The subarachnoid space separates the arachnoid membrane from the underlying pia mater membrane. It contains a clear fluid (cerebrospinal fluid or CSF) as well as the small blood vessels that supply the outer surface of the brain. In a subarachnoid hemorrhage, one of the small arteries within the subarachnoid space bursts, flooding the area with blood and contaminating the cerebrospinal fluid. Since the CSF flows throughout the cranium, within the spaces of the brain, subarachnoid hemorrhage can lead to extensive damage throughout the brain. In fact, subarachnoid hemorrhage is the most deadly of all strokes.

Transient Ischemic Attacks

A transient ischemic attack (TIA), sometimes called a mini-stroke, starts just like a stroke but then resolves leaving no noticeable symptoms or deficits. The occurrence of a TIA is a warning that the person is at risk for a more serious and debilitating stroke. Of the approximately 50,000 Americans who have a TIA each year, about one-third will have an acute stroke sometime in the future. The addition of other risk factors compounds a person's risk for a recurrent stroke. The average duration of a TIA is a few minutes. For almost all TIAs, the symptoms go away within an hour. There is no way to tell whether symptoms will be just a TIA or persist and lead to death or disability. The patient should assume that all stroke symptoms signal an emergency and should not wait to see if they go away.

Recurrent Stroke

Recurrent stroke is frequent; about 25 percent of people who recover from their first stroke will have another stroke within 5 years. Recurrent stroke is a major contributor to stroke disability and death, with the risk of severe disability or death from stroke increasing with each stroke recurrence. The risk of a recurrent stroke is greatest right after a stroke, with the risk decreasing with time. About 3 percent of stroke patients will have another stroke within 30 days of their first stroke and one-third of recurrent strokes take place within 2 years of the first stroke.

Imaging for the Diagnosis of Acute Stroke

Health care professionals also use a variety of imaging devices to evaluate stroke patients. The most widely used imaging procedure is the computed tomography (CT) scan. Also known as a CAT scan or computed axial tomography, CT creates a series of cross-sectional images of the head and brain. Because it is readily available at all hours at most major hospitals and produces images quickly, CT is the preferred diagnostic technique for acute stroke. CT also has unique diagnostic benefits. It will quickly rule out a hemorrhage, can occasionally show a tumor that might mimic a stroke, and may even show evidence of early infarction. Infarctions generally show up on a CT scan about 6 to 8 hours after the start of stroke symptoms.

If a stroke is caused by hemorrhage, a CT can show evidence of bleeding into the brain almost immediately after stroke symptoms appear. Hemorrhage is the primary reason for avoiding certain drug treatments for stroke, such as thrombolytic therapy, the only proven acute stroke therapy for ischemic stroke. Thrombolytic therapy cannot be used until the doctor can confidently diagnose the patient as suffering from an ischemic stroke because this treatment might increase bleeding and could make a hemorrhagic stroke worse.

Another imaging device used for stroke patients is the magnetic resonance imaging (MRI) scan. MRI uses magnetic fields to detect subtle changes in brain tissue content. One effect of stroke is an increase of water content in the cells of brain tissue, a condition called cytotoxic edema. MRI can detect edema as soon as a few hours after the onset of stroke. The benefit of MRI over CT imaging is that MRI is better able to detect small infarcts soon after stroke onset. Unfortunately, not every hospital has access to an MRI device and the procedure is time-consuming and expensive. It also is not as accurate in determining when hemorrhage is present. Finally, because MRI takes longer to perform than CT, it should not be used if it delays treatment.

Other types of MRI scans, often used for the diagnosis of cerebrovascular disease and to predict the risk of stroke, are magnetic resonance angiography (MRA) and functional magnetic resonance imaging (fMRI). Neurosurgeons use MRA to detect stenosis (blockage) of the brain arteries inside the skull by mapping flowing blood. Functional MRI uses a magnet to pick up signals from oxygenated blood and can show brain activity through increases in local blood flow. Duplex Doppler ultrasound and arteriography are two diagnostic imaging techniques used to decide if an individual would benefit from a surgical procedure called carotid endarterectomy. This surgery is used to remove fatty deposits from the carotid arteries and can help prevent stroke.

Doppler ultrasound is a painless, noninvasive test in which sound waves above the range of human hearing are sent into the neck. Echoes bounce off the moving blood and the tissue in the artery and can be formed into an image. Ultrasound is fast, painless, risk-free, and relatively inexpensive compared to MRA and arteriography, but it is not considered to be as accurate as arteriography. Arteriography is an X-ray of the carotid artery taken when a special dye is injected into the artery. The procedure carries its own small risk of causing a stroke and is costly to perform. The benefits of arteriography over MR techniques and ultrasound are that it is extremely reliable and still the best way to measure stenosis of the carotid arteries. Even so, significant advances are being made every day involving noninvasive imaging techniques such as fMRI.

Who Is at Risk for Stroke?

Some people are at a higher risk for stroke than others. Unmodifiable risk factors include age, gender, race/ethnicity, and stroke family history. In contrast, other risk factors for stroke, like high blood pressure or cigarette smoking, can be changed or controlled by the person at risk.

Unmodifiable Risk Factors

It is a myth that stroke occurs only in elderly adults. In actuality, stroke strikes all age groups, from fetuses still in the womb to centenarians. It is true, however, that older people have a higher risk for stroke than the general population and that the risk for stroke increases with age. For every decade after the age of 55, the risk of stroke doubles, and two-thirds of all strokes occur in people over 65 years old. People over 65 also have a seven-fold greater risk of dying from stroke than the general population. And the incidence of stroke is increasing proportionately with the increase in the elderly population. When the baby boomers move into the over-65 age group, stroke and other diseases will take on even greater significance in the health care field.

Gender also plays a role in risk for stroke. Men have a higher risk for stroke, but more women die from stroke. The stroke risk for men is 1.25 times that for women. But men do not live as long as women, so men are usually younger when they have their strokes and therefore have a higher rate of survival than women. In other words, even though women have fewer strokes than men, women are generally older when they have their strokes and are more likely to die from them. Stroke seems to run in some families. Several factors might contribute to familial stroke risk. Members of a family might have a genetic tendency for stroke risk factors, such as an inherited predisposition for hypertension or diabetes. The influence of a common lifestyle among family members could also contribute to familial stroke.

The risk for stroke varies among different ethnic and racial groups. The incidence of stroke among African-Americans is almost double that of white Americans, and twice as many African-Americans who have a stroke die from the event compared to white Americans. African-Americans between the ages of 45 and 55 have four to five times the stroke death rate of whites. After age 55 the stroke mortality rate for whites increases and is equal to that of African-Americans.

Compared to white Americans, African-Americans have a higher incidence of stroke risk factors, including high blood pressure and cigarette smoking. African-Americans also have a higher incidence and prevalence of some genetic diseases, such as diabetes and sickle cell anemia, that predispose them to stroke.

Hispanics and Native Americans have stroke incidence and mortality rates more similar to those of white Americans. In Asian-Americans stroke incidence and mortality rates are also similar to those in white Americans, even though Asians in Japan, China, and other countries of the Far East have significantly higher stroke incidence and mortality rates than white Americans. This suggests that environment and lifestyle factors play a large role in stroke risk.

The "Stroke Belt"

Several decades ago, scientists and statisticians noticed that people in the southeastern United States had the highest stroke mortality rate in the country. They named this region the stroke belt. For many years, researchers believed that the increased risk was due to the higher percentage of African-Americans and an overall lower socio-economic status (SES) in the southern states. A low SES is associated with an overall lower standard of living, leading to a lower standard of health care and therefore an increased risk of stroke. But researchers now know that the higher percentage of African-Americans and the overall lower SES in the southern states does not adequately account for the higher incidence of, and mortality from, stroke in those states. This means that other factors must be contributing to the higher incidence of and mortality from stroke in this region.

Recent studies have also shown that there is a stroke buckle in the stroke belt. Three southeastern states, North Carolina, South Carolina, and Georgia, have an extremely high stroke mortality rate, higher than the rate in other stroke belt states and up to two times the stroke mortality rate of the United States overall. The increased risk could be due to geographic or environmental factors or to regional differences in lifestyle, including higher rates of cigarette smoking and a regional preference for salty, high-fat foods.

Other Risk Factors

The most important risk factors for stroke are hypertension, heart disease, diabetes, and cigarette smoking. Others include heavy alcohol consumption, high blood cholesterol levels, illicit drug use, and genetic or congenital conditions, particularly vascular abnormalities. People with more than one risk factor have what is called "amplification of risk." This means that the multiple risk factors compound their destructive effects and create an overall risk greater than the simple cumulative effect of the individual risk factors.

Hypertension

Of all the risk factors that contribute to stroke, the most powerful is hypertension, or high blood pressure. People with hypertension have a risk for stroke that is four to six times higher than the risk for those without hypertension. One-third of the adult U.S. population, about 50 million people (including 40-70 percent of those over age 65) have high blood pressure. Forty to 90 percent of stroke patients have high blood pressure before their stroke event.

A systolic pressure of 120 mm of Hg over a diastolic pressure of 80 mm of Hg is generally considered normal. Persistently high blood pressure greater than 140 over 90 leads to the diagnosis of the disease called hypertension. The impact of hypertension on the total risk for stroke decreases with increasing age, therefore factors other than hypertension play a greater role in the overall stroke risk in elderly adults. For people without hypertension, the absolute risk of stroke increases over time until around the age of 90, when the absolute risk becomes the same as that for people with hypertension.

Like stroke, there is a gender difference in the prevalence of hypertension. In younger people, hypertension is more common among men than among women. With increasing age, however, more women than men have hypertension. This hypertension gender-age difference probably has an impact on the incidence and prevalence of stroke in these populations.

Antihypertensive medication can decrease a person's risk for stroke. Recent studies suggest that treatment can decrease the stroke incidence rate by 38 percent and decrease the stroke fatality rate by

40 percent. Common hypertensive agents include adrenergic agents, beta-blockers, angiotensin converting enzyme inhibitors, calcium channel blockers, diuretics, and vasodilators.

Heart Disease

After hypertension, the second most powerful risk factor for stroke is heart disease, especially a condition known as atrial fibrillation. Atrial fibrillation is irregular beating of the left atrium, or left upper chamber, of the heart. In people with atrial fibrillation, the left atrium beats up to four times faster than the rest of the heart. This leads to an irregular flow of blood and the occasional formation of blood clots that can leave the heart and travel to the brain, causing a stroke.

Atrial fibrillation, which affects as many as 2.2 million Americans, increases an individual's risk of stroke by 4 to 6 percent, and about 15 percent of stroke patients have atrial fibrillation before they experience a stroke. The condition is more prevalent in the upper age groups, which means that the prevalence of atrial fibrillation in the United States will increase proportionately with the growth of the elderly population. Unlike hypertension and other risk factors that have a lesser impact on the ever-rising absolute risk of stroke that comes with advancing age, the influence of atrial fibrillation on total risk for stroke increases powerfully with age. In people over 80 years old, atrial fibrillation is the direct cause of one in four strokes.

Other forms of heart disease that increase stroke risk include malformations of the heart valves or the heart muscle. Some valve diseases, like mitral valve stenosis or mitral annular calcification, can double the risk for stroke, independent of other risk factors.

Heart muscle malformations can also increase the risk for stroke. Patent foramen ovale (PFO) is a passage or a hole (sometimes called a "shunt") in the heart wall separating the two atria, or upper chambers, of the heart. Clots in the blood are usually filtered out by the lungs, but PFO could allow emboli or blood clots to bypass the lungs and go directly through the arteries to the brain, potentially causing a stroke. Research is currently under way to determine how important PFO is as a cause for stroke. Atrial septal aneurysm (ASA), a congenital (present from birth) malformation of the heart tissue, is a bulging of the septum or heart wall into one of the atria of the heart.

Researchers do not know why this malformation increases the risk for stroke. PFO and ASA frequently occur together and therefore amplify the risk for stroke. Two other heart malformations that seem to increase the risk for stroke for unknown reasons are left atrial enlargement and left ventricular hypertrophy. People with left atrial enlargement have a larger than normal left atrium of the heart; those with left ventricular hypertrophy have a thickening of the wall of the left ventricle.

Another risk factor for stroke is cardiac surgery to correct heart malformations or reverse the effects of heart disease. Strokes occurring in this situation are usually the result of surgically dislodged plaques from the aorta that travel through the bloodstream to the arteries in the neck and head, causing stroke. Cardiac surgery increases a person's risk of stroke by about 1 percent. Other types of surgery can also increase the risk of stroke.

Diabetes

Diabetes is another disease that increases a person's risk for stroke. People with diabetes have three times the risk of stroke compared to people without diabetes. The relative risk of stroke from diabetes is highest in the fifth and sixth decades of life and decreases after that. Like hypertension, the relative risk of stroke from diabetes is highest for men at an earlier age and highest for women at an older age. People with diabetes may also have other contributing risk factors that can amplify the overall risk for stroke. For example, the prevalence of hypertension is 40 percent higher in the diabetic population compared to the general population.

Blood Cholesterol Levels

Most people know that high cholesterol levels contribute to heart disease. But many don't realize that a high cholesterol level also contributes to stroke risk. Cholesterol, a waxy substance produced by the liver, is a vital body product. It contributes to the production of hormones and vitamin D and is an integral component of cell membranes. The liver makes enough cholesterol to fuel the body's needs and this natural production of cholesterol alone is not a large contributing factor to atherosclerosis, heart disease, and stroke. Research has shown that the danger from cholesterol comes from a dietary intake of foods that contain high levels of cholesterol. Foods high in saturated fat and cholesterol, like meats, eggs, and dairy products, can increase the amount of total cholesterol in the body to alarming levels, contributing to the risk of atherosclerosis and thickening of the arteries.

Cholesterol is classified as a lipid, meaning that it is fat-soluble rather than water-soluble. Other lipids include fatty acids, glycerides, alcohol, waxes, steroids, and fat-soluble vitamins A, D, and E. Lipids and water, like oil and water, do not mix. Blood is a water-based liquid, therefore cholesterol does not mix with blood. In order to travel through the blood without clumping together, cholesterol needs to be covered by a layer of protein. The cholesterol and protein together are called a lipoprotein.

There are two kinds of cholesterol, commonly called the "good" and the "bad." Good cholesterol is high-density lipoprotein, or HDL; bad cholesterol is low-density lipoprotein, or LDL. Together, these two forms of cholesterol make up a person's total serum cholesterol level. Most cholesterol tests measure the level of total cholesterol in the blood and don't distinguish between good and bad cholesterol. For these total serum cholesterol tests, a level of less than 200 mg/dL is considered safe, while a level of more than 240 is considered dangerous and places a person at risk for heart disease and stroke.

Most cholesterol in the body is in the form of LDL. LDLs circulate through the bloodstream, picking up excess cholesterol and depositing cholesterol where it is needed (for example, for the production and maintenance of cell membranes). But when too much cholesterol starts circulating in the blood, the body cannot handle the excessive LDLs, which build up along the inside of the arterial walls. The buildup of LDL coating on the inside of the artery walls hardens and turns into arterial plaque, leading to stenosis and atherosclerosis. This plaque blocks blood vessels and contributes to the formation of blood clots. A person's LDL level should be less than 130 mg/dL to be safe. LDL levels between 130 and 159 put a person at a slightly higher risk for atherosclerosis, heart disease, and stroke. A score over 160 puts a person at great risk for a heart attack or stroke.

The other form of cholesterol, HDL, is beneficial and contributes to stroke prevention. HDL carries a small percentage of the cholesterol in the blood, but instead of depositing its cholesterol on the inside of artery walls, HDL returns to the liver to unload its cholesterol. The liver then eliminates the excess cholesterol by passing it along to the kidneys. Currently, any HDL score higher than 35 is considered desirable. Recent studies have shown that high levels of HDL are associated with a reduced risk for heart disease and stroke and that low levels (less than 35 mg/dL), even in people with normal levels of LDL, lead to an increased risk for heart disease and stroke.

A person may lower his risk for atherosclerosis and stroke by improving his cholesterol levels. A healthy diet and regular exercise are the best ways to lower total cholesterol levels. In some cases, physicians may prescribe cholesterol-lowering medication, and recent

studies have shown that the newest types of these drugs, called re-
ductase inhibitors or statin drugs, significantly reduce the risk for
stroke in most patients with high cholesterol. Scientists believe that
statins may work by reducing the amount of bad cholesterol the body
produces and by reducing the body's inflammatory immune reaction
to cholesterol plaque associated with atherosclerosis and stroke.

Using a stethoscope and a cuff that is wrapped around the patient's
upper arm, a health professional listens to the sounds of blood rush-
ing through an artery. The first sound registered on the instrument
gauge (which measures the pressure of the blood in millimeters on a
column of mercury) is called the systolic pressure. This is the maximum pressure produced as the left ventricle of the heart contracts
and the blood begins to flow through the artery. The second sound is
the diastolic pressure and is the lowest pressure in the artery when
the left ventricle is relaxing.

Modifiable Lifestyle Risk Factors

Cigarette smoking is the most powerful modifiable stroke risk factor. Smoking almost doubles a person's risk for ischemic stroke, independent of other risk factors, and it increases a person's risk for
subarachnoid hemorrhage by up to 3.5 percent. Smoking is directly
responsible for a greater percentage of the total number of strokes in
young adults than in older adults. Risk factors other than smoking—
like hypertension, heart disease, and diabetes—account for more of
the total number of strokes in older adults.

Heavy smokers are at greater risk for stroke than light smokers.
The relative risk of stroke decreases immediately after quitting smoking, with a major reduction of risk seen after 2 to 4 years. Unfortunately, it may take several decades for a former smoker's risk to drop
to the level of someone who never smoked.

Smoking increases the risk of stroke by promoting atherosclerosis
and increasing the levels of blood-clotting factors, such as fibrinogen.
In addition to promoting conditions linked to stroke, smoking also
increases the damage that results from stroke by weakening the en-
dothelial wall of the cerebrovascular system. This leads to greater
damage to the brain from events that occur in the secondary stage of
stroke.

High alcohol consumption is another modifiable risk factor for
stroke. Generally, an increase in alcohol consumption leads to an increase in blood pressure. While scientists agree that heavy drinking
is a risk for both hemorrhagic and ischemic stroke, in several research

studies daily consumption of smaller amounts of alcohol has been found to provide a protective influence against ischemic stroke, perhaps because alcohol decreases the clotting ability of platelets in the blood.

Moderate alcohol consumption may act in the same way as aspirin to decrease blood clotting and prevent ischemic stroke. Heavy alcohol consumption, though, may seriously deplete platelet numbers and compromise blood clotting and blood viscosity, leading to hemorrhage. In addition, heavy drinking or binge drinking can lead to a rebound effect after the alcohol is purged from the body. The consequences of this rebound effect are that blood viscosity (thickness) and platelet levels skyrocket after heavy drinking, increasing the risk for ischemic stroke.

The use of illicit drugs, such as cocaine and crack cocaine, can cause stroke. Cocaine may act on other risk factors, such as hypertension, heart disease, and vascular disease, to trigger a stroke. It decreases relative cerebrovascular blood flow by up to 30 percent, causes vascular constriction, and inhibits vascular relaxation, leading to narrowing of the arteries. Cocaine also affects the heart, causing arrhythmias and rapid heart rate that can lead to the formation of blood clots.

Marijuana smoking may also be a risk factor for stroke. Marijuana decreases blood pressure and may interact with other risk factors, such as hypertension and cigarette smoking, to cause rapidly fluctuating blood pressure levels, damaging blood vessels.

Other drugs of abuse, such as amphetamines, heroin, and anabolic steroids (and even some common, legal drugs, such as caffeine and L-asparaginase and pseudoephedrine found in over-the-counter decongestants), have been suspected of increasing stroke risk. Many of these drugs are vasoconstrictors, meaning that they cause blood vessels to constrict and blood pressure to rise.

Head and Neck Injuries

Injuries to the head or neck may damage the cerebrovascular system and cause a small number of strokes. Head injury or traumatic brain injury may cause bleeding within the brain leading to damage akin to that caused by a hemorrhagic stroke. Neck injury, when associated with spontaneous tearing of the vertebral or carotid arteries caused by sudden and severe extension of the neck, neck rotation, or pressure on the artery, is a contributing cause of stroke, especially in young adults. This type of stroke is often called "beauty-parlor syndrome," which refers to the practice of extending the neck backwards over a sink for hair washing in beauty parlors. Neck calisthenics, "bottoms-up" drinking, and improperly performed chiropractic manipulation of the neck can also put strain on the vertebral and carotid arteries, possibly leading to ischemic stroke.

Infections

Recent viral and bacterial infections may act with other risk factors to add a small risk for stroke. The immune system responds to infection by increasing inflammation and increasing the infection-fighting properties of the blood. Unfortunately, this immune response increases the number of clotting factors in the blood, leading to an increased risk of embolic-ischemic stroke.

Genetic Risk Factors

Although there may not be a single genetic factor associated with stroke, genes do play a large role in the expression of stroke risk factors such as hypertension, heart disease, diabetes, and vascular malformations. It is also possible that an increased risk for stroke within a family is due to environmental factors, such as a common sedentary lifestyle or poor eating habits, rather than hereditary factors.

Vascular malformations that cause stroke may have the strongest genetic link of all stroke risk factors. A vascular malformation is an abnormally formed blood vessel or group of blood vessels. One genetic vascular disease called CADASIL, which stands for cerebral autosomal dominant arteriopathy with subcortical infarcts and leukoencephalopathy. CADASIL is a rare, genetically inherited, congenital vascular disease of the brain that causes strokes, subcortical dementia, migraine-like headaches, and psychiatric disturbances. CADASIL is very debilitating and symptoms usually surface around the age of 45. Although CADASIL can be treated with surgery to repair the defective blood vessels, patients often die by the age of 65. The exact incidence of CADASIL in the United States is unknown.

What Stroke Therapies are Available?

Physicians have a wide range of therapies to choose from when determining a stroke patient's best therapeutic plan. The type of stroke therapy a patient should receive depends upon the stage of disease. Generally there are three treatment stages for stroke: prevention, therapy immediately after stroke, and post-stroke rehabilitation. Therapies to prevent a first or recurrent stroke are based on treating an individual's underlying risk factors for stroke, such as hypertension, atrial fibrillation, and diabetes, or preventing the widespread formation of blood clots that can cause ischemic stroke in everyone, whether or not risk factors are present. Acute stroke therapies try to stop a stroke while it is happening by quickly dissolving a blood clot causing the stroke or by stopping the bleeding of a hemorrhagic stroke. The purpose of post-stroke rehabilitation is to overcome disabilities that result from stroke damage.

Therapies for stroke include medications, surgery, or rehabilitation.

Medications

Medication or drug therapy is the most common treatment for stroke. The most popular classes of drugs used to prevent or treat stroke are antithrombotics (antiplatelet agents and anticoagulants), thrombolytics, and neuroprotective agents.

Antithrombotics prevent the formation of blood clots that can become lodged in a cerebral artery and cause strokes. Antiplatelet drugs prevent clotting by decreasing the activity of platelets, blood cells that contribute to the clotting property of blood. These drugs reduce the risk of blood-clot formation, thus reducing the risk of ischemic stroke. In the context of stroke, physicians prescribe antiplatelet drugs mainly for prevention. The most widely known and used antiplatelet drug is aspirin. Other antiplatelet drugs include clopidogrel and ticlopidine. The NINDS sponsors a wide range of clinical trials to determine the effectiveness of antiplatelet drugs for stroke prevention.

Anticoagulants reduce stroke risk by reducing the clotting property of the blood. The most commonly used anticoagulants include warfarin (also known as Coumadin®) and heparin. The NINDS has sponsored several trials to test the efficacy of anticoagulants versus antiplatelet drugs.

The Stroke Prevention in Atrial Fibrillation (SPAF) trial found that, although aspirin is an effective therapy for the prevention of a second stroke in most patients with atrial fibrillation, some patients with additional risk factors do better on warfarin therapy. Another study, the Trial of Org 10127 in Acute Stroke Treatment (TOAST), tested the effectiveness of low-molecular weight heparin (Org 10172) in stroke prevention. TOAST showed that heparin anticoagulants are not generally effective in preventing recurrent stroke or improving outcome.

Thrombolytic agents are used to treat an ongoing, acute ischemic stroke caused by an artery blockage. These drugs halt the stroke by dissolving the blood clot that is blocking blood flow to the brain. Recombinant tissue plasminogen activator (rt-PA) is a genetically engineered form of t-PA, a thombolytic substance made naturally by the body. It can be effective if given intravenously within 3 hours of stroke symptom onset, but it should be used only after a physician has confirmed that the patient has suffered an ischemic stroke. Thrombolytic agents can increase bleeding and therefore must be used only after careful patient screening. The NINDS rt-PA Stroke Study showed the efficacy of t-PA and in 1996 led to the first FDA-approved treatment for acute ischemic stroke. Other thrombolytics are currently being tested in clinical trials.

Neuroprotectants are medications that protect the brain from secondary injury caused by stroke. Although only a few neuroprotectants are FDA-approved for use at this time, many are in clinical trials. There are several different classes of neuroprotectants that show promise for future therapy, including calcium antagonists, glutamate antagonists, opiate antagonists, antioxidants, apoptosis inhibitors, and many others. One of the calcium antagonists, nimodipine, also called a calcium channel blocker, has been shown to decrease the risk of the neurological damage that results from subarachnoid hemorrhage. Calcium channel blockers, such as nimodipine, act by reducing the risk of cerebral vasospasm, a dangerous side effect of subarachnoid hemorrhage in which the blood vessels in the subarachnoid space constrict erratically, cutting off blood flow.

Surgery

Surgery can be used to prevent stroke, to treat acute stroke, or to repair vascular damage or malformations in and around the brain. There are two prominent types of surgery for stroke prevention and treatment: carotid endarterectomy and extracranial/intracranial (EC/IC) bypass. Carotid endarterectomy is a surgical procedure in which a doctor removes fatty deposits (plaque) from the inside of one of the carotid arteries, which are located in the neck and are the main suppliers of blood to the brain. As mentioned earlier, the disease atherosclerosis is characterized by the buildup of plaque on the inside of large arteries, and the blockage of an artery by this fatty material is called stenosis. The NINDS has sponsored two large clinical trials to test the efficacy of carotid endarterectomy: the North American Symptomatic Carotid Endarterectomy Trial (NASCET) and the Asymptomatic Carotid Atherosclerosis Trial

(ACAS). These trials showed that carotid endarterectomy is a safe and effective stroke prevention therapy for most people with greater than 50 percent stenosis of the carotid arteries when performed by a qualified and experienced neurosurgeon or vascular surgeon.

Currently, the NINDS is sponsoring the Carotid Revascularization Endarterectomy vs. Stenting Trial (CREST), a large clinical trial designed to test the effectiveness of carotid endarterectomy versus a newer surgical procedure for carotid stenosis called stenting. The procedure involves inserting a long, thin catheter tube into an artery in the leg and threading the catheter through the vascular system into the narrow stenosis of the carotid artery in the neck. Once the catheter is in place in the carotid artery, the radiologist expands the stent with a balloon on the tip of the catheter. The CREST trial will test the effectiveness of the new surgical technique versus the established standard technique of carotid endarterectomy surgery.

EC/IC bypass surgery is a procedure that restores blood flow to a blood-deprived area of brain tissue by rerouting a healthy artery in the scalp to the area of brain tissue affected by a blocked artery. The NINDS-sponsored EC/IC Bypass Study tested the ability of this surgery to prevent recurrent strokes in stroke patients with atherosclerosis. The study showed that, in the long run, EC/IC does not seem to benefit these patients. The surgery is still performed occasionally for patients with aneurysms, some types of small artery disease, and certain vascular abnormalities.

One useful surgical procedure for treatment of brain aneurysms that cause subarachnoid hemorrhage is a technique called "clipping." Clipping involves clamping off the aneurysm from the blood vessel, which reduces the chance that it will burst and bleed.

A new therapy that is gaining wide attention is the detachable coil technique for the treatment of high-risk intracranial aneurysms. A small platinum coil is inserted through an artery in the thigh and threaded through the arteries to the site of the aneurysm. The coil is then released into the aneurysm, where it evokes an immune response from the body. The body produces a blood clot inside the aneurysm, strengthening the artery walls and reducing the risk of rupture. Once the aneurysm is stabilized, a neurosurgeon can clip the aneurysm with less risk of hemorrhage and death to the patient.

Rehabilitation Therapy

Stroke is the number one cause of serious adult disability in the United States. Stroke disability is devastating to the stroke patient and family, but therapies are available to help rehabilitate post-stroke patients.

For most stroke patients, physical therapy (PT) is the cornerstone of the rehabilitation process. A physical therapist uses training, exercises, and physical manipulation of the stroke patient's body with the intent of restoring movement, balance, and coordination. The aim of PT is to have the stroke patient relearn simple motor activities such as walking, sitting, standing, lying down, and the process of switching from one type of movement to another.

Another type of therapy involving relearning daily activities is occupational therapy (OT). OT also involves exercise and training to help the stroke patient relearn everyday activities such as eating, drinking and swallowing, dressing, bathing, cooking, reading and writing, and toileting. The goal of OT is to help the patient become independent or semi-independent.

Speech and language problems arise when brain damage occurs in the language centers of the brain. Due to the brain's great ability to learn and change (called brain plasticity), other areas can adapt to take over some of the lost functions. Speech therapy helps stroke patients relearn language and speaking skills, or learn other forms of communication. Speech therapy is appropriate for patients who have no deficits in cognition or thinking, but have problems understanding speech or written words, or problems forming speech. A speech therapist helps stroke patients help themselves by working to improve language skills, develop alternative ways of communicating, and develop coping skills to deal with the frustration of not being able to communicate fully. With time and patience, a stroke survivor should be able to regain some, and sometimes all, language and speaking abilities.

Many stroke patients require psychological or psychiatric help after a stroke. Psychological problems, such as depression, anxiety, frustration, and anger, are common post-stroke disabilities. Talk therapy, along with appropriate medication, can help alleviate some of the mental and emotional problems that result from stroke. Sometimes it is also beneficial for family members of the stroke patient to seek psychological help as well.

What Disabilities Can Result from a Stroke?

Although stroke is a disease of the brain, it can affect the entire body. Some of the disabilities that can result from a stroke include paralysis, cognitive deficits, speech problems, emotional difficulties, daily living problems, and pain.

Paralysis

A common disability that results from stroke is paralysis on one side of the body, called hemiplegia. A related disability that is not as debilitating as paralysis is one-sided weakness or hemiparesis. The paralysis or weakness may affect only the face, an arm, or a leg or may affect one entire side of the body and face. A person who suffers a stroke in the left hemisphere of the brain will show right-sided paralysis or paresis. Conversely, a person with a stroke in the right hemisphere of the brain will show deficits on the left side of the body. A stroke patient may have problems with the simplest of daily activities, such as walking, dressing, eating, and using the bathroom. Motor deficits can result from damage to the motor cortex in the frontal lobes of the brain or from damage to the lower parts of the brain, such as the cerebellum, which controls balance and coordination. Some stroke patients also have trouble eating and swallowing, called dysphagia.

Cognitive Deficits

Stroke may cause problems with thinking, awareness, attention, learning, judgment, and memory. If the cognitive problems are severe, the stroke patient may be said to have apraxia, agnosia, or "neglect." In the context of stroke, neglect means that a stroke patient has no knowledge of one side of his or her body, or one side of the visual field, and is unaware of the deficit. A stroke patient may be unaware of his or her surroundings, or may be unaware of the mental deficits that resulted from the stroke.

Language Deficits

Stroke victims often have problems understanding or forming speech. A deficit in understanding speech is called aphasia. Trouble speaking or forming words is called dysarthria. Language problems usually result from damage to the left temporal and parietal lobes of the brain.

Emotional Deficits

A stroke can lead to emotional problems. Stroke patients may have difficulty controlling their emotions or may express inappropriate emotions in certain situations. One common disability that occurs with many stroke patients is depression. Post-stroke depression may be more than a general sadness resulting from the stroke incident. It is a clinical behavioral problem that can hamper recovery and rehabilitation and may even lead to suicide. Post-stroke depression is treated as any depression is treated, with antidepressant medications and therapy.

Pain

Stroke patients may experience pain, uncomfortable numbness, or strange sensations after a stroke. These sensations may be due to many factors including damage to the sensory regions of the brain, stiff joints, or a disabled limb. An uncommon type of pain resulting from stroke is called central stroke pain or central pain syndrome (CPS). CPS results from damage to an area in the mid-brain called the thalamus. The pain is a mixture of sensations, including heat and cold, burning, tingling, numbness, and sharp stabbing and underlying aching pain. The pain is often worse in the extremities—the hands and feet—and is made worse by movement and temperature changes, especially cold temperatures. Unfortunately, since most pain medications provide little relief from these sensations, very few treatments or therapies exist to combat CPS.

What Special Risks Do Women Face?

Some risk factors for stroke apply only to women. Primary among these are pregnancy, childbirth, and menopause. These risk factors are tied to hormonal fluctuations and changes that affect a woman in different stages of life. Research in the past few decades has shown that high-dose oral contraceptives, the kind used in the 1960s and 1970s, can increase the risk of stroke in women. Fortunately, oral contraceptives with high doses of estrogen are no longer used and have been replaced with safer and more effective oral contraceptives with lower doses of estrogen. Some studies have shown the newer low-dose oral contraceptives may not significantly increase the risk of stroke in women.

Other studies have demonstrated that pregnancy and childbirth can put a woman at an increased risk for stroke. Pregnancy increases the risk of stroke as much as three to 13 times. Of course, the risk of stroke in young women of childbearing years is very small to begin with, so a moderate increase in risk during pregnancy is still a relatively small risk. Pregnancy and childbirth cause strokes in approximately eight in 100,000 women. Unfortunately, 25 percent of strokes during pregnancy end in death, and hemorrhagic strokes, although rare, are still the leading cause of maternal death in the United States. Subarachnoid hemorrhage, in particular, causes one to five maternal deaths per 10,000 pregnancies.

A study sponsored by the NINDS showed that the risk of stroke during pregnancy is greatest in the post-partum period—the 6 weeks following childbirth. The risk of ischemic stroke after pregnancy is about nine times higher and the risk of hemorrhagic stroke is more than 28 times higher for post-partum women than for women who are not pregnant or post-partum. The cause is unknown.

In the same way that the hormonal changes during pregnancy and childbirth are associated with increased risk of stroke, hormonal changes at the end of the childbearing years can increase the risk of stroke. Several studies have shown that menopause, the end of a woman's reproductive ability marked by the termination of her menstrual cycle, can increase a woman's risk of stroke.

Fortunately, some studies have suggested that hormone replacement therapy can reduce some of the effects of menopause and decrease stroke risk. Currently, the NINDS is sponsoring the Women's Estrogen for Stroke Trial (WEST), a randomized, placebo-controlled, double-blind trial, to determine whether estrogen therapy can reduce the risk of death or recurrent stroke in postmenopausal women who have a history of a recent TIA or non-disabling stroke. The mechanism by which estrogen can prove beneficial to postmenopausal women could include its role in cholesterol control. Studies have shown that estrogen acts to increase levels of HDL while decreasing LDL levels.

Are Children at Risk For Stroke?

The young have several risk factors unique to them. Young people seem to suffer from hemorrhagic strokes more than ischemic strokes, a significant difference from older age groups where ischemic strokes make up the majority of stroke cases. Hemorrhagic strokes represent 20 percent of all strokes in the United States and young people account for many of these.

Clinicians often separate the "young" into two categories: those younger than 15 years of age, and those 15 to 44 years of age. People 15 to 44 years of age are generally considered young adults and have many of the risk factors mentioned above, such as drug use, alcohol abuse, pregnancy, head and neck injuries, heart disease or heart malformations, and infections. Some other causes of stroke in the young are linked to genetic diseases.

271

Medical complications that can lead to stroke in children include intracranial infection, brain injury, vascular malformations such as moyamoya syndrome, occlusive vascular disease, and genetic disorders such as sickle cell anemia, tuberous sclerosis, and Marfan's syndrome.

The symptoms of stroke in children are different from those in adults and young adults. A child experiencing a stroke may have seizures, a sudden loss of speech, a loss of expressive language (including body language and gestures), hemiparesis (weakness on one side of the body), hemiplegia (paralysis on one side of the body), dysarthria (impairment of speech), convulsions, headache, or fever. It is a medical emergency when a child shows any of these symptoms.

In children with stroke the underlying conditions that led to the stroke should be determined and managed to prevent future strokes. For example, a recent clinical study sponsored by the National Heart, Lung, and Blood Institute found that giving blood transfusions to young children with sickle cell anemia greatly reduces the risk of stroke. The Institute even suggests attempting to prevent stroke in high-risk children by giving them blood transfusions before they experience a stroke.

Most children who experience a stroke will do better than most adults after treatment and rehabilitation. This is due in part to the immature brain's great plasticity, the ability to adapt to deficits and injury. Children who experience seizures along with stroke do not recover as well as children who do not have seizures. Some children may experience residual hemiplegia, though most will eventually learn how to walk.

Chapter 32

Brain Tumors and Headache Pain

Symptoms of Brain Tumors

The symptoms of brain tumors depend mainly on their size and their location in the brain. Symptoms are caused by damage to vital tissue and by pressure on the brain as the tumor grows within the limited space in the skull. They also may be caused by swelling and a buildup of fluid around the tumor, a condition called edema. Symptoms may also be due to hydrocephalus, which occurs when the tumor blocks the flow of cerebrospinal fluid and causes it to build up in the ventricles. If a brain tumor grows very slowly, its symptoms may appear so gradually that they are overlooked for a long time.

The most frequent symptoms of brain tumors include:

- Headaches that tend to be worse in the morning and ease during the day,
- Seizures (convulsions),
- Nausea or vomiting,
- Weakness or loss of feeling in the arms or legs,
- Stumbling or lack of coordination in walking (ataxic gait),
- Abnormal eye movements or changes in vision,
- Drowsiness,

Excerpted from "Brain Tumors," National Cancer Institute (NCI), NIH Pub. No. 95-1558, September 1998.

- Changes in personality or memory, and

- Changes in speech.

These symptoms may be caused by brain tumors or by other problems. Only a doctor can make a diagnosis.

Diagnosis

To find the cause of a person's symptoms, the doctor asks about the patient's personal and family medical history and performs a complete physical examination. In addition to checking general signs of health, the doctor does a neurologic exam. This includes checks for alertness, muscle strength, coordination, reflexes, and response to pain. The doctor also examines the eyes to look for swelling caused by a tumor pressing on the nerve that connects the eye and the brain.

Depending on the results of the physical and neurologic examinations, the doctor may request one or both of the following:

- A CT (or CAT) scan is a series of detailed pictures of the brain. The pictures are created by a computer linked to an x-ray machine. In some cases, a special dye is injected into a vein before the scan. The dye helps to show differences in the tissues of the brain.

- MRI (magnetic resonance imaging) gives pictures of the brain, using a powerful magnet linked to a computer. MRI is especially useful in diagnosing brain tumors because it can "see" through the bones of the skull to the tissue underneath. A special dye may be used to enhance the likelihood of detecting a brain tumor.

The doctor may also request other tests such as:

- A skull x-ray can show changes in the bones of the skull caused by a tumor. It can also show calcium deposits, which are present in some types of brain tumors.

- A brain scan reveals areas of abnormal growth in the brain and records them on special film. A small amount of a radioactive material is injected into a vein. This dye is absorbed by the tumor, and the growth shows up on the film. (The radiation leaves the body within 6 hours and is not dangerous.)

- An angiogram, or arteriogram, is a series of x-rays taken after a special dye is injected into an artery (usually in the area where the abdomen joins the top of the leg). The dye, which flows through the blood vessels of the brain, can be seen on the x-rays. These x-rays can show the tumor and blood vessels that lead to it.

- A myelogram is an x-ray of the spine. A special dye is injected into the cerebrospinal fluid in the spine, and the patient is tilted to allow the dye to mix with the fluid. This test may be done when the doctor suspects a tumor in the spinal cord.

About Brain Tumors

The body is made up of many types of cells. Each type of cell has special functions. Most cells in the body grow and then divide in an orderly way to form new cells as they are needed to keep the body healthy and working properly. When cells lose the ability to control their growth, they divide too often and without any order. The extra cells form a mass of tissue called a tumor. Tumors are benign or malignant.

Benign brain tumors do not contain cancer cells. Usually these tumors can be removed, and they are not likely to recur. Benign brain tumors have clear borders. Although they do not invade nearby tissue, they can press on sensitive areas of the brain and cause symptoms.

Malignant brain tumors contain cancer cells. They interfere with vital functions and are life threatening. Malignant brain tumors are likely to grow rapidly and crowd or invade the tissue around them. Like a plant, these tumors may put out "roots" that grow into healthy brain tissue. If a malignant tumor remains compact and does not have roots, it is said to be encapsulated. When an otherwise benign tumor is located in a vital area of the brain and interferes with vital functions, it may be considered malignant (even though it contains no cancer cells).

Doctors refer to some brain tumors by grade—from low grade (grade I) to high grade (grade IV). The grade of a tumor refers to the way the cells look under a microscope. Cells from higher grade tumors are more abnormal looking and generally grow faster than cells from lower grade tumors; higher grade tumors are more malignant than lower grade tumors.

Possible Causes

The causes of brain tumors are not known. Researchers are trying to solve this problem. The more they can find out about the causes of brain tumors, the better the chances of finding ways to prevent them. Doctors cannot explain why one person gets a brain tumor and another doesn't, but they do know that no one can "catch" a brain tumor from another person. Brain tumors are not contagious.

Although brain tumors can occur at any age, studies show that they are most common in two age groups. The first group is children 3 to 12 years old; the second is adults 40 to 70 years old.

By studying large numbers of patients, researchers have found certain risk factors that increase a person's chance of developing a brain tumor. People with these risk factors have a higher-than-average risk of getting a brain tumor. For example, studies show that some types of brain tumors are more frequent among workers in certain industries, such as oil refining, rubber manufacturing, and drug manufacturing. Other studies have shown that chemists and embalmers have a higher incidence of brain tumors. Researchers also are looking at exposure to viruses as a possible cause.

Because brain tumors sometimes occur in several members of the same family, researchers are studying families with a history of brain tumors to see whether heredity is a cause. At this time, scientists do not believe that head injuries cause brain tumors to develop.

In most cases, patients with a brain tumor have no clear risk factors. The disease is probably the result of several factors acting together.

Treatment

Treatment for a brain tumor depends on a number of factors. Among these are the type, location, and size of the tumor, as well as the patient's age and general health. Treatment methods and schedules often vary for children and adults. The doctor develops a treatment plan to fit each patient's needs.

The patient's doctor may want to discuss the case with other doctors who treat brain tumors. Also, the patient may want to talk with the doctor about taking part in a research study of new treatment methods. Many patients want to learn all they can about their disease and their treatment choices so they can take an active part in decisions about their medical care. A person with a brain tumor will have many questions, and the doctor is the best person to answer them. Most patients want to know what kind of tumor they have, how it can be treated, how effective the treatment is likely to be, and how much it's likely to cost.

Here are some important questions to ask the doctor:

- What type of treatment will I receive?

- What are the expected benefits of treatment?

- What are the risks and possible side effects of treatment?

- What can be done about side effects?

- Would a clinical trial be appropriate for me?

- Will I need to change my normal activities? If so, for how long?

- How often will I need to have checkups?

Many people find it helpful to make a list of their questions before they see the doctor. Taking notes can make it easier to remember what the doctor says. Some patients find that it also helps to have a family member or friend with them when they talk with the doctor—either to take part in the discussion or just to listen.

Patients and their families have a lot to learn about brain tumors and their treatment. They should not feel that they need to understand everything the first time they hear it. They will have other chances to ask the doctor to explain things that are not clear.

Living with a Brain Tumor

The diagnosis of a brain tumor can change the lives of patients and the people who care about them. These changes can be hard to handle. Patients and their families and friends may have many different and sometimes confusing emotions.

At times, patients and those close to them may feel frightened, angry, or depressed. These are normal reactions when people face a serious health problem. Most patients, including children and teenagers, find it helps to share their thoughts and feelings with loved ones. Sharing can help everyone feel more at ease and can open the way for others to show their concern and offer their support.

Worries about tests, treatments, hospital stays, rehabilitation, and medical bills are common. Parents may worry about whether their children will be able to take part in normal school or social activities. Doctors, nurses, social workers, and other members of the health care team may be able to calm fears and ease confusion. They can also provide information and suggest helpful resources.

Patients and their families are naturally concerned about what the future holds. Sometimes they use statistics to try to figure out whether the patient will be cured or how long he or she will live. It is important to remember, however, that statistics are averages based on large numbers of patients. They cannot be used to predict what will happen to a certain patient because no two cancer patients are alike. The doctor who takes care of the patient and knows that person's medical history is in the best position to discuss the patient's outlook (prognosis).

People should feel free to ask the doctor about their prognosis, but it is important to keep in mind that not even the doctor can tell exactly what will happen. When doctors talk about recovering from a brain tumor, they may use the term remission rather than cure. Even though many people recover completely, doctors use this term because a brain tumor can recur.

Part Five

Additional Help and Information

Chapter 33

Glossary

Abdominal Migraine: A type of migraine that mainly occurs in childhood, characterized by abdominal pain, nausea, vomiting, and sometimes diarrhea, but with little or no headache. Later in life, children with abdominal migraine may develop more typical migraine attacks.

Abortive Medication: Medication taken to "abort" or stop a headache after it already begins.

Acetaminophen: An aspirin substitute. Like aspirin, acetaminophen works as a pain killer and fever reducer, but it does not have anti-inflammatory properties and does not produce the side effects associated with aspirin, such as stomach irritation.

ACHE: American Council for Headache Education, an organization affiliated with AHS, and made up of both headache patients and professionals who treat headache. The purpose of the organization is to educate patients and the public about headache, and to advocate up-to-date treatment for headache sufferers.

Acupressure: Derived from traditional Chinese medicine, this is a form of treatment for pain that involves pressure on particular points in the body know as "acupressure points."

Text in this chapter is from "Glossary of Headache Terms," American Council for Headache Education (ACHE) © 2000. Reprinted from the web site of the American Council for Headache Education (www.achenet.org); reprinted with permission.

Acupuncture: Derived from traditional Chinese medicine, this is a form of treatment for pain that involves insertion of fine needles into particular points in the body known as "acupuncture points."

AHS: American Headache Society, a professional organization of physicians, dentists, physician's assistants, nurses, and other health professionals and scientists interested in the study of headache and its treatment.

Amitriptyline: An anti-depressant medication useful in treating migraine and tension type headaches.

Analgesic: Medication for the relief of pain. An analgesic works to increase the patient's pain threshold, thereby decreasing the sensation of pain. Analgesics range from aspirin and acetaminophen to narcotics.

Aneurysm: A congenital weak point in the wall of an artery that may bulge outwards, and may occasionally rupture and bleed, causing what is called a "subarachnoid hemorrhage," which produces a severe headache and stiff neck and sometimes can be fatal.

Anticonvulsant: A class of drugs used to treat convulsive seizures, or epilepsy. Some of these medications, such as Valproic Acid or Depakote, are also used in prevention of headache, even when headaches are not associated with seizures.

Antidepressant: A class of drugs used primarily to treat depression. Some of these drugs have also been found to be useful in the prevention of headache, even when headaches are not associated with depression.

Antiemetics: A class of drugs used to treat nausea and/or vomiting.

Anti-inflammatory: A class of drugs that reduces inflammation in the body, and that are often used to treat arthritis. These drugs can also be useful in reducing the inflammation associated with certain types of headaches, but may cause gastrointestinal upset.

Aspartame: Artificial sweetener known to act as a migraine trigger in some vulnerable people.

Aura: The warning symptoms, usually visual, that may sometimes occur shortly before a migraine headache begins. The word "aura" comes from the Greek word for wind, and just as a strong wind may precede a storm, an aura may precede the storm of migraine. Auras may occur without head pain.

Barbiturate: A class of drugs that causes sedation and relaxation. Barbiturates may be found in combination abortive medications used to treat the symptoms of headache. If used too frequently (more than a couple of days per week), they may be habit-forming.

Basilar Migraine: A type of migraine that mainly affects children and adolescents. Associated with the headache are a number of symptoms related to the part of the brain supplied by the basilar artery. These include vertigo (spinning sensations), loss of balance, and sometimes, loss of consciousness as well as prominent nausea and vomiting.

Benzodiazepines: A category of potentially addictive tranquilizers that may increase depression at the same time that they reduce anxiety.

Beta Blockers: A class of drugs used to treat heart disease and high blood pressure. These drugs lower blood pressure and slow the heart rate. They were discovered accidentally to also be useful for preventing migraine headaches.

Biofeedback: A form of treatment for headache that uses electronic feedback of hand temperature and/or muscle tension to rapidly teach patients how to deeply relax. Acquiring and regularly practicing these skills has been shown to often reduce the frequency and severity of both migraine and tension-type headaches.

Caffeine: A stimulating drug found in coffee, tea, and cola beverages. After a headache begins, caffeine may be helpful in aborting headaches, so it is widely used in combination drugs prescribed for relief of headache. Paradoxically, using caffeine to excess or too rapid withdrawal from caffeine, may cause headaches in some individuals.

Caffeine Withdrawal Headache: A headache caused by dilation of the blood vessels once the constrictive effects of caffeine are no longer present.

Calcium Channel Blocker: A type of medication that may prevent migraine headaches by acting on the blood vessels, the brain, or both.

CAT Scan: "Computerized Axial Tomographic" scan, a type of X-ray scan utilized for diagnostic purposes which can be useful in identifying causes of headache that may masquerade as migraine.

Chiropractic: A philosophic system of mechanical therapeutics that associates many diseases on poor alignment of the vertebrae. Chiropractors treat disease with manipulation of the vertebrae in order to relieve pressure on the nerves, "so that nerve force may flow freely from the brain to the rest of the body."

Chlorpromazine: A powerful major tranquilizer that relieves the pain and nausea of migraine.

Chronic Headache: Headache that occurs frequently over a period of time, generally at least every other day or 15 days per month for a period of at least six months.

Chronic Paroxysmal Hemicrania: (CPH) A very rare headache syndrome which can resemble cluster headache as it presents itself as multiple, short, severe headaches that occurs on a daily basis. They can also be associated with tearing, nasal stuffiness, etc. CPH differs from cluster headache in that the patients are almost always female, the headache attacks are shorter (1-2 minutes) and much more frequent with attacks occurring on average of 14 times per day. This condition responds almost 100% of the time to treatment with Indomethacin.

Classic Migraine: An older term for what is now called "migraine with aura."

Cluster Headache: A particular type of headache that mainly affects men by a 6 to 1 ratio. It is characterized by intense but brief (30 minutes to 2 hours) pain in and around one eye occurring daily or several times per day in "clusters" that typically last for a couple of months. The patient then may go for many months with no headaches at all. Along with the headache, there are usually other phenomena such as tearing and redness of the affected eye, or stuffy nose.

Cognitive Behavioral Therapy: An approach to psychotherapy that helps patients take control of their illness, and their lives, through insight, self knowledge and planning.

Common Migraine: An older term for what is now called "migraine without aura."

Daily Headache: Headache that occurs either daily or almost daily, at least 20 days per month.

Depression: Not just temporary or situational sadness, but a persistent and pervasive feeling of sadness or hopelessness that is often associated with weight loss (or gain), sleep disturbances, constipation, disturbances of sexual function, and feelings of guilt or self-blame.

Dexamethasone: A steroid drug used to treat inflammation.

DHE: Abbreviation for Dihydroergotamine, a drug used, usually by injection or nasal spray, to treat migraine, rebound and cluster headaches.

Diagnosis: The process of taking a history and performing an examination in order to decide what is causing a particular symptom, such as headache, so that a correct treatment can be chosen.

D.O.: Abbreviation for a doctor of osteopathy, a degree indicating medical training approximately the same as that for a doctor of medicine or M.D. Practitioners of osteopathy or osteopaths, use the diagnostic and therapeutic measures of ordinary medicine in addition to having training in manipulative measures.

Dopamine: One of several chemicals called "neurotransmitters" that transmit or send messages from one nerve cell to another in the nervous system.

Dysrhythmia: A disturbance in the normal pattern of brain waves as recorded in encephalography (EEG). Dysrhythmias of different kinds may show up during migraine, sleep, overexcitement, etc.

EEG: Electroencephalography is a test used to detect and record the electrical activity generated by the brain.

EMG: Electromyography is a test used to discover diseases of the muscles, spinal cord, and peripheral nerves.

Endorphins: Hormone-like substances produced in the brain that have analgesic properties.

Episodic: Describing occurrences that come and go, with or without a regular pattern.

Ergotamine: A drug originally derived from the ergot fungus that constricts blood vessels and has been used since the 1920's to treat migraine headaches.

Exercise: Many headache specialists believe that regular physical exercise can reduce the frequency and severity of headaches, although, not many research studies have been done to prove or disprove this widespread belief. If true, exercise may help by reducing stress.

Feverfew: An herb (plant of the chrysanthemum family) used for the prevention of migraine headaches. It is more widely used in England than in this country. Potency varies from one preparation to another since this herb is not regulated by the Federal Food and Drug Administration. There are anecdotal reports in the medical literature that it is helpful, but no carefully controlled scientific studies.

Glaucoma: An eye disease that can eventually cause blindness. Glaucoma is sometimes the cause of headache pain.

Hangover Headache: A headache linked to the consumption of alcohol, which dilates and irritates the brain's blood vessels.

Head Trauma: Injury to the head, which may in some cases lead to what are called "post-traumatic headaches."

Headache: Generally refers to a persistent or lasting pain in the head region, as contrasted with a "head pain," such as trigeminal neuralgia, which is quite brief.

Homeopathy: The practice of the use of active ingredients in minute dosages along with naturally occurring substances in order to provide a healthier balance of internal chemistry. These minute dosages would be viewed in traditional medicine as ineffective.

Hormone Replacement Therapy: The therapeutic use of synthetic hormones, usually estrogen and progesterone after menopause or following a hysterectomy.

Hormones: Powerful substances secreted by the endocrine glands in the body that are carried through the blood stream to have effects on other parts of the body distant from where they are produced.

Hydrocephalus: An uncharacteristic swelling in the amount of cerebrospinal fluid within the skull, causing dangerous expansion of the cerebral ventricles.

Hypertension Headache: A headache that strikes people who have very high blood pressure. Its "hatband" type pain can be most severe in the morning.

Hypnosis: A sleep-like state usually induced by another person in which the subject retains awareness of the presence of the hypnotist and where the subject is susceptible to heightened suggestibility. After training by a hypnotist, some migraine patients can be taught to hypnotize themselves in order to reduce stress and related symptoms.

Ice Cream Headache: A painful condition in the roof of the mouth produced by eating ice cream too quickly.

Idiopathic: Occurring spontaneously, not traceable to a direct cause.

Imitrex: Brand name for Sumatriptan, a fairly new migraine abortive medication available as a self-administered injection or as a tablet.

Indomethacin: A nonsteroidal anti-inflammatory medication which can be effective for the relief of migraine and other types of headaches.

International Headache Society: An international professional organization of physicians and other health professionals and scientists interested in the study of headache and its' treatment. In 1988, the International Headache Society, or IHS, developed definitions of the different types of headaches that are widely accepted by physicians and others who treat headache worldwide.

Intractable Migraine: A migraine headache that "just won't stop." By definition, any migraine that persists longer than 72 hours is referred to as "status migrainosus." Migraines may often become transformed into a chronic daily headache by too frequent use of either painkillers or ergots.

Letdown Migraine: Migraine may often occur after times of stress, as after a big exam, or on weekends after a hectic week at work. These are referred to as "letdown" attacks.

Light Sensitivity: People with migraine may become very sensitive to light, a condition known as "photophobia," or literally "fear of light." A similar sensitivity to sound may also occur, and is known as "phonophobia."

Magnesium: An element found in trace amounts in the body, in certain foods, and believed to possibly play a role in the cause of migraine headaches, according to some recent research.

MAO Inhibitors: Monoamine Oxidase Inhibitors are a class of drugs used for treating depression and also have been found useful in treatment of migraine. Persons taking MAO inhibitors may not eat certain foods containing tyramine because of the danger of increase in blood pressure and, therefore, must be closely monitored during treatment.

Massage: A method of manipulation of the body by rubbing, pinching, kneading, tapping, etc., that can be helpful in producing relaxation.

M.D.: Abbreviation for "medical doctor."

Menstrual Migraine: The terms "pure menstrual migraine" or "true menstrual migraine" refers to migraine attacks that occur only with menses. If attacks occur mainly but not exclusively with menses, this may be referred to as "mainly menstrual migraine."

Migraine: A particular form of recurrent headache that often runs in families. According to the International Headache Society, migraine headache pain must have four of the following characteristics: one-sided, pulsating or throbbing, at least moderate if not severe, and worsened by ordinary daily activities such as climbing stairs or housework. In addition, the pain must be accompanied by either nausea or else sensitivity to light and noise. There must be no evidence of other disease and at least 4-5 attacks before a physician can be confident of the diagnosis.

Migraine Equivalents: Symptoms such as unexplained flashing lights or visual disturbances, transient numbness, unexplained bouts of abdominal pain or nausea, etc., all of which are considered to be fragments of a full-blown migraine attack. Migraine equivalents tend to occur most commonly in either children or older persons. Other disorders that might explain these symptoms must be ruled out by appropriate tests.

Migraineur: A designation sometimes used for people with migraine.

Monoamine Oxidase: A family of enzymes involved in the breakdown of certain neurotransmitters. MAO inhibitors act to block these enzymes.

MRI: An acronym for "magnetic resonance imaging," a computerized way of making pictures or images without the use of X-rays, but instead with the help of a powerful magnet.

MSG: Abbreviation for "monosodium glutamate," often found in seasonings or Chinese food. MSG may sometimes trigger migraine attacks in susceptible individuals.

Naproxen: A nonsteroidal anti-inflammatory medication.

Narcotics: Strong prescription painkillers such as Demerol, Stadol, or Codeine, all of which are habit-forming if taken too often for too long at a time.

Naturopathy: The practice of the use of natural substances to provide a healthier balance of internal chemistry.

Neuralgia: The pain spasms of a major nerve. The pain can be jabbing, sudden and repetitive. There are several different types of neuralgia's, and each affects a different area. Trigeminal neuralgia, for example, affects the nerves of the face.

Neurologic: Relating to neurology or to the nervous system itself.

Neurologist: A medical specialist with advanced training in diagnosis and treatment of diseases of the brain, spinal cord, nerves and muscles, including such common disorders as headache, dizziness, stroke and back pain.

Neurology: The branch of medical science that specializes in the nervous system.

Neurotransmitters: Naturally occurring chemicals in the brain which transmit messages from one nerve cell to another.

Neurovascular: Pertaining to the relationship between nerves and the blood vessels they supply.

Nitrites: Chemical preservatives used in meats, various processed foods and, because they are known to dilate blood vessels, they can cause headaches in some people.

Nondrug Therapy: A treatment that does not involve the use of drugs or medications. In the case of headache, such nondrug therapies might include: biofeedback, acupuncture, dietary counseling, stress management training, physical therapy, etc.

Ocular Migraine: A type of migraine with aura or "classical" migraine in which visual symptoms are prominent, sometimes with little or no headache component.

Ophthalmoplegic Migraine: A very rare type of migraine in which there is weakness of one or more of the muscles that moves the eye.

This is said to occur mainly in young people, and other, more common causes for painful paralysis of the eye muscles, must be excluded by appropriate diagnostic testing.

Oxygen Therapy: Breathing of oxygen from a tank which is sometimes very helpful for cluster headaches.

Pain Rating System: Since pain is an internal and private experience, various scales have been devised for rating pain. One of the most common, rates pain on a zero to ten scale, with ten being the most severe pain a person has ever experienced. Yet another assigns the number one to mild pain, two to moderate pain, three to severe pain, and four to pain that causes incapacity.

Personality: In the past, it was thought that there was a typical "migraine personality." Now, this is no longer felt to be the case, as the primary factor determining whether or not a person will have migraine or not is heredity, not personality. Nevertheless, hurrying, worrying, and stress can all aggravate migraine.

Phonophobia: Abnormal sensitivity to sound.

Phosphenes: Tiny, brilliant sparks often seen during the first stage of migraine.

Photophobia: Abnormal sensitivity to light.

Postdrome: The period following a bad migraine headache during which a person feels "hung over," tired, and "beaten up" is referred to as the headache postdrome.

Posttraumatic Headache: Headache which follows an injury or trauma. There does not have to be loss of consciousness for an injury to cause significant headache in some cases.

Premenstrual Syndrome: (PMS) Combination of symptoms experienced by some women prior to menstruation.

Prodrome: The period of time preceding a migraine headache during which a person may feel irritable, out of sorts, moody, unusually sensitive to light or noise, and may notice some fluid retention. This may go on for one or two days or just a few hours before the actual headache begins.

Prophylactic Medication: Preventative medication taken on a regular schedule to prevent the onset of an ailment such as migraine.

Prophylaxis: Measures taken to prevent the development of headache. These measures may include daily use of medication or nondrug therapies.

Propranolol: Beta blocker medication widely prescribed for hypertension and other chronic conditions, and effective in preventing migraine.

Rebound Headache: A chronic form of headache brought about by taking painkillers to excess (usually at least two days out of three). This is thought to be due to suppression of the body's own painfighting mechanisms.

Referred Pain: Pain perceived as occurring in a part of the body other than its true source.

Scintillation: The perception of twinkling light of varying intensity that can occur during the migraine aura.

Scotoma: An area of decreased or lost vision. Scotoma can be a characteristic symptom of migraine auras.

Serotonin: A neurotransmitter thought to be important in the mechanism of migraine headaches.

Sinus Headache: A headache caused by a clogged sinus cavity.

Sinusitis: Infection or inflammation of the sinuses. When the sinuses are infected, there is usually a low-grade fever, tenderness to touch over the sinuses, and a thick, colored nasal or post-nasal drainage.

Status Migrainosus: A severe unrelenting migraine headache associated with nausea and vomiting which lasts for several days and may not be manageable under outpatient care.

Stress: An emotionally disruptive or upsetting condition occurring in response to adverse external influences and capable of affecting physical health which can be characterized by increased heart rate, a rise in blood pressure, muscular tension, irritability and depression. Stress does not cause migraine but can be a migraine "trigger."

Sumatriptan: Refer to "Imitrex."

Synapse: The junction between nerve cells where a nerve impulse is transferred from one neuron to another.

Syncope: A brief loss of consciousness (a blackout).

Temporal Arteritis: A headache caused by inflamed arteries in the head and neck. It requires immediate medical attention.

TENS: Acronym for "transcutaneous electrical nerve stimulation." A TENS unit is a small battery powered device with wires that attach to electrodes pasted to the skin. Small electrical stimuli are applied to the skin in order to "tie up" nerve pathways that carry pain messages. This interferes with the transmission of pain messages to the brain, and can be helpful in certain chronic pain problems.

Tension Headache: As defined by the International Headache Society, a tension type headache is just the opposite of migraine. That is, the pain is on both sides of the head, is pressing and steady, rather than pulsating, is usually mild and does not cause incapacity and, is not worsened by ordinary daily activities. There is no associated nausea or sensitivity to light and noise.

TMJ: Acronym for "temporomandibular joint," or the joints where the jaw attaches to the skull just in front of the ears. It is sometimes linked to headache pain.

Trigeminal Nerve: The fifth cranial nerve, a major nerve of the face and head. It is related to nerve impulses that direct the muscles for jaw movement.

Trigger: Anything that can set off a migraine headache in a genetically predisposed individual is referred to as a "trigger." Common triggers include (but are not limited to) stress, changes in female hormone levels, skipping meals, certain odors such as perfume, sleeping late on weekends, sleep loss, alcohol, and some foods including cheese, chocolate and MSG.

Tumor Headache: A headache caused by a tumor, or growth, that presses on the brain. Symptoms can include seizures, loss of consciousness, projectile vomiting and speech disturbances. While migraine sufferers can experience severe pain (making them feel as though they may have a tumor), of those persons suffering from migraine, less than 0.004% actually suffer from a brain tumor.

Tyramine: A substance found in meats, cheese and red wine, which can trigger migraine in a susceptible individual.

Unilateral: Affecting or relating to only one side.

Vascular: Relating to the channels that carry body fluids, usually used in connection with the blood vessels.

Vascular Pain: Pain caused by the dilation or constriction of blood vessels. Dilating (enlarging) the blood vessels in the head causes pain when the vessels exert pressure on surrounding nerves. Constructing (narrowing) the blood vessels reduces the supply of blood to the brain. The tissue around the blood vessels may become inflamed, and chemical irritants build up in the area.

Vasoactive: Affecting the dilation or constriction of blood vessels.

Verapamil: A type of calcium channel blocker medication which can be effective in preventing migraine.

Vertigo: The sensation of spinning or whirling.

Chapter 34

Clinical Trials

Choosing to participate in a clinical trial is an important personal decision. The following frequently asked questions will provide you with detailed information about clinical trials. In addition, it is often helpful to talk to your health care provider, family members, or friends about deciding to join a trial. After you have identified some trial options, the next step is to contact the study research staff and ask questions about specific trials.

What is a clinical trial?

A clinical trial is a research study to answer specific questions about vaccines or new therapies or new ways of using known treatments. Clinical trials (also called medical research and research studies) are used to determine whether new drugs or treatments are both safe and effective. Carefully conducted clinical trials are the fastest and safest way to find treatments that work.

Ideas for clinical trials usually come from researchers. Once researchers test new therapies or procedures in the laboratory and get promising results, they begin planning Phase I clinical trials. New therapies are tested on people only after laboratory and animal studies show promising results.

The National Institutes of Health (NIH), an undated fact sheet available at www.ClinicalTrials.gov, cited September 2001. For information about clinical trials currently recruiting headache patients, visit www.ClinicalTrials.gov and enter the search term "headache."

What is a protocol?

All clinical trials are based on a set of rules called a protocol. A protocol describes what types of people may participate in the trial; the schedule of tests, procedures, medications, and dosages; and the length of the study. While in a clinical trial, participants are seen regularly by the research staff to monitor their health and to determine the safety and effectiveness of their treatment.

What are clinical trial phases?

Clinical trials of experimental drugs proceed through four phases:

- In Phase I clinical trials, researchers test a new drug or treatment in a small group of people (20-80) for the first time to evaluate its safety, determine a safe dosage range, and identify side effects.

- In Phase II clinical trials, the study drug or treatment is given to a larger group of people (100-300) to see if it is effective and to further evaluate its safety.

- In Phase III studies, the study drug or treatment is given to large groups of people (1,000-3,000) to confirm its effectiveness, monitor side effects, compare it to commonly used treatments, and collect information that will allow the drug or treatment to be used safely.

- Phase IV studies are done after the drug or treatment has been marketed. These studies continue testing the study drug or treatment to collect information about their effect in various populations and any side effects associated with long-term use.

What protections are there for people who participate in clinical trials?

The government has strict guidelines and safeguards to protect people who choose to participate in clinical trials. Every clinical trial in the U.S. must be approved and monitored by an Institutional Review Board (IRB) to make sure the risks are as low as possible and are worth any potential benefits.

An IRB is an independent committee of physicians, statisticians, community advocates, and others that ensures that a clinical trial is ethical and the rights of study participants are protected. All institutions that conduct or support biomedical research involving people must, by federal regulation, have an IRB that initially approves and periodically reviews the research.

What is informed consent?

Informed consent is the process of learning the key facts about a clinical trial before you decide whether or not to participate. These facts include:

- Why the research is being done.

- What the researchers want to accomplish.

- What will be done during the trial and for how long.

- What risks are involved in the trial.

- What benefits can be expected from the trial.

- What other treatments are available.

- The fact that you have the right to leave the trial at any time.

If you are considering joining a clinical trial, the research staff will give you informed consent documents that include the details about the study. If English is not your native language, you can ask for the consent documents in languages other than English. Since joining a clinical trial is an important decision, you should ask the research team any questions you may have about the study and the consent forms before you make a decision.

It is also a good idea to take the consent documents home and discuss them with family members or friends. Talking about your options can help you to feel comfortable with your decision. If you decide to join the clinical trial, be sure to ask for a copy of the informed consent documents so you can review them at any time.

Remember informed consent is more than signing a form. It is a process that continues through the study. You should feel free to ask the research team questions before, during, and after the study. Informed consent continues as long as you are in the study.

Who can participate in a clinical trial?

All clinical trials have guidelines about who can get into the program. Guidelines are based on such factors as age, type of disease, medical history, and current medical condition. Before you join a clinical trial, you must qualify for the study. Some research studies seek volunteers with illnesses or conditions to be studied in the clinical trial, while others need healthy volunteers. Healthy volunteers participate in Phase I trials, vaccine studies, and trials on research on preventive care for children or adults.

The factors that allow you to participate in a clinical trial are called inclusion criteria and the factors that keep you from participating are called exclusion criteria. It is important to note that inclusion and exclusion criteria are not used to reject people personally. Instead, the criteria are used to identify appropriate participants and keep them safe. The criteria help ensure that researchers will be able to answer the questions they plan to study.

Who sponsors clinical trials?

Clinical trials are sponsored by government agencies: such as the National Institutes of Health (NIH); pharmaceutical companies; individual physician-investigators; health care institutions such as health maintenance organizations (HMOs); and organizations that develop medical devices or equipment. Trials can take place in a variety of locations, such as hospitals, universities, doctors' offices, or community clinics.

What happens during a clinical trial?

The clinical trial process depends on the kind of trial you participate in. The team will include doctors and nurses as well as social workers and other health care professionals. They will check your health at the beginning of the trial, give you specific instructions for participating in the trial, monitor you carefully during the trial, and stay in touch with you after the study.

Some clinical trials involve more tests and doctor visits than you would normally have for your illness or condition. For all types of trials, you will work with a research team. Your participation will be most successful if you follow the protocol carefully and stay in contact with the research staff. Some terms that will help you understand what happens in a trial are defined below.

What is a placebo?

A placebo is an inactive pill, liquid, or powder that has no treatment value. In clinical trials, experimental treatments are often compared with placebos to assess the treatment's effectiveness. In some studies, the participants in the control group will receive a placebo instead of an active drug or treatment.

What is a control or control group?

A control is the standard by which experimental observations are evaluated. In many clinical trials, one group of patients will be given an experimental drug or treatment, while the control group is given either a standard treatment for the illness or a placebo.

What is a blinded or masked study?

A blinded or masked study is one in which participants do not know whether they are in the experimental or control group in a research study. Those in the experimental group get the medications or treatments being tested, while those in the control group get a standard treatment or no treatment.

What is a double-blind or double-masked study?

A double-blind or double-masked study is one in which neither the participants nor the study staff know which participants are receiving the experimental treatment and which ones are getting either a standard treatment or a placebo. These studies are performed so neither the patients' nor the doctors' expectations about the experimental drug can influence the outcome.

What are side effects and adverse reactions?

Side effects are any undesired actions or effects of drug or treatment. Negative or adverse effects may include headache, nausea, hair loss, skin irritation, or other physical problems. Experimental treatments must be evaluated for both immediate and long-term side effects.

What are the benefits and risks associated with clinical trials?

There are both benefits and risks associated with clinical trials. By participating in a clinical trial, you can:

* Take an active role in your own health care.

* Gain access to new treatments that are not available to the public.

- Obtain expert medical care at leading health care facilities during the trial.

- Help others by contributing to medical research.

Clinical trials have risks:

- There may be side effects or adverse reactions to medications or treatments.

- The treatment may not be effective for you.

- The protocol may require a lot of your time for trips to the study site, treatments, hospital stays, or complex dosage requirements.

What should I know before I join a clinical trial?

You should know as much as possible about the research study. It is important for you to feel very comfortable asking questions and the staff should answer them in a way you can understand.

How should I prepare for the meeting with the research coordinator or doctor?

- Plan ahead and write down the questions you want to ask.

- Ask a friend or relative to come with you for support and to hear the responses to your questions.

- Bring a tape recorder so you can replay the discussion after you get home.

What questions should I ask?

Some questions you might ask about the research include:

- Why is this research being done?

- What is the purpose of the study?

- Who is sponsoring the study?

- Who has reviewed and approved this study?

- Why does the research team think the treatment, drug, or medical device will work?

Some questions about your participation in the study include:

- Where is the study site?
- What kinds of therapies, procedures, and/or tests will I have during the trial?
- Will they hurt? If so, for how long?
- How will the tests in the study compare to tests I would have outside the study?
- How long will the study last?
- How often will I have to go to the study site?
- Who will provide my medical care after the study ends?
- Will I be able to take my regular medications during the trial?
- What medications, procedures, or treatments must I avoid while in the study?
- What are my responsibilities during the study?
- Will I have to be in the hospital during the study?
- Will the study researchers work with my doctor while I am in the study?
- Can anyone find out that I am participating in a study?
- Can I talk to other people in the study?
- Will I be able to find out the results of the trial?

Questions about risks and benefits include:

- How do the possible risks and benefits of the study compare with approved treatments for me?
- What are the possible immediate and long-term side effects?

Other questions include:

- What other treatment options do I have?
- Will I have to pay anything to participate in the study?
- What are the charges likely to be?
- Is my insurance likely to cover those expenses?

Should I continue working with my primary health care provider if I participate in a trial?

Yes. Most clinical trials provide short-term treatments related to a designated illness or condition, but not extended or complete primary health care. In addition, by having your health care provider work with the research team, you can ensure that your other medications or treatments will not conflict with the clinical trial protocol.

Can I leave a clinical trial after it has begun?

Yes. You can leave a clinical trial at any time. If you plan to stop participating, let the research team know why you are leaving the study.

Will I be paid for participating in a clinical trial?

Some clinical trials will pay you for joining the trial, while others will not. In some programs, researchers will reimburse you for expenses associated with participating in the research. Such expenses may include transportation costs, child care, meals, and accommodations.

Chapter 35

Getting Good Care from Managed Care

As businesses cut back on employee benefits, managed care increasingly is the way healthcare is delivered. For those who do not have health insurance through their employer, membership in an HMO or managed care organization (MCO) usually offers the only affordable access to routine and emergency healthcare.

Managed care organizations work to control the costs of healthcare by reducing the number of unnecessary medications, procedures, and consultations with specialists. Those cost controls can be health promoting in themselves by protecting patients from possible side effects and complications of avoidable treatments. Many MCOs also focus on providing excellent preventive care-prenatal care for expectant mothers, well-baby examinations, vaccinations, disease screening, and education in better self-care.

But, MCOs' cost-cutting measures can work against the best interests of patients with chronic but benign conditions such as headache. Headache sufferers who do not get adequate relief from standard medications too often find that their MCO is reluctant to authorize referrals to headache specialists or refuses to pay for more expensive headache medications.

If you are in a managed care organization now or thinking of joining one, you need to be sure you will get the care you need for your headaches—now and in the future if the severity of your headaches changes.

© 2000 American Headache Society (AHS), available online at http://www.ahsnet.org; reprinted with permission.

303

Most people wouldn't sign a lease or buy a car without questions and research. Healthcare decisions that impact your health and your quality of life are at least as important. As with any other service or product, you will get more from managed care if you are an active and educated consumer. It is worth the time and effort to understand your options, and to appeal decisions that affect your health and well-being.

What to Ask Before Joining a Managed Care Plan

If your employer offers you a choice of healthcare plans, a little bit of research at enrollment time may save you aggravation and out-of-pocket expenses if you should need to see a specialist or change to a more expensive medication.

1. Is it a closed network plan, or a point-of-service or preferred provider plan? If it is a closed network plan, your choice of specialists is restricted to the network; with the other plans, you can access specialists outside the network for a higher co-payment.

2. Can I choose my primary care physician or is one assigned to me?

3. Can I choose to see a specialist or must all referrals to specialists be authorized by my primary care physician?

4. Does the plan cover home injection of medications?

5. Does the plan cover non-drug therapies such as biofeedback or acupuncture?

6. What is the appeals process if referral or reimbursement is denied to me?

7. How are the physicians in the plan paid-on a fee-for-service basis or by capitation?

Under capitation, physicians are paid a fixed amount per patient regardless of how much care that individual needs. This creates an incentive to limit the amount of care provided. Headache patients often need longer and more frequent consultations to establish a successful treatment plan.

Denials—Don't Take "No" for an Answer

If you are denied a needed referral to a specialist or reimbursement for medication or other medical care, there is much you can do to try to reverse that decision.

Step One. Be sure you follow all the steps in the appeals procedure used by your managed care organization (MCO). Save copies of all forms and all correspondence and keep a log for tracking the dates of correspondence, following up if you don't get a reply. Log any phone conversations you have with the MCO's staff. Keep careful records of the names, job titles, and phone numbers of all your contacts as you make your appeals.

Step Two. Speak to your company's benefits representative, if your coverage is through your employer and the business is large enough to have a person in charge of benefits.

Step Three. Ask your doctor to write a letter in your behalf, addressed to the medical director of the managed care organization (MCO).

Step Four. Write to the medical director yourself.

Step Five. If there is no response, send a second certified letter enclosing the first one and asking for an appeal hearing.

Step Six. Contact the insurance executive of your state, your state representative and senator, and U.S. senator and representative. Send copies of these letters to the medical director of the MCO.

Step Seven. Consider whether you wish to consult an attorney; if yes, send another certified letter announcing your intention to retain an attorney. If the response is still unsatisfactory, have your attorney write or call the MCO to state your case and your determination to seek legal remedies.

Step Eight. Publicize your case. Send a letter detailing the repeated denials to the local newspaper. Send letters to local and national patient support and advocacy organizations (including ACHE). Again, send copies of these letters to the medical director of the MCO.

Put It in Writing—to Everyone

If your managed care organization (MCO) is denying you needed care for your headaches, you can do something about it. You may feel that it's useless to struggle against managed care rules and bureaucracy, but you do have three important tools at your disposal: persistence, political pressure, and publicity. Don't hesitate to use them. All they will cost you is stationery, stamps and a few hours of your time.

Send a letter to the medical director of your managed care company. (Ask your company's benefit manager or call the MCO to get the medical director's name and address.) Use this letter to appeal a denial of referral to a headache specialist outside the company's network of healthcare providers.

If an appeal to the medical director is unsuccessful, you may send a letter to your state insurance commissioner and/or your state representative and senator, and your US representative and senator, detailing the denial of referral you experienced. Be sure to send copies of these letters to the medical director of your managed care company.

To obtain names and addresses elected officials, look in your telephone directory for the local number of the League of Women Voters and ask for the name and address of your representatives. If you have Internet access, you can find up-to-date contact information on the "Vote Smart" website, http://www.vote-smart.org.

If your managed care company has refused to pay for medication or other headache treatments that your doctor considers necessary, send a letter appealing the denial of reimbursement to the medical director of your managed care organization.

If your appeal to the medical director is unsuccessful, you may then send a letter to your state insurance commissioner and/or your state representative and senator, and your US representative and senator, detailing the denial of reimbursement you experienced. Be sure to send copies of these letters to the medical director of your managed care organization.

If your medical plan is provided by your employer, you may wish to notify your benefits manager of the problems you've encountered with the healthcare plan and enlist his/her help in appealing the denial as a first step. If you are in a smaller company that does not have a benefits manager, you can consider whether you should also inform your human resources/personnel director or employer of the denials. This is an individual decision based on your standing in the company and your sense of your employer's readiness to help with such an issue.

If your current doctor is supportive of your efforts to appeal the MCO's decision, you may ask him or her to write a letter to support your case, or to sign one that you have prepared or ask him or her to write to the Medical Director of the MCO in your behalf.

Bear in mind that your doctor may feel uncomfortable with your request and say no. In some areas, a single HMO or MCO may control a large portion of the doctor's practice. He or she may be legitimately worried about being decertified-dropped from the company's list of approved providers. Or your doctor may just feel too pressured for time to fight every denial. If so, don't press the point, but continue with your own letter-writing campaign.

Chapter 36

Headache Clinics

Alabama

The Ford Headache Clinic
Montclair Road, Suite 102
Birmingham, AL
Toll Free: 800-307-PAIN
Tel: 205-871-2243
Internet: http://
www.fordheadacheclinic.com

California

The California Medical Clinic for Headache
16500 Ventura Blvd., Suite 245
Encino, CA 91436
Tel: 818-986-4248
Tel: 310-289-9440
Internet: http://
www.headachedoc.com
E-Mail: info@headachedoc.com

Neurological Associates
1020 29th Street, #360
Sacramento, CA 95816
Tel: 916-733-8915

San Francisco Headache Clinic
909 Hyde Street, Suite 322
San Francisco, CA 94109
Tel: 415-673-4600
Fax: 415-673-9532
Internet: http://www.sfcrc.com

Headache and Facial Pain Clinic
Department of Neurology
Kaiser Permanente Medical Center
27400 Hesperian Boulevard
Hayward, CA 94545-4297
Tel: 510-784-4607

Information in this chapter was compiled from several sources deemed reliable; all contact information was verified and updated in October 2001.

Colorado

Colorado Neuro and Headache Center
1155 E. 18th Avenue
Denver, CO 80218
Tel: 303-839-9900
Fax: 303-839-5470

Connecticut

New England Center for Headache
778 Long Ridge Road
Stamford, CT 06902
Tel: 203-968-1799
Fax: 203 968 8303

Florida

The Hyde Park Headache Center, Inc.
210 West Platt Street
Tampa, FL 33606
Tel: 813-254-8878
Fax: 813-258-2610
Internet: http://
www.hpheadachecenter.com
E-Mail:
info@hpheadachecenter.com

Georgia

Neurology & Headache Specialists of Atlanta
2665 North Decatur Road
Suite 630
Decatur, GA 30033
Tel: 404-294-3040

Illinois

Diamond Headache Clinic
467 West Deming Place
Chicago, IL 60614
Toll Free: 800-432-3224
Tel: 773-878-5558
Internet: http://
www.diamondheadache.com
E-Mail:
clinic@diamondheadache.com

The Robbins Headache Clinic
1535 Lake Cook Road, Suite 506
Northbrook, IL 60062
Tel: 847-480-9399
Internet: http://
www.headachedrugs.com
E-Mail: headachedrugs@aol.com

Kansas

Headache Clinic
Department of Neurology
University of Kansas Medical Center
3901 Rainbow Boulevard
Kansas City, KS 66160-7314
Tel: 913-588-6970
Fax: 913-588-6965
Internet: http://kumc.edu

Louisiana

The Neurology Clinic
1415 Tulane Avenue
New Orleans, LA 70112
Tel: 504-588-5231
Fax: 504-584-1727

New Orleans Headache and Neurology Clinic
120 Meadowcrest Street, #420
Gretna, LA 70056
Tel: 504-391-7547
Fax: 504-391-7541

Maryland

Headache Management Center
10780 Hickory Ridge Road
Columbia, MD 21044
Tel: 410-997-3113
Fax: 410-997-1828

University of Maryland Pediatric Headache Clinic
22 South Greene Street
Baltimore, MD 21201
Toll Free: 800-492-5539
Internet: http://www.umm.edu/peds-neuro

Michigan

Headache Clinic
Department of Neurology
Henry Ford Health System
2799 West Grand Blvd.
Detroit, MI 48202
Tel: 313-916-3396
Fax: 313-916-3014

Michigan Head Pain & Neurological Institute
3120 Professional Drive
Ann Arbor, MI 48104-5199
Tel: 734-973-1155
Fax: 734-677-2422
Internet: http://www.mhni.com

Minnesota

Head and Neck Pain Centers of Minnesota
2365 Ariel Street
St. Paul, MN 55109
Tel: 651-777-8987
Fax: 651-777-2366
Internet: http://minnesotaheadache.neurohub.net

Missouri

Chronic Headache Program
Saint Louis University Health Sciences Center
1129 Macklind
St. Louis, MO 63110
Tel: 314-534-0200
Fax: 314 534 7996
Internet: http://www.slbmi.com

Ryan Headache Center
1585 Woodlake Drive, Suite 200
St. Louis, MO 63017
Tel: 314-205-0007
Fax: 314-205-8849

The Saint Louis Behavioral Medicine Institute
Chronic Headache Program
1129 Macklind Avenue
St. Louis, MO 63110
Tel: 314-534-0200
Fax: 314-534-7996
Internet: http://www.slbmi.com/othersrvcs.htm
E-Mail: info@slbmi.com

New Hampshire

Dartmouth-Hitchcock Medical Center (DHMC)
Department of Neurology, Headache Center
One Medical Center Drive
Lebanon, NH 03756
Tel: 603-650-5000
Internet: http://www.hitchcock.org

New Jersey

University Headache Center
513 S. Lenola Rd.
Moorestown, NJ 08057
Tel: 856-234-7421
Internet: http://som.umdnj.edu

Pain Management Center
Holy Name Hospital
718 Teaneck Road
Teaneck, NJ 07666
Tel: 201-833-3000
Internet: http://www.holyname.org

The Princeton Headache Clinic
11 State Road, Suite 300
Princeton, NJ 08540
Tel: 609-863-5404
Internet: http://www.princetonheadache.com

New York

The Coddon Headache Institute
Neurology Faculty Associates
1031 5th Ave Box 1139
5 East 98th Street
New York, NY 10029
Tel: 212-369-5888

Headache Clinic
The Mount Sinai Medical Center
One Gustave Levy Place
New York, NY 10029
Tel: 212-241-7138
Fax: 212-876-7775

Montefiore Headache Unit
111 East 210th Street
Bronx, NY 10467
Tel: 718-920-4203
Fax: 718-920-8341
Internet: http://www.montefiore.org

The New York Headache Center
30 East 76th Street
New York, NY 10021
Tel: 212-794-3350
Fax: 212-794-3550
Internet: http://nyheadache.com
E-Mail: nyheadache@aol.com

Ohio

University Hospital Cleveland
11100 Euclid Avenue
Hannah House 5
Cleveland, OH 44106
Tel: 216-844-1476
Internet: http://www.uhhs.com

Ohio University Headache Project
Institute of Health and Behavioral Sciences
Ohio University
032 Porter Hal
Athens, OH 45701
Tel: 740-593-1060
Fax: 740-593-0110
Internet: http://www.ohiou.edu

Oklahoma

Headache & Neurological Center of Oklahoma, Inc.
6585 S. Yale, Suite 620
Tulsa, OK 74136
Tel: 918-481-4781
Fax: 918-481-4796

Oregon

The Oregon Headache Clinic
1001 Molalla Avenue, Suite 111
Oregon City, OR 97045
Tel: 503-656-9844
Internet: http://
migrainesurvival.com/
clinic.html
E-Mail:
noheadaches@migrainesurvival.com

Pennsylvania

Comprehensive Headache Center at Thomas Jefferson University
8130 Gibbon Building
111 South 11th Street
Philadelphia, PA 19107
Tel: 215-955-2243
Fax: 215-955-1960
Internet: http://
www.jeffersonhospital.org

Tennessee

Memphis Area Headache Center
3960 Knight Arnold, Suite 302
Memphis, TN 38118
Tel: 901-366-0558
Fax: 901-363-3235

Texas

Anodyne Pain Care
5446 Glen Lakes Drive
Dallas, TX 75231
Tel: 214-750-6664
Fax: 214-750-6671

Dallas Headache Clinic
8226 Douglas Avenue, Suite 325
Dallas, TX 75225
Tel: 214-902-0800

Texas Headache Institute
1804 N.E. Loop 410, Suite 100
San Antonio, TX 78217
Tel: 210-805-8484

Houston Headache Clinic

1213 Hermann Drive, Suite 350
Houston, TX 77004
Tel: 713-528-1916
Fax: 713-526-6369

Virginia

The Neurology and Headache Treatment Center

4660 Kenmore Avenue
Suite 900
Alexandria, VA 22304
Tel: 703-212-0700
Fax: 703-212-0705
Internet: http://
www.neurologychannel.com/
neuro-headache

Washington

The Headache Clinic

116 107th Avenue, N.E.
Bellevue, WA 98004
Toll Free: 800-868-4545
Internet: http://
www.halcyon.com/headache

Virginia Mason Clinic

1100 Ninth Avenue
Seattle, WA 98111
Tel: 206-341-0420
Fax: 206-625-7240

Wisconsin

University of Wisconsin Headache Clinic

1552 University Avenue
Madison, WI 53705
Tel: 608-262-0519
Fax: 608-262-9160

Chapter 37

Headache Resources on the Internet

American Academy of Pain Medicine
http://www.painmed.org

The American Academy of Pain Medicine (AAPM) is an organization that provides for quality care to patients suffering with pain, through the education and training of all physicians, through research, and through the advancement of the specialty of pain medicine.

American Council for Headache Education (ACHE)
http://www.ache.net

The American Council for Headache Education (ACHE) was created in 1990 through an initiative of the American Headache Society (AHS). ACHE is a nonprofit patient-health professional partnership dedicated to advancing the treatment and management of headache and raising the public awareness of headache as a valid, biologically based illness.

American Academy of Neurology (AAN)
http://www.aan.com

The American Academy of Neurology is a medical specialty society established to advance the art and science of neurology, and thereby promote the best possible care for patients with neurological disorders.

American Pain Society

http://www.ampainsoc.org

The American Pain Society (APS) is a multidisciplinary organization of basic and clinical scientists, practicing clinicians, policy analysts, and others working to advance pain-related research, education, treatment and professional practice.

The Brain Matters

http://www.thebrainmatters.org

A group of sixty advocacy and patient support groups has teamed up to focus public attention on the personal and societal impacts of neurological diseases.

British Association for the Study of Headache

http://www.bash.org.uk

The British Association for the Study of Headache (BASH) is an organization whose objectives are to relieve persons suffering from headache by the advancement of scientific study.

Headache Impact Test

http://www.headachetest.com

The Headache Impact Test(tm) (HIT) is a tool to measure the impact headaches have on a person's ability to function on the job, at school, at home, and in social situations. The score indicates the impact that headaches have on normal daily life and the ability to function. After taking the HIT survey, you can print a report for yourself and one to share with your doctor.

International Headache Society

http://www.i-h-s.org

The International Headache Society (IHS) is an organization whose strategic objective is to alleviate the burden of headache worldwide, in particular by promoting research into causes, mechanisms, diagnosis, treatment and other aspects of headache.

JAMA Migraine Information Center

http://www.ama-assn.org/special/migraine.htm

The *JAMA* Migraine Information Center is designed as a resource for physicians and other health professionals. The site is produced and maintained by *JAMA* editors and staff under the direction of an editorial review board of leading migraine authorities.

Journal of the American Medical Association *(JAMA)*
http://www.ama-assn.org/public/journals/jama/jamahome.htm

The *Journal of the American Medical Association (JAMA)* is an international peer-reviewed general medical journal designed to promote the science and art of medicine and the betterment of the public health.

MAGNUM
http://www.migraines.org

MAGNUM (Migraine Awareness Group: A National Understanding for Migraineurs) was created to bring public awareness, utilizing the electronic, print, and artistic media, to the fact that Migraine is a true organic neurologic disease, to assist Migraine sufferers, their families, and co-workers, and to help improve the quality of life of Migraine sufferers worldwide.

MEDLINEplus
http://www.nlm.nih.gov/medlineplus

MEDLINEplus is a service that provides access to extensive information about specific diseases and conditions and also has links to consumer health information from the National Institutes of Health, dictionaries, lists of hospitals and physicians, health information in Spanish and other languages, and clinical trials.

The Migraine Trust
http://www.migrainetrust.org

The Migraine Trust aims to help people with migraine and other headaches, as well as organizations, groups, and individuals who work to support them through research and care.

PainLink
http://www.edc.org/PainLink

PainLink is a virtual community if health professionals working in institutions that are committed to alleviating pain.

PubMed

http://www.ncbi.nlm.nih.gov/PubMed

PubMed is the National Library of Medicine's search service that provides access to over 10 million citations in MEDLINE, PreMEDLINE, and other related databases, with links to participating online journals.

Trigeminal Neuralgia Association

http://neurosurgery.mgh.harvard.edu/tna/#services

The Trigeminal Neuralgia Association (TNA) is a nonprofit organization founded in 1990 by individuals who had been directly affected by the pain of trigeminal neuralgia, as patients or as family members of a patient. TNA provides help and support for trigeminal neuralgia patients and other face pain patients, care givers, and medical professionals.

World Headache Alliance

http://www.w-h-a.org

The World Headache Alliance (WHA) is a global alliance of lay organizations whose aim is to provide a comprehensive, and frequently updated, information service for people who suffer from severe headache or migraine, and their families and friends.

Worldwide Congress of Pain

http://www.pain.com

Chapter 38

Recommended Reading

Basics of Acupuncture
Gabriel Stux (Editor) and Bruce Pomerantz
Published by Springer Verlag, Berlin, Germany, 4th Edition, 1998
ISBN: 3540632352

Between Heaven and Earth:
A Guide to Chinese Medicine
Harriet Beinfield and Efrem Korngold
Published by Ballantine Books, New York, NY, 1991; reprint 1992
ISBN: 0345379748

Complete Idiot's Guide to Migraines and Other Headaches
Jeanne Rejaunier; Dennis Fox, M.D.
Published by Alpha Books, 2000
ISBN: 0028639464

Conquering Your Migraine:
The Essential Guide to Understanding and Treating
Migraines for All Sufferers and Their Families
Seymour Diamond, M.D.
Published by Fireside, 2001
ISBN: 0684873109

References in this list were compiled from various sources in December 2001. Check your local library or favorite bookstore for availablitiy.

Diets to Help Migraine
Martin Budd
Published by Thorsons Publishing, 1998
ISBN: 0722533268

Headache Help:
A Complete Guide to Understanding Headaches and the Medications That Relieve Them
Lawrence Robbins, M.D. and Susan S. Lang
Published by Houghton Mifflin Company, 2000
ISBN: 0618044361

Headaches in Children:
Practical Informative Guide for Parents, Teachers and Paramedical Personnel
Leonardo Garcia-Mendez, M.D.
Published by Lemar Publishers, 1996
ISBN: 0963926918

Headache Relief for Women:
How You Can Manage and Prevent Pain
Alan M. Rapoport; Fred D. Sheftell
Published by Little Brown & Co., 1996
ISBN: 0316733911

Management of Headache and Headache Medications
Lawrence Robbins, M.D.
Published by Springer Verlag, 2000
ISBN: 0387989447

A Manual of Acupuncture
Peter Deadman and Mazin Al-Khafaji
Published by Eastland Press, 1998
ISBN: 0951054678

Migraine
Oliver Sacks
Published by Vintage Books, 1999
ISBN: 037570406X

Migraines—Everything You Need to Know about Their
Cause and Cure
Arthur Elkind, M.D.
Published by Avon Books, 1997
ISBN: 0380790777

Migraine Headaches and the Foods You Eat:
200 Recipes for Relief
Agnes Peg Hartnell; G. Scott Tyler
Published by Chronimed Publishers, 1997
ISBN: 0471346861

No More Headaches No More Migraines
Zuzana Bic; Frances Bic; L. Francis Bic
Published by Avery Penguin Putnam, 1999
ISBN: 0895299240

Principles and Practice of Contemporary Acupuncture
Sung J. Liao, Matthew Lee, and Lorenz K.Y. Ng
Published by Marcel Dekker, New York, NY, 1994
ISBN: 0824792912

Taking Control of Your Headaches—How to Get the
Treatment You Need
Paul Duckro, Ph.D.; William Richardson, M.D.; Janet E. Marshall,
R.N.
Published by The Guilford Press, 1999
ISBN: 1572304715

The Chinese Way to Healing:
Many Paths to Wholeness
Misha Ruth Cohen
Published by The Berkeley Publishing Group, New York, NY, 1996
ISBN: 0399522328

The Headache Prevention Cookbook:
Eating Right to Prevent Migraines and Other Headaches
David R. Marks, M.D.; Laura Marks.
Published by Houghton Mifflin Co., 2000
ISBN: 039597163

The Web That Has No Weaver:
Understanding Chinese Medicine, 2ⁿᵈ Edition
Ted Kaptchuk
Published by McGraw-Hill, New York, NY, 2000
0809228408

The Yellow Emperor's Classic of Internal Medicine:
A New Translation of the Neijing Suwen With Commentary
Maoshing Ni
Published by Shambhala Publications, 1995
ISBN: 1570620806

Wolff's Headache and Other Head Pain
Stephen D. Silberstein (Editor); Richard B. Lipton (Editor); and Don Dalessio
Published by Oxford University Press, 2001
ISBN: 0195435180

Index

Index

Page numbers followed by 'n' indicate a footnote. Page numbers in *italics* indicate a table or illustration.

A

325

"Cluster Headache" (National Headache Foundation) 47n
cocaine hydrochloride, cluster headache 15
The Coddon Headache Institute, contact information 312
codeine
 combination analgesics 110
 opioid drugs 115
 pregnancy *217*
Cognex (tacrine) 172
cognition restructuring, described 17
cognitive-behavioral therapy
 defined 284
 migraine prevention 78, 79
 see also behavior modification
Colorado Neuro and Headache Center, contact information 310
common migraine
 defined 284
 described 7
Compazine (prochlorperazine)
 migraine headache 111
 pregnancy *218*
complementary medicine 163–66
Complete Idiot's Guide to Migraines and Other Headaches (Rejaunier, Fox) 319
Comprehensive Headache Center at Thomas Jefferson University, contact information 313
computed tomography (CT scan)
 brain tumor 274
 headache diagnosis 6
  children 69
 stroke diagnosis 254–55
computerized axial tomography (CAT scan), defined 283
computer use 28
congeners 56
Conquering Your Migraine (Diamond) 319
control group, defined 299
Cooke, David A. 23n
cordotomy, described 190
coronary artery disease, hormone replacement therapy 230–31
corticosteroids
 cluster headache 49
 migraine headache 34

cortisone, pregnancy *219*
Coumadin (warfarin) 265
Council of Colleges of Acupuncture and Oriental Medicine, contact information 146
counseling, migraine headache 33
CPH *see* chronic paroxysmal hemicrania
cyclizine, pregnancy *218*
cyproheptadine
 postpartum migraine 224
 pregnancy *218*

D

daily headache, defined 284
Dallas Headache Clinic, contact information 313
Dartmouth-Hitchcock Medical Center, contact information 312
Darvocet 116
Darvon 116
ddI 171
Debakote (divalproex) 117
deep breathing, headache management 152
deep relaxation, headache management 151–54
Demerol (meperidine) 117
Depakote (divalproex)
 birth defects 216
 frequent headaches 112, 117
depression
 defined 285
 headache 20, 56, 91–94, 209
 migraine headache 237
"Depression and Headaches" (National Headache Foundation) 91n
desipramine, pregnancy *219*
dexamethasone
 defined 285
 pregnancy *219*
DHE *see* dihydroergotamine
DHE-45 (dihydroergotamine) 109, 116
diabetes mellitus, stroke risk 260
diagnosis, defined 285
Diamond Headache Clinic, contact information 310

Health Reference Series
COMPLETE CATALOG

Adolescent Health Sourcebook

Basic Consumer Health Information about Common Medical, Mental, and Emotional Concerns in Adolescents, Including Facts about Acne, Body Piercing, Mononucleosis, Nutrition, Eating Disorders, Stress, Depression, Behavior Problems, Peer Pressure, Violence, Gangs, Drug Use, Puberty, Sexuality, Pregnancy, Learning Disabilities, and More

Along with a Glossary of Terms and Other Resources for Further Help and Information

Edited by Chad T. Kimball. 700 pages. 2002. 0-7808-0248-9. $78.

■

AIDS Sourcebook, 1st Edition

Basic Information about AIDS and HIV Infection, Featuring Historical and Statistical Data, Current Research, Prevention, and Other Special Topics of Interest for Persons Living with AIDS

Along with Source Listings for Further Assistance

Edited by Karen Bellenir and Peter D. Dresser. 831 pages. 1995. 0-7808-0031-1. $78.

"One strength of this book is its practical emphasis. The intended audience is the lay reader . . . useful as an educational tool for health care providers who work with AIDS patients. Recommended for public libraries as well as hospital or academic libraries that collect consumer materials."
— *Bulletin of the Medical Library Association, Jan '96*

"This is the most comprehensive volume of its kind on an important medical topic. Highly recommended for all libraries." — *Reference Book Review, '96*

"Very useful reference for all libraries."
— *Choice, Association of College and Research Libraries, Oct '95*

"There is a wealth of information here that can provide much educational assistance. It is a must book for all libraries and should be on the desk of each and every congressional leader. Highly recommended."
— *AIDS Book Review Journal, Aug '95*

"Recommended for most collections."
— *Library Journal, Jul '95*

■

AIDS Sourcebook, 2nd Edition

Basic Consumer Health Information about Acquired Immune Deficiency Syndrome (AIDS) and Human Immunodeficiency Virus (HIV) Infection, Featuring Updated Statistical Data, Reports on Recent Research and Prevention Initiatives, and Other Special Topics of Interest for Persons Living with AIDS, Including New Antiretroviral Treatment Options, Strategies for Com-

bating Opportunistic Infections, Information about Clinical Trials, and More

Along with a Glossary of Important Terms and Resource Listings for Further Help and Information

Edited by Karen Bellenir. 751 pages. 1999. 0-7808-0225-X. $78.

"Highly recommended."
— *American Reference Books Annual, 2000*

"Excellent sourcebook. This continues to be a highly recommended book. There is no other book that provides as much information as this book provides."
— *AIDS Book Review Journal, Dec-Jan 2000*

"Recommended reference source."
— *Booklist, American Library Association, Dec '99*

"A solid text for college-level health libraries."
— *The Bookwatch, Aug '99*

Cited in *Reference Sources for Small and Medium-Sized Libraries, American Library Association, 1999*

■

Alcoholism Sourcebook

Basic Consumer Health Information about the Physical and Mental Consequences of Alcohol Abuse, Including Liver Disease, Pancreatitis, Wernicke-Korsakoff Syndrome (Alcoholic Dementia), Fetal Alcohol Syndrome, Heart Disease, Kidney Disorders, Gastrointestinal Problems, and Immune System Compromise and Featuring Facts about Addiction, Detoxification, Alcohol Withdrawal, Recovery, and the Maintenance of Sobriety

Along with a Glossary and Directories of Resources for Further Help and Information

Edited by Karen Bellenir. 613 pages. 2000. 0-7808-0325-6. $78.

"This title is one of the few reference works on alcoholism for general readers. For some readers this will be a welcome complement to the many self-help books on the market. Recommended for collections serving general readers and consumer health collections."
— *E-Streams, Mar '01*

"This book is an excellent choice for public and academic libraries."
— *American Reference Books Annual, 2001*

"Recommended reference source."
— *Booklist, American Library Association, Dec '00*

"Presents a wealth of information on alcohol use and abuse and its effects on the body and mind, treatment, and prevention." — *SciTech Book News, Dec '00*

"Important new health guide which packs in the latest consumer information about the problems of alcoholism." — *Reviewer's Bookwatch, Nov '00*

SEE ALSO Drug Abuse Sourcebook, Substance Abuse Sourcebook

Allergies Sourcebook, 1st Edition

Basic Information about Major Forms and Mechanisms of Common Allergic Reactions, Sensitivities, and Intolerances, Including Anaphylaxis, Asthma, Hives and Other Dermatologic Symptoms, Rhinitis, and Sinusitis

Along with Their Usual Triggers Like Animal Fur, Chemicals, Drugs, Dust, Foods, Insects, Latex, Pollen, and Poison Ivy, Oak, and Sumac; Plus Information on Prevention, Identification, and Treatment

Edited by Allan R. Cook. 611 pages. 1997. 0-7808-0036-2. $78.

Allergies Sourcebook, 2nd Edition

Basic Consumer Health Information about Allergic Disorders, Triggers, Reactions, and Related Symptoms, Including Anaphylaxis, Rhinitis, Sinusitis, Asthma, Dermatitis, Conjunctivitis, and Multiple Chemical Sensitivity

Along with Tips on Diagnosis, Prevention, and Treatment, Statistical Data, a Glossary, and a Directory of Sources for Further Help and Information

Edited by Annemarie S. Muth. 598 pages. 2002. 0-7808-0376-0. $78.

Alternative Medicine Sourcebook

Basic Consumer Health Information about Alternatives to Conventional Medicine, Including Acupressure, Acupuncture, Aromatherapy, Ayurveda, Bioelectromagnetics, Environmental Medicine, Essence Therapy, Food and Nutrition Therapy, Herbal Therapy, Homeopathy, Imaging, Massage, Naturopathy, Reflexology, Relaxation and Meditation, Sound Therapy, Vitamin and Mineral Therapy, and Yoga, and More

Edited by Allan R. Cook. 737 pages. 1999. 0-7808-0200-4. $78.

"Recommended reference source."
—Booklist, American Library Association, Feb '00

"A great addition to the reference collection of every type of library." *—American Reference Books Annual, 2000*

Alzheimer's, Stroke & 29 Other Neurological Disorders Sourcebook, 1st Edition

Basic Information for the Layperson on 31 Diseases or Disorders Affecting the Brain and Nervous System, First Describing the Illness, Then Listing Symptoms, Diagnostic Methods, and Treatment Options, and Including Statistics on Incidences and Causes

Edited by Frank E. Bair. 579 pages. 1993. 1-55888-748-2. $78.

"Nontechnical reference book that provides reader-friendly information."
—Family Caregiver Alliance Update, Winter '96

"Should be included in any library's patient education section." *—American Reference Books Annual, 1994*

"Written in an approachable and accessible style. Recommended for patient education and consumer health collections in health science center and public libraries." *—Academic Library Book Review, Dec '93*

"It is very handy to have information on more than thirty neurological disorders under one cover, and there is no recent source like it." *—Reference Quarterly, American Library Association, Fall '93*

SEE ALSO Brain Disorders Sourcebook

Alzheimer's Disease Sourcebook, 2nd Edition

Basic Consumer Health Information about Alzheimer's Disease, Related Disorders, and Other Dementias, Including Multi-Infarct Dementia, AIDS-Related Dementia, Alcoholic Dementia, Huntington's Disease, Delirium, and Confusional States

Along with Reports Detailing Current Research Efforts in Prevention and Treatment, Long-Term Care Issues, and Listings of Sources for Additional Help and Information

Edited by Karen Bellenir. 524 pages. 1999. 0-7808-0223-3. $78.

"Provides a wealth of useful information not otherwise available in one place. This resource is recommended for all types of libraries."
—American Reference Books Annual, 2000

"Recommended reference source."
—Booklist, American Library Association, Oct '99

Arthritis Sourcebook

Basic Consumer Health Information about Specific Forms of Arthritis and Related Disorders, Including Rheumatoid Arthritis, Osteoarthritis, Gout, Polymyalgia Rheumatica, Psoriatic Arthritis, Spondyloarthropathies, Juvenile Rheumatoid Arthritis, and Juvenile Ankylosing Spondylitis

Along with Information about Medical, Surgical, and Alternative Treatment Options, and Including Strategies for Coping with Pain, Fatigue, and Stress

Edited by Allan R. Cook. 550 pages. 1998. 0-7808-0201-2. $78.

". . . accessible to the layperson."
—Reference and Research Book News, Feb '99

Asthma Sourcebook

Basic Consumer Health Information about Asthma, Including Symptoms, Traditional and Nontraditional Remedies, Treatment Advances, Quality-of-Life Aids, Medical Research Updates, and the Role of Allergies, Exercise, Age, the Environment, and Genetics in the Development of Asthma

344

Along with Statistical Data, a Glossary, and Directories of Support Groups, and Other Resources for Further Information

Edited by Annemarie S. Muth. 628 pages. 2000. 0-7808-0381-7. $78.

"A worthwhile reference acquisition for public libraries and academic medical libraries whose readers desire a quick introduction to the wide range of asthma information." — *Choice, Association of College & esearch Libraries, Jun '01*

"Recommended reference source."
— *Booklist, American Library Association, Feb '01*

"Highly recommended." — *The Bookwatch, Jan '01*

"There is much good information for patients and their families who deal with asthma daily."
— *American Medical Writers Association Journal, Winter '01*

"This informative text is recommended for consumer health collections in public, secondary school, and community college libraries and the libraries of universities with a large undergraduate population."
— *American Reference Books Annual, 2001*

Back & Neck Disorders Sourcebook

Basic Information about Disorders and Injuries of the Spinal Cord and Vertebrae, Including Facts on Chiropractic Treatment, Surgical Interventions, Paralysis, and Rehabilitation

Along with Advice for Preventing Back Trouble

Edited by Karen Bellenir. 548 pages. 1997. 0-7808-0202-0. $78.

"The strength of this work is its basic, easy-to-read format. Recommended."
— *Reference and User Services Quarterly, American Library Association, Winter '97*

Blood & Circulatory Disorders Sourcebook

Basic Information about Blood and Its Components, Anemias, Leukemias, Bleeding Disorders, and Circulatory Disorders, Including Aplastic Anemia, Thalassemia, Sickle-Cell Disease, Hemochromatosis, Hemophilia, Von Willebrand Disease, and Vascular Diseases

Along with a Special Section on Blood Transfusions and Blood Supply Safety, a Glossary, and Source Listings for Further Help and Information

Edited by Karen Bellenir and Linda M. Shin. 554 pages. 1998. 0-7808-0203-9. $78.

"Recommended reference source."
— *Booklist, American Library Association, Feb '99*

"An important reference sourcebook written in simple language for everyday, non-technical users. "
— *Reviewer's Bookwatch, Jan '99*

Brain Disorders Sourcebook

Basic Consumer Health Information about Strokes, Epilepsy, Amyotrophic Lateral Sclerosis (ALS/Lou Gehrig's Disease), Parkinson's Disease, Brain Tumors, Cerebral Palsy, Headache, Tourette Syndrome, and More

Along with Statistical Data, Treatment and Rehabilitation Options, Coping Strategies, Reports on Current Research Initiatives, a Glossary, and Resource Listings for Additional Help and Information

Edited by Karen Bellenir. 481 pages. 1999. 0-7808-0229-2. $78.

"Belongs on the shelves of any library with a consumer health collection." — *E-Streams, Mar '00*

"Recommended reference source."
— *Booklist, American Library Association, Oct '99*

SEE ALSO *Alzheimer's, Stroke & 29 Other Neurological Disorders Sourcebook, 1st Edition*

Breast Cancer Sourcebook

Basic Consumer Health Information about Breast Cancer, Including Diagnostic Methods, Treatment Options, Alternative Therapies, Self-Help Information, Related Health Concerns, Statistical and Demographic Data, and Facts for Men with Breast Cancer

Along with Reports on Current Research Initiatives, a Glossary of Related Medical Terms, and a Directory of Sources for Further Help and Information

Edited by Edward J. Prucha and Karen Bellenir. 580 pages. 2001. 0-7808-0244-6. $78.

"Recommended reference source."
— *Booklist, American Library Association, Jan '02*

"This reference source is highly recommended. It is quite informative, comprehensive and detailed in nature, and yet it offers practical advice in easy-to-read language. It could be thought of as the 'bible' of breast cancer for the consumer." — *E-Streams, Jan '02*

"From the pros and cons of different screening methods and results to treatment options, *Breast Cancer Sourcebook* provides the latest information on the subject."
— *Library Bookwatch, Dec '01*

"This thoroughgoing, very readable reference covers all aspects of breast health and cancer.... Readers will find much to consider here. Recommended for all public and patient health collections."
— *Library Journal, Sep '01*

SEE ALSO *Cancer Sourcebook for Women, 1st and 2nd Editions, Women's Health Concerns Sourcebook*

Breastfeeding Sourcebook

Basic Consumer Health Information about the Benefits of Breastmilk, Preparing to Breastfeed, Breastfeeding as a Baby Grows, Nutrition, and More, Including Information on Special Situations and Concerns Such as Mastitis, Illness, Medications, Allergies, Multiple Births, Prematurity, Special Needs, and Adoption

Along with a Glossary and Resources for Additional Help and Information

Edited by Jenni Lynn Colson. 350 pages. 2002. 0-7808-0332-9. $78.

SEE ALSO Pregnancy & Birth Sourcebook

Burns Sourcebook

Basic Consumer Health Information about Various Types of Burns and Scalds, Including Flame, Heat, Cold, Electrical, Chemical, and Sun Burns

Along with Information on Short-Term and Long-Term Treatments, Tissue Reconstruction, Plastic Surgery, Prevention Suggestions, and First Aid

Edited by Allan R. Cook. 604 pages. 1999. 0-7808-0204-7. $78.

"This is an exceptional addition to the series and is highly recommended for all consumer health collections, hospital libraries, and academic medical centers."
—*E-Streams, Mar '00*

"This key reference guide is an invaluable addition to all health care and public libraries in confronting this ongoing health issue."
—*American Reference Books Annual, 2000*

"Recommended reference source."
—*Booklist, American Library Association, Dec '99*

SEE ALSO Skin Disorders Sourcebook

Cancer Sourcebook, 1st Edition

Basic Information on Cancer Types, Symptoms, Diagnostic Methods, and Treatments, Including Statistics on Cancer Occurrences Worldwide and the Risks Associated with Known Carcinogens and Activities

Edited by Frank E. Bair. 932 pages. 1990. 1-55888-888-8. $78.

Cited in Reference Sources for Small and Medium-Sized Libraries, American Library Association, 1999

"Written in nontechnical language. Useful for patients, their families, medical professionals, and librarians."
—*Guide to Reference Books, 1996*

"Designed with the non-medical professional in mind. Libraries and medical facilities interested in patient education should certainly consider adding the *Cancer Sourcebook* to their holdings. This compact collection of reliable information . . . is an invaluable tool for helping patients and patients' families and friends to take the first steps in coping with the many difficulties of cancer."
—*Medical Reference Services Quarterly, Winter '91*

"Specifically created for the nontechnical reader . . . an important resource for the general reader trying to understand the complexities of cancer."
—*American Reference Books Annual, 1991*

"This publication's nontechnical nature and very comprehensive format make it useful for both the general public and undergraduate students."
—*Choice, Association of College and Research Libraries, Oct '90*

New Cancer Sourcebook, 2nd Edition

Basic Information about Major Forms and Stages of Cancer, Featuring Facts about Primary and Secondary Tumors of the Respiratory, Nervous, Lymphatic, Circulatory, Skeletal, and Gastrointestinal Systems, and Specific Organs; Statistical and Demographic Data; Treatment Options; and Strategies for Coping

Edited by Allan R. Cook. 1,313 pages. 1996. 0-7808-0041-9. $78.

"An excellent resource for patients with newly diagnosed cancer and their families. The dialogue is simple, direct, and comprehensive. Highly recommended for patients and families to aid in their understanding of cancer and its treatment."
—*Booklist Health Sciences Supplement, American Library Association, Oct '97*

"The amount of factual and useful information is extensive. The writing is very clear, geared to general readers. Recommended for all levels."
—*Choice, Association of College and Research Libraries, Jan '97*

Cancer Sourcebook, 3rd Edition

Basic Consumer Health Information about Major Forms and Stages of Cancer, Featuring Facts about Primary and Secondary Tumors of the Respiratory, Nervous, Lymphatic, Circulatory, Skeletal, and Gastrointestinal Systems, and Specific Organs

Along with Statistical and Demographic Data, Treatment Options, Strategies for Coping, a Glossary, and a Directory of Sources for Additional Help and Information

Edited by Edward J. Prucha. 1,069 pages. 2000. 0-7808-0227-6. $78.

"This title is recommended for health sciences and public libraries with consumer health collections."
—*E-Streams, Feb '01*

". . . can be effectively used by cancer patients and their families who are looking for answers in a language they can understand. Public and hospital libraries should have it on their shelves."
—*American Reference Books Annual, 2001*

"Recommended reference source."
—*Booklist, American Library Association, Dec '00*

Cancer Sourcebook for Women, 1st Edition

Basic Information about Specific Forms of Cancer That Affect Women, Featuring Facts about Breast Cancer, Cervical Cancer, Ovarian Cancer, Cancer of the Uterus and Uterine Sarcoma, Cancer of the Vagina, and Cancer of the Vulva; Statistical and Demographic Data; Treatments, Self-Help Management Suggestions, and Current Research Initiatives

Edited by Allan R. Cook and Peter D. Dresser. 524 pages. 1996. 0-7808-0076-1. $78.

". . . written in easily understandable, non-technical language. Recommended for public libraries or hospital and academic libraries that collect patient education or consumer health materials."
— *Medical Reference Services Quarterly, Spring '97*

"Would be of value in a consumer health library. . . . written with the health care consumer in mind. Medical jargon is at a minimum, and medical terms are explained in clear, understandable sentences."
— *Bulletin of the Medical Library Association, Oct '96*

"The availability under one cover of all these pertinent publications, grouped under cohesive headings, makes this certainly a most useful sourcebook."
— *Choice, Association of College and Research Libraries, Jun '96*

"Presents a comprehensive knowledge base for general readers. Men and women both benefit from the gold mine of information nestled between the two covers of this book. Recommended."
— *Academic Library Book Review, Summer '96*

"This timely book is highly recommended for consumer health and patient education collections in all libraries."
— *Library Journal, Apr '96*

SEE ALSO *Breast Cancer Sourcebook, Women's Health Concerns Sourcebook*

■

Cancer Sourcebook for Women, 2nd Edition

Basic Consumer Health Information about Gynecologic Cancers and Related Concerns, Including Cervical Cancer, Endometrial Cancer, Gestational Trophoblastic Tumor, Ovarian Cancer, Uterine Cancer, Vaginal Cancer, Vulvar Cancer, Breast Cancer, and Common Non-Cancerous Uterine Conditions, with Facts about Cancer Risk Factors, Screening and Prevention, Treatment Options, and Reports on Current Research Initiatives

Along with a Glossary of Cancer Terms and a Directory of Resources for Additional Help and Information

Edited by Karen Bellenir. 604 pages. 2002. 0-7808-0226-8. $78.

SEE ALSO *Breast Cancer Sourcebook, Women's Health Concerns Sourcebook*

Cardiovascular Diseases & Disorders Sourcebook, 1st Edition

Basic Information about Cardiovascular Diseases and Disorders, Featuring Facts about the Cardiovascular System, Demographic and Statistical Data, Descriptions of Pharmacological and Surgical Interventions, Lifestyle Modifications, and a Special Section Focusing on Heart Disorders in Children

Edited by Karen Bellenir and Peter D. Dresser. 683 pages. 1995. 0-7808-0032-X. $78.

". . . comprehensive format provides an extensive overview on this subject." — *Choice, Association of College & Research Libraries, Jun '96*

". . . an easily understood, complete, up-to-date resource. This well executed public health tool will make valuable information available to those that need it most, patients and their families. The typeface, sturdy non-reflective paper, and library binding add a feel of quality found wanting in other publications. Highly recommended for academic and general libraries. "
— *Academic Library Book Review, Summer '96*

SEE ALSO *Healthy Heart Sourcebook for Women, Heart Diseases & Disorders Sourcebook, 2nd Edition*

■

Caregiving Sourcebook

Basic Consumer Health Information for Caregivers, Including a Profile of Caregivers, Caregiving Responsibilities and Concerns, Tips for Specific Conditions, Care Environments, and the Effects of Caregiving

Along with Facts about Legal Issues, Financial Information, and Future Planning, a Glossary, and a Listing of Additional Resources

Edited by Joyce Brennfleck Shannon. 600 pages. 2001. 0-7808-0331-0. $78.

"An ideal addition to the reference collection of any public library. Health sciences information professionals may also want to acquire the *Caregiving Sourcebook* for their hospital or academic library for use as a ready reference tool by health care workers interested in aging and caregiving." — *E-Streams, Jan '02*

"Recommended reference source."
— *Booklist, American Library Association, Oct '01*

■

Colds, Flu & Other Common Ailments Sourcebook

Basic Consumer Health Information about Common Ailments and Injuries, Including Colds, Coughs, the Flu, Sinus Problems, Headaches, Fever, Nausea and Vomiting, Menstrual Cramps, Diarrhea, Constipation, Hemorrhoids, Back Pain, Dandruff, Dry and Itchy Skin, Cuts, Scrapes, Sprains, Bruises, and More

Along with Information about Prevention, Self-Care, Choosing a Doctor, Over-the-Counter Medications, Folk Remedies, and Alternative Therapies, and Including a Glossary of Important Terms and a Directory of Resources for Further Help and Information

Edited by Chad T. Kimball. 638 pages. 2001. 0-7808-0435-X. $78.

"Will prove valuable to any library seeking to maintain a current, comprehensive reference collection of health resources. . . . Excellent reference."
— *The Bookwatch, Aug '01*

"Recommended reference source."
— *Booklist, American Library Association, July '01*

Communication Disorders Sourcebook

Basic Information about Deafness and Hearing Loss, Speech and Language Disorders, Voice Disorders, Balance and Vestibular Disorders, and Disorders of Smell, Taste, and Touch

Edited by Linda M. Ross. 533 pages. 1996. 0-7808-0077-X. $78.

"This is skillfully edited and is a welcome resource for the layperson. It should be found in every public and medical library." — *Booklist Health Sciences Supplement, American Library Association, Oct '97*

Congenital Disorders Sourcebook

Basic Information about Disorders Acquired during Gestation, Including Spina Bifida, Hydrocephalus, Cerebral Palsy, Heart Defects, Craniofacial Abnormalities, Fetal Alcohol Syndrome, and More

Along with Current Treatment Options and Statistical Data

Edited by Karen Bellenir. 607 pages. 1997. 0-7808-0205-5. $78.

"Recommended reference source."
— *Booklist, American Library Association, Oct '97*

SEE ALSO Pregnancy & Birth Sourcebook

Consumer Issues in Health Care Sourcebook

Basic Information about Health Care Fundamentals and Related Consumer Issues, Including Exams and Screening Tests, Physician Specialties, Choosing a Doctor, Using Prescription and Over-the-Counter Medications Safely, Avoiding Health Scams, Managing Common Health Risks in the Home, Care Options for Chronically or Terminally Ill Patients, and a List of Resources for Obtaining Help and Further Information

Edited by Karen Bellenir. 618 pages. 1998. 0-7808-0221-7. $78.

"Both public and academic libraries will want to have a copy in their collection for readers who are interested in self-education on health issues."
— *American Reference Books Annual, 2000*

"The editor has researched the literature from government agencies and others, saving readers the time and

effort of having to do the research themselves. Recommended for public libraries."
— *Reference and User Services Quarterly, American Library Association, Spring '99*

"Recommended reference source."
— *Booklist, American Library Association, Dec '98*

Contagious & Non-Contagious Infectious Diseases Sourcebook

Basic Information about Contagious Diseases like Measles, Polio, Hepatitis B, and Infectious Mononucleosis, and Non-Contagious Infectious Diseases like Tetanus and Toxic Shock Syndrome, and Diseases Occurring as Secondary Infections Such as Shingles and Reye Syndrome

Along with Vaccination, Prevention, and Treatment Information, and a Section Describing Emerging Infectious Disease Threats

Edited by Karen Bellenir and Peter D. Dresser. 566 pages. 1996. 0-7808-0075-3. $78.

Death & Dying Sourcebook

Basic Consumer Health Information for the Layperson about End-of-Life Care and Related Ethical and Legal Issues, Including Chief Causes of Death, Autopsies, Pain Management for the Terminally Ill, Life Support Systems, Insurance, Euthanasia, Assisted Suicide, Hospice Programs, Living Wills, Funeral Planning, Counseling, Mourning, Organ Donation, and Physician Training

Along with Statistical Data, a Glossary, and Listings of Sources for Further Help and Information

Edited by Annemarie S. Muth. 641 pages. 1999. 0-7808-0230-6. $78.

"Public libraries, medical libraries, and academic libraries will all find this sourcebook a useful addition to their collections."
— *American Reference Books Annual, 2001*

"An extremely useful resource for those concerned with death and dying in the United States."
— *Respiratory Care, Nov '00*

"Recommended reference source."
— *Booklist, American Library Association, Aug '00*

"This book is a definite must for all those involved in end-of-life care." — *Doody's Review Service, 2000*

Diabetes Sourcebook, 1st Edition

Basic Information about Insulin-Dependent and Non-insulin-Dependent Diabetes Mellitus, Gestational Diabetes, and Diabetic Complications, Symptoms, Treatment, and Research Results, Including Statistics on Prevalence, Morbidity, and Mortality

Along with Source Listings for Further Help and Information

Edited by Karen Bellenir and Peter D. Dresser. 827 pages. 1994. 1-55888-751-2. $78.

". . . very informative and understandable for the layperson without being simplistic. It provides a comprehensive overview for laypersons who want a general understanding of the disease or who want to focus on various aspects of the disease."
— *Bulletin of the Medical Library Association, Jan '96*

■

Diabetes Sourcebook, 2nd Edition

Basic Consumer Health Information about Type 1 Diabetes (Insulin-Dependent or Juvenile-Onset Diabetes), Type 2 (Noninsulin-Dependent or Adult-Onset Diabetes), Gestational Diabetes, and Related Disorders, Including Diabetes Prevalence Data, Management Issues, the Role of Diet and Exercise in Controlling Diabetes, Insulin and Other Diabetes Medicines, and Complications of Diabetes Such as Eye Diseases, Periodontal Disease, Amputation, and End-Stage Renal Disease

Along with Reports on Current Research Initiatives, a Glossary, and Resource Listings for Further Help and Information

Edited by Karen Bellenir. 688 pages. 1998. 0-7808-0224-1. $78.

"An invaluable reference." — *Library Journal, May '00*

Selected as one of the 250 "Best Health Sciences Books of 1999."   — *Doody's Rating Service, Mar-Apr 2000*

"This comprehensive book is an excellent addition for high school, academic, medical, and public libraries. This volume is highly recommended."
—*American Reference Books Annual, 2000*

"Provides useful information for the general public."
— *Healthlines, University of Michigan Health Management Research Center, Sep/Oct '99*

". . . provides reliable mainstream medical information . . . belongs on the shelves of any library with a consumer health collection."   — *E-Streams, Sep '99*

"Recommended reference source."
— *Booklist, American Library Association, Feb '99*

■

Diet & Nutrition Sourcebook, 1st Edition

Basic Information about Nutrition, Including the Dietary Guidelines for Americans, the Food Guide Pyramid, and Their Applications in Daily Diet, Nutritional Advice for Specific Age Groups, Current Nutritional Issues and Controversies, the New Food Label and How to Use It to Promote Healthy Eating, and Recent Developments in Nutritional Research

Edited by Dan R. Harris. 662 pages. 1996. 0-7808-0084-2. $78.

"Useful reference as a food and nutrition sourcebook for the general consumer." — *Booklist Health Sciences Supplement, American Library Association, Oct '97*

"Recommended for public libraries and medical libraries that receive general information requests on nutrition. It is readable and will appeal to those interested in learning more about healthy dietary practices."
—*Medical Reference Services Quarterly, Fall '97*

"An abundance of medical and social statistics is translated into readable information geared toward the general reader."   — *Bookwatch, Mar '97*

"With dozens of questionable diet books on the market, it is so refreshing to find a reliable and factual reference book. Recommended to aspiring professionals, librarians, and others seeking and giving reliable dietary advice. An excellent compilation."   — *Choice, Association of College and Research Libraries, Feb '97*

SEE ALSO *Digestive Diseases & Disorders Sourcebook, Gastrointestinal Diseases & Disorders Sourcebook*

■

Diet & Nutrition Sourcebook, 2nd Edition

Basic Consumer Health Information about Dietary Guidelines, Recommended Daily Intake Values, Vitamins, Minerals, Fiber, Fat, Weight Control, Dietary Supplements, and Food Additives

Along with Special Sections on Nutrition Needs throughout Life and Nutrition for People with Such Specific Medical Concerns as Allergies, High Blood Cholesterol, Hypertension, Diabetes, Celiac Disease, Seizure Disorders, Phenylketonuria (PKU), Cancer, and Eating Disorders, and Including Reports on Current Nutrition Research and Source Listings for Additional Help and Information

Edited by Karen Bellenir. 650 pages. 1999. 0-7808-0228-4. $78.

"This book is an excellent source of basic diet and nutrition information."   — *Booklist Health Sciences Supplement, American Library Association, Dec '00*

"This reference document should be in any public library, but it would be a very good guide for beginning students in the health sciences. If the other books in this publisher's series are as good as this, they should all be in the health sciences collections."
—*American Reference Books Annual, 2000*

"This book is an excellent general nutrition reference for consumers who desire to take an active role in their health care for prevention. Consumers of all ages who select this book can feel confident they are receiving current and accurate information."   — *Journal of Nutrition for the Elderly, Vol. 19, No. 4, '00*

"Recommended reference source."
—*Booklist, American Library Association, Dec '99*

SEE ALSO *Digestive Diseases & Disorders Sourcebook, Gastrointestinal Diseases & Disorders Sourcebook*

Digestive Diseases & Disorders Sourcebook

Basic Consumer Health Information about Diseases and Disorders that Impact the Upper and Lower Digestive System, Including Celiac Disease, Constipation, Crohn's Disease, Cyclic Vomiting Syndrome, Diarrhea, Diverticulosis and Diverticulitis, Gallstones, Heartburn, Hemorrhoids, Hernias, Indigestion (Dyspepsia), Irritable Bowel Syndrome, Lactose Intolerance, Ulcers, and More

Along with Information about Medications and Other Treatments, Tips for Maintaining a Healthy Digestive Tract, a Glossary, and Directory of Digestive Diseases Organizations

Edited by Karen Bellenir. 335 pages. 2000. 0-7808-0327-2. $78.

"This title would be an excellent addition to all public or patient-research libraries."
— *American Reference Books Annual, 2001*

"This title is recommended for public, hospital, and health sciences libraries with consumer health collections." — *E-Streams, Jul-Aug '00*

"Recommended reference source."
— *Booklist, American Library Association, May '00*

SEE ALSO *Diet & Nutrition Sourcebook, 1st and 2nd Editions, Gastrointestinal Diseases & Disorders Sourcebook*

Disabilities Sourcebook

Basic Consumer Health Information about Physical and Psychiatric Disabilities, Including Descriptions of Major Causes of Disability, Assistive and Adaptive Aids, Workplace Issues, and Accessibility Concerns

Along with Information about the Americans with Disabilities Act, a Glossary, and Resources for Additional Help and Information

Edited by Dawn D. Matthews. 616 pages. 2000. 0-7808-0389-2. $78.

"A much needed addition to the Omnigraphics *Health Reference Series.* A current reference work to provide people with disabilities, their families, caregivers or those who work with them, a broad range of information in one volume, has not been available until now. . . . It is recommended for all public and academic library reference collections." — *E-Streams, May '01*

"An excellent source book in easy-to-read format covering many current topics; highly recommended for all libraries." — *Choice, Association of College and Research Libraries, Jan '01*

"Recommended reference source."
— *Booklist, American Library Association, Jul '00*

"An involving, invaluable handbook."
— *The Bookwatch, May '00*

Domestic Violence & Child Abuse Sourcebook

Basic Consumer Health Information about Spousal/ Partner, Child, Sibling, Parent, and Elder Abuse, Covering Physical, Emotional, and Sexual Abuse, Teen Dating Violence, and Stalking; Includes Information about Hotlines, Safe Houses, Safety Plans, and Other Resources for Support and Assistance, Community Initiatives, and Reports on Current Directions in Research and Treatment

Along with a Glossary, Sources for Further Reading, and Governmental and Non-Governmental Organizations Contact Information

Edited by Helene Henderson. 1,064 pages. 2001. 0-7808-0235-7. $78.

"This is important information. The Web has many resources but this sourcebook fills an important societal need. I am not aware of any other resources of this type." — *Doody's Review Service, Sep '01*

"Recommended for all libraries, scholars, and practitioners." — *Choice, Association of College & Research Libraries, Jul '01*

"Recommended reference source."
— *Booklist, American Library Association, Apr '01*

"Important pick for college-level health reference libraries." — *The Bookwatch, Mar '01*

"Because this problem is so widespread and because this book includes a lot of issues within one volume, this work is recommended for all public libraries."
— *American Reference Books Annual, 2001*

Drug Abuse Sourcebook

Basic Consumer Health Information about Illicit Substances of Abuse and the Diversion of Prescription Medications, Including Depressants, Hallucinogens, Inhalants, Marijuana, Narcotics, Stimulants, and Anabolic Steroids

Along with Facts about Related Health Risks, Treatment Issues, and Substance Abuse Prevention Programs, a Glossary of Terms, Statistical Data, and Directories of Hotline Services, Self-Help Groups, and Organizations Able to Provide Further Information

Edited by Karen Bellenir. 629 pages. 2000. 0-7808-0242-X. $78.

"Containing a wealth of information, this book will be useful to the college student just beginning to explore the topic of substance abuse. This resource belongs in libraries that serve a lower-division undergraduate or community college clientele as well as the general public." — *Choice, Association of College and Research Libraries, Jun '01*

"Recommended reference source."
— *Booklist, American Library Association, Feb '01*

"Highly recommended." — *The Bookwatch, Jan '01*

"Even though there is a plethora of books on drug abuse, this volume is recommended for school, public, and college libraries."
— *American Reference Books Annual, 2001*

SEE ALSO *Alcoholism Sourcebook, Substance Abuse Sourcebook*

Ear, Nose & Throat Disorders Sourcebook

Basic Information about Disorders of the Ears, Nose, Sinus Cavities, Pharynx, and Larynx, Including Ear Infections, Tinnitus, Vestibular Disorders, Allergic and Non-Allergic Rhinitis, Sore Throats, Tonsillitis, and Cancers That Affect the Ears, Nose, Sinuses, and Throat

Along with Reports on Current Research Initiatives, a Glossary of Related Medical Terms, and a Directory of Sources for Further Help and Information

Edited by Karen Bellenir and Linda M. Shin. 576 pages. 1998. 0-7808-0206-3. $78.

"Overall, this sourcebook is helpful for the consumer seeking information on ENT issues. It is recommended for public libraries."
— *American Reference Books Annual, 1999*

"Recommended reference source."
— *Booklist, American Library Association, Dec '98*

Eating Disorders Sourcebook

Basic Consumer Health Information about Eating Disorders, Including Information about Anorexia Nervosa, Bulimia Nervosa, Binge Eating, Body Dysmorphic Disorder, Pica, Laxative Abuse, and Night Eating Syndrome

Along with Information about Causes, Adverse Effects, and Treatment and Prevention Issues, and Featuring a Section on Concerns Specific to Children and Adolescents, a Glossary, and Resources for Further Help and Information

Edited by Dawn D. Matthews. 322 pages. 2001. 0-7808-0335-3. $78.

"This volume is another convenient collection of excerpted articles. Recommended for school and public library patrons; lower-division undergraduates; and two-year technical program students."
— *Choice, Association of College & Research Libraries, Jan '02*

"Recommended reference source." — *Booklist, American Library Association, Oct '01*

Endocrine & Metabolic Disorders Sourcebook

Basic Information for the Layperson about Pancreatic and Insulin-Related Disorders Such as Pancreatitis, Diabetes, and Hypoglycemia; Adrenal Gland Disorders Such as Cushing's Syndrome, Addison's Disease, and Congenital Adrenal Hyperplasia; Pituitary Gland Disorders Such as Growth Hormone Deficiency, Acromegaly, and Pituitary Tumors; Thyroid Disorders Such as Hypothyroidism, Graves' Disease, Hashimoto's

Disease, and Goiter; Hyperparathyroidism; and Other Diseases and Syndromes of Hormone Imbalance or Metabolic Dysfunction

Along with Reports on Current Research Initiatives

Edited by Linda M. Shin. 574 pages. 1998. 0-7808-0207-1. $78.

"Omnigraphics has produced another needed resource for health information consumers."
— *American Reference Books Annual, 2000*

"Recommended reference source."
— *Booklist, American Library Association, Dec '98*

Environmentally Induced Disorders Sourcebook

Basic Information about Diseases and Syndromes Linked to Exposure to Pollutants and Other Substances in Outdoor and Indoor Environments Such as Lead, Asbestos, Formaldehyde, Mercury, Emissions, Noise, and More

Edited by Allan R. Cook. 620 pages. 1997. 0-7808-0083-4. $78.

"Recommended reference source."
— *Booklist, American Library Association, Sep '98*

"This book will be a useful addition to anyone's library." — *Choice Health Sciences Supplement, Association of College and Research Libraries, May '98*

". . . a good survey of numerous environmentally induced physical disorders . . . a useful addition to anyone's library."
— *Doody's Health Sciences Book Reviews, Jan '98*

". . . provide[s] introductory information from the best authorities around. Since this volume covers topics that potentially affect everyone, it will surely be one of the most frequently consulted volumes in the *Health Reference Series.*" — *Rettig on Reference, Nov '97*

Ethnic Diseases Sourcebook

Basic Consumer Health Information for Ethnic and Racial Minority Groups in the United States, Including General Health Indicators and Behaviors, Ethnic Diseases, Genetic Testing, the Impact of Chronic Diseases, Women's Health, Mental Health Issues, and Preventive Health Care Services

Along with a Glossary and a Listing of Additional Resources

Edited by Joyce Brennfleck Shannon. 664 pages. 2001. 0-7808-0336-1. $78.

"Recommended for health sciences libraries where public health programs are a priority."
— *E-Streams, Jan '02*

"Recommended reference source."
— *Booklist, American Library Association, Oct '01*

"Will prove valuable to any library seeking to maintain

a current, comprehensive reference collection of health resources.... An excellent source of health information about genetic disorders which affect particular ethnic and racial minorities in the U.S."

—The Bookwatch, Aug '01

Family Planning Sourcebook

Basic Consumer Health Information about Planning for Pregnancy and Contraception, Including Traditional Methods, Barrier Methods, Hormonal Methods, Permanent Methods, Future Methods, Emergency Contraception, and Birth Control Choices for Women at Each Stage of Life

Along with Statistics, a Glossary, and Sources of Additional Information

Edited by Amy Marcaccio Keyzer. 520 pages. 2001. 0-7808-0379-5. $78.

"Recommended reference source."
— Booklist, American Library Association, Oct '01

"Will prove valuable to any library seeking to maintain a current, comprehensive reference collection of health resources. . . . Excellent reference."
— The Bookwatch, Aug '01

SEE ALSO *Pregnancy & Birth Sourcebook*

Fitness & Exercise Sourcebook, 1st Edition

Basic Information on Fitness and Exercise, Including Fitness Activities for Specific Age Groups, Exercise for People with Specific Medical Conditions, How to Begin a Fitness Program in Running, Walking, Swimming, Cycling, and Other Athletic Activities, and Recent Research in Fitness and Exercise

Edited by Dan R. Harris. 663 pages. 1996. 0-7808-0186-5. $78.

"A good resource for general readers." *— Choice,* Association of College and Research Libraries, Nov '97

"The perennial popularity of the topic . . . make this an appealing selection for public libraries."
— Rettig on Reference, Jun/Jul '97

Fitness & Exercise Sourcebook, 2nd Edition

Basic Consumer Health Information about the Fundamentals of Fitness and Exercise, Including How to Begin and Maintain a Fitness Program, Fitness as a Lifestyle, the Link between Fitness and Diet, Advice for Specific Groups of People, Exercise as It Relates to Specific Medical Conditions, and Recent Research in Fitness and Exercise

Along with a Glossary of Important Terms and Resources for Additional Help and Information

Edited by Kristen M. Gledhill. 646 pages. 2001. 0-7808-0334-5. $78.

"Highly recommended for public, consumer, and school grades fourth through college."
—E-Streams, Nov '01

"Recommended reference source." *— Booklist, American Library Association, Oct '01*

"The information appears quite comprehensive and is considered reliable. . . . This second edition is a welcomed addition to the series."
—Doody's Review Service, Sep '01

"This reference is a valuable choice for those who desire a broad source of information on exercise, fitness, and chronic-disease prevention through a healthy lifestyle." *—American Medical Writers Association Journal, Fall '01*

"Will prove valuable to any library seeking to maintain a current, comprehensive reference collection of health resources. . . . Excellent reference."
— The Bookwatch, Aug '01

Food & Animal Borne Diseases Sourcebook

Basic Information about Diseases That Can Be Spread to Humans through the Ingestion of Contaminated Food or Water or by Contact with Infected Animals and Insects, Such as Botulism, E. Coli, Hepatitis A, Trichinosis, Lyme Disease, and Rabies

Along with Information Regarding Prevention and Treatment Methods, and Including a Special Section for International Travelers Describing Diseases Such as Cholera, Malaria, Travelers' Diarrhea, and Yellow Fever, and Offering Recommendations for Avoiding Illness

Edited by Karen Bellenir and Peter D. Dresser. 535 pages. 1995. 0-7808-0033-8. $78.

"Targeting general readers and providing them with a single, comprehensive source of information on selected topics, this book continues, with the excellent caliber of its predecessors, to catalog topical information on health matters of general interest. Readable and thorough, this valuable resource is highly recommended for all libraries."
— Academic Library Book Review, Summer '96

"A comprehensive collection of authoritative information." *— Emergency Medical Services, Oct '95*

Food Safety Sourcebook

Basic Consumer Health Information about the Safe Handling of Meat, Poultry, Seafood, Eggs, Fruit Juices, and Other Food Items, and Facts about Pesticides, Drinking Water, Food Safety Overseas, and the Onset, Duration, and Symptoms of Foodborne Illnesses, Including Types of Pathogenic Bacteria, Parasitic Protozoa, Worms, Viruses, and Natural Toxins

Along with the Role of the Consumer, the Food Handler, and the Government in Food Safety; a Glossary, and Resources for Additional Help and Information

Edited by Dawn D. Matthews. 339 pages. 1999. 0-7808-0326-4. $78.

"This book is recommended for public libraries and universities with home economic and food science programs." —*E-Streams, Nov '00*

"Recommended reference source."
—*Booklist, American Library Association, May '00*

"This book takes the complex issues of food safety and foodborne pathogens and presents them in an easily understood manner. [It does] an excellent job of covering a large and often confusing topic."
—*American Reference Books Annual, 2000*

■

Forensic Medicine Sourcebook

Basic Consumer Information for the Layperson about Forensic Medicine, Including Crime Scene Investigation, Evidence Collection and Analysis, Expert Testimony, Computer-Aided Criminal Identification, Digital Imaging in the Courtroom, DNA Profiling, Accident Reconstruction, Autopsies, Ballistics, Drugs and Explosives Detection, Latent Fingerprints, Product Tampering, and Questioned Document Examination

Along with Statistical Data, a Glossary of Forensics Terminology, and Listings of Sources for Further Help and Information

Edited by Annemarie S. Muth. 574 pages. 1999. 0-7808-0232-2. $78.

"Given the expected widespread interest in its content and its easy to read style, this book is recommended for most public and all college and university libraries."
—*E-Streams, Feb '01*

"Recommended for public libraries."
—*Reference & User Services Quarterly, American Library Association, Spring 2000*

"Recommended reference source."
—*Booklist, American Library Association, Feb '00*

"A wealth of information, useful statistics, references are up-to-date and extremely complete. This wonderful collection of data will help students who are interested in a career in any type of forensic field. It is a great resource for attorneys who need information about types of expert witnesses needed in a particular case. It also offers useful information for fiction and nonfiction writers whose work involves a crime. A fascinating compilation. All levels." —*Choice, Association of College and Research Libraries, Jan 2000*

"There are several items that make this book attractive to consumers who are seeking certain forensic data. . . . This is a useful current source for those seeking general forensic medical answers."
—*American Reference Books Annual, 2000*

■

Gastrointestinal Diseases & Disorders Sourcebook

Basic Information about Gastroesophageal Reflux Disease (Heartburn), Ulcers, Diverticulosis, Irritable Bowel Syndrome, Crohn's Disease, Ulcerative Colitis, Diarrhea, Constipation, Lactose Intolerance, Hemorrhoids, Hepatitis, Cirrhosis, and Other Digestive Problems, Featuring Statistics, Descriptions of Symptoms,

and Current Treatment Methods of Interest for Persons Living with Upper and Lower Gastrointestinal Maladies

Edited by Linda M. Ross. 413 pages. 1996. 0-7808-0078-8. $78.

". . . very readable form. The successful editorial work that brought this material together into a useful and understandable reference makes accessible to all readers information that can help them more effectively understand and obtain help for digestive tract problems."
—*Choice, Association of College and Research Libraries, Feb '97*

SEE ALSO Diet & Nutrition Sourcebook, 1st and 2nd Editions, Digestive Diseases & Disorders

■

Genetic Disorders Sourcebook, 1st Edition

Basic Information about Heritable Diseases and Disorders Such as Down Syndrome, PKU, Hemophilia, Von Willebrand Disease, Gaucher Disease, Tay-Sachs Disease, and Sickle-Cell Disease, Along with Information about Genetic Screening, Gene Therapy, Home Care, and Including Source Listings for Further Help and Information on More Than 300 Disorders

Edited by Karen Bellenir. 642 pages. 1996. 0-7808-0034-6. $78.

"Recommended for undergraduate libraries or libraries that serve the public."
—*Science & Technology Libraries, Vol. 18, No. 1, '99*

"Provides essential medical information to both the general public and those diagnosed with a serious or fatal genetic disease or disorder." —*Choice, Association of College and Research Libraries, Jan '97*

"Geared toward the lay public. It would be well placed in all public libraries and in those hospital and medical libraries in which access to genetic references is limited." —*Doody's Health Sciences Book Review, Oct '96*

■

Genetic Disorders Sourcebook, 2nd Edition

Basic Consumer Health Information about Hereditary Diseases and Disorders, Including Cystic Fibrosis, Down Syndrome, Hemophilia, Huntington's Disease, Sickle Cell Anemia, and More; Facts about Genes, Gene Research and Therapy, Genetic Screening, Ethics of Gene Testing, Genetic Counseling, and Advice on Coping and Caring

Along with a Glossary of Genetic Terminology and a Resource List for Help, Support, and Further Information

Edited by Kathy Massimini. 768 pages. 2001. 0-7808-0241-1. $78.

"Recommended for public libraries and medical and hospital libraries with consumer health collections."
—*E-Streams, May '01*

"Recommended reference source."
—*Booklist, American Library Association, Apr '01*

Head Trauma Sourcebook

Basic Information for the Layperson about Open-Head and Closed-Head Injuries, Treatment Advances, Recovery, and Rehabilitation

Along with Reports on Current Research Initiatives

Edited by Karen Bellenir. 414 pages. 1997. 0-7808-0208-X. $78.

Headache Sourcebook

Basic Consumer Health Information about Migraine, Tension, Cluster, Rebound and Other Types of Headaches, with Facts about the Cause and Prevention of Headaches, the Effects of Stress and the Environment, Headaches during Pregnancy and Menopause, and Childhood Headaches

Along with a Glossary and Other Resources for Additional Help and Information

Edited by Dawn D. Matthews. 362 pages. 2002. 0-7808-0337-X. $78.

Health Insurance Sourcebook

Basic Information about Managed Care Organizations, Traditional Fee-for-Service Insurance, Insurance Portability and Pre-Existing Conditions Clauses, Medicare, Medicaid, Social Security, and Military Health Care

Along with Information about Insurance Fraud

Edited by Wendy Wilcox. 530 pages. 1997. 0-7808-0222-5. $78.

Health Reference Series Cumulative Index 1999

A Comprehensive Index to the Individual Volumes of the Health Reference Series, Including a Subject Index, Name Index, Organization Index, and Publication Index

Along with a Master List of Acronyms and Abbreviations

Edited by Edward J. Prucha, Anne Holmes, and Robert Rudnick. 990 pages. 2000. 0-7808-0382-5. $78.

Healthy Aging Sourcebook

Basic Consumer Health Information about Maintaining Health through the Aging Process, Including Advice on Nutrition, Exercise, and Sleep, Help in Making Decisions about Midlife Issues and Retirement, and Guidance Concerning Practical and Informed Choices in Health Consumerism

Along with Data Concerning the Theories of Aging, Different Experiences in Aging by Minority Groups, and Facts about Aging Now and Aging in the Future; and Featuring a Glossary, a Guide to Consumer Help, Additional Suggested Reading, and Practical Resource Directory

Edited by Jenifer Swanson. 536 pages. 1999. 0-7808-0390-6. $78.

SEE ALSO *Physical & Mental Issues in Aging Sourcebook*

Healthy Heart Sourcebook for Women

Basic Consumer Health Information about Cardiac Issues Specific to Women, Including Facts about Major Risk Factors and Prevention, Treatment and Control Strategies, and Important Dietary Issues

Along with a Special Section Regarding the Pros and Cons of Hormone Replacement Therapy and Its Impact on Heart Health, and Additional Help, Including Recipes, a Glossary, and a Directory of Resources

Edited by Dawn D. Matthews. 336 pages. 2000. 0-7808-0329-9. $78.

SEE ALSO *Cardiovascular Diseases & Disorders Sourcebook, 1st Edition, Heart Diseases & Disorders Sourcebook, 2nd Edition, Women's Health Concerns Sourcebook*

Heart Diseases & Disorders Sourcebook, 2nd Edition

Basic Consumer Health Information about Heart Attacks, Angina, Rhythm Disorders, Heart Failure, Valve Disease, Congenital Heart Disorders, and More, Including Descriptions of Surgical Procedures and Other Interventions, Medications, Cardiac Rehabilitation, Risk Identification, and Prevention Tips

Along with Statistical Data, Reports on Current Research Initiatives, a Glossary of Cardiovascular Terms, and Resource Directory

Edited by Karen Bellenir. 612 pages. 2000. 0-7808-0238-1. $78.

SEE ALSO *Cardiovascular Diseases & Disorders Sourcebook, 1st Edition; Healthy Heart Sourcebook for Women*

Household Safety Sourcebook

Basic Consumer Health Information about Household Safety, Including Information about Poisons, Chemicals, Fire, and Water Hazards in the Home

Along with Advice about the Safe Use of Home Maintenance Equipment, Choosing Toys and Nursery Furniture, Holiday and Recreation Safety, a Glossary, and Resources for Further Help and Information

Edited by Dawn D. Matthews. 606 pages. 2002. 0-7808-0338-8. $78.

Immune System Disorders Sourcebook

Basic Information about Lupus, Multiple Sclerosis, Guillain-Barré Syndrome, Chronic Granulomatous Disease, and More

Along with Statistical and Demographic Data and Reports on Current Research Initiatives

Edited by Allan R. Cook. 608 pages. 1997. 0-7808-0209-8. $78.

Infant & Toddler Health Sourcebook

Basic Consumer Health Information about the Physical and Mental Development of Newborns, Infants, and Toddlers, Including Neonatal Concerns, Nutrition Recommendations, Immunization Schedules, Common Pediatric Disorders, Assessments and Milestones, Safety Tips, and Advice for Parents and Other Caregivers

Along with a Glossary of Terms and Resource Listings for Additional Help

Edited by Jenifer Swanson. 585 pages. 2000. 0-7808-0246-2. $78.

Injury & Trauma Sourcebook

Basic Consumer Health Information about the Impact of Injury, the Diagnosis and Treatment of Common and Traumatic Injuries, Emergency Care, and Specific Injuries Related to Home, Community, Workplace, Transportation, and Recreation

Along with Guidelines for Injury Prevention, a Glossary, and a Directory of Additional Resources

Edited by Joyce Brennfleck Shannon. 700 pages. 2002. 0-7808-0421-X. $78.

Kidney & Urinary Tract Diseases & Disorders Sourcebook

Basic Information about Kidney Stones, Urinary Incontinence, Bladder Disease, End Stage Renal Disease, Dialysis, and More

Along with Statistical and Demographic Data and Reports on Current Research Initiatives

Edited by Linda M. Ross. 602 pages. 1997. 0-7808-0079-6. $78.

Learning Disabilities Sourcebook

Basic Information about Disorders Such as Dyslexia, Visual and Auditory Processing Deficits, Attention Deficit/Hyperactivity Disorder, and Autism

Along with Statistical and Demographic Data, Reports on Current Research Initiatives, an Explanation of the Assessment Process, and a Special Section for Adults with Learning Disabilities

Edited by Linda M. Shin. 579 pages. 1998. 0-7808-0210-1. $78.

"An excellent candidate for inclusion in a public library reference section. It's a great source of information. Teachers will also find the book useful. Definitely worth reading."
—*Journal of Adolescent & Adult Literacy, Feb 2000*

"Readable . . . provides a solid base of information regarding successful techniques used with individuals who have learning disabilities, as well as practical suggestions for educators and family members. Clear language, concise descriptions, and pertinent information for contacting multiple resources add to the strength of this book as a useful tool." — *Choice, Association of College and Research Libraries, Feb '99*

"Recommended reference source."
—*Booklist, American Library Association, Sep '98*

"A useful resource for libraries and for those who don't have the time to identify and locate the individual publications." — *Disability Resources Monthly, Sep '98*

Liver Disorders Sourcebook

Basic Consumer Health Information about the Liver and How It Works; Liver Diseases, Including Cancer, Cirrhosis, Hepatitis, and Toxic and Drug Related Diseases; Tips for Maintaining a Healthy Liver; Laboratory Tests, Radiology Tests, and Facts about Liver Transplantation

Along with a Section on Support Groups, a Glossary, and Resource Listings

Edited by Joyce Brennfleck Shannon. 591 pages. 2000. 0-7808-0383-3. $78.

"A valuable resource."
—*American Reference Books Annual, 2001*

"This title is recommended for health sciences and public libraries with consumer health collections."
— *E-Streams, Oct '00*

"Recommended reference source."
—*Booklist, American Library Association, Jun '00*

Lung Disorders Sourcebook

Basic Consumer Health Information about Emphysema, Pneumonia, Tuberculosis, Asthma, Cystic Fibrosis, and Other Lung Disorders, Including Facts about Diagnostic Procedures, Treatment Strategies, Disease Prevention Efforts, and Such Risk Factors as Smoking, Air Pollution, and Exposure to Asbestos, Radon, and Other Agents

Along with a Glossary and Resources for Additional Help and Information

Edited by Dawn D. Matthews. 678 pages. 2002. 0-7808-0339-6. $78.

Medical Tests Sourcebook

Basic Consumer Health Information about Medical Tests, Including Periodic Health Exams, General Screening Tests, Tests You Can Do at Home, Findings of the U.S. Preventive Services Task Force, X-ray and Radiology Tests, Electrical Tests, Tests of Blood and Other Body Fluids and Tissues, Scope Tests, Lung Tests, Genetic Tests, Pregnancy Tests, Newborn Screening Tests, Sexually Transmitted Disease Tests, and Computer Aided Diagnoses

Along with a Section on Paying for Medical Tests, a Glossary, and Resource Listings

Edited by Joyce Brennfleck Shannon. 691 pages. 1999. 0-7808-0243-8. $78.

"Recommended for hospital and health sciences libraries with consumer health collections."
—*E-Streams, Mar '00*

"This is an overall excellent reference with a wealth of general knowledge that may aid those who are reluctant to get vital tests performed."
— *Today's Librarian, Jan 2000*

"A valuable reference guide."
—*American Reference Books Annual, 2000*

Men's Health Concerns Sourcebook

Basic Information about Health Issues That Affect Men, Featuring Facts about the Top Causes of Death in Men, Including Heart Disease, Stroke, Cancers, Prostate Disorders, Chronic Obstructive Pulmonary Disease, Pneumonia and Influenza, Human Immunodeficiency Virus and Acquired Immune Deficiency Syndrome, Diabetes Mellitus, Stress, Suicide, Accidents and Homicides; and Facts about Common Concerns for Men, Including Impotence, Contraception, Circumcision, Sleep Disorders, Snoring, Hair Loss, Diet, Nutrition, Exercise, Kidney and Urological Disorders, and Backaches

Edited by Allan R. Cook. 738 pages. 1998. 0-7808-0212-8. $78.

"This comprehensive resource and the series are highly recommended."
—*American Reference Books Annual, 2000*

"Recommended reference source."
— *Booklist, American Library Association, Dec '98*

Mental Health Disorders Sourcebook, 1st Edition

Basic Information about Schizophrenia, Depression, Bipolar Disorder, Panic Disorder, Obsessive-Compulsive Disorder, Phobias and Other Anxiety Disorders, Paranoia and Other Personality Disorders, Eating Disorders, and Sleep Disorders

Along with Information about Treatment and Therapies

Edited by Karen Bellenir. 548 pages. 1995. 0-7808-0040-0. $78.

"This is an excellent new book . . . written in easy-to-understand language."
— *Booklist Health Sciences Supplement, American Library Association, Oct '97*

". . . useful for public and academic libraries and consumer health collections."
— *Medical Reference Services Quarterly, Spring '97*

"The great strengths of the book are its readability and its inclusion of places to find more information. Especially recommended." — *Reference Quarterly, American Library Association, Winter '96*

". . . a good resource for a consumer health library."
— *Bulletin of the Medical Library Association, Oct '96*

"The information is data-based and couched in brief, concise language that avoids jargon. . . . a useful reference source." — *Readings, Sep '96*

"The text is well organized and adequately written for its target audience." — *Choice, Association of College and Research Libraries, Jun '96*

". . . provides information on a wide range of mental disorders, presented in nontechnical language."
— *Exceptional Child Education Resources, Spring '96*

"Recommended for public and academic libraries."
— *Reference Book Review, 1996*

Mental Health Disorders Sourcebook, 2nd Edition

Basic Consumer Health Information about Anxiety Disorders, Depression and Other Mood Disorders, Eating Disorders, Personality Disorders, Schizophrenia, and More, Including Disease Descriptions, Treatment Options, and Reports on Current Research Initiatives

Along with Statistical Data, Tips for Maintaining Mental Health, a Glossary, and Directory of Sources for Additional Help and Information

Edited by Karen Bellenir. 605 pages. 2000. 0-7808-0240-3. $78.

"Well organized and well written."
— *American Reference Books Annual, 2001*

"Recommended reference source."
— *Booklist, American Library Association, Jun '00*

Mental Retardation Sourcebook

Basic Consumer Health Information about Mental Retardation and Its Causes, Including Down Syndrome, Fetal Alcohol Syndrome, Fragile X Syndrome, Genetic Conditions, Injury, and Environmental Sources

Along with Preventive Strategies, Parenting Issues, Educational Implications, Health Care Needs, Employment and Economic Matters, Legal Issues, a Glossary, and a Resource Listing for Additional Help and Information

Edited by Joyce Brennfleck Shannon. 642 pages. 2000. 0-7808-0377-9. $78.

"Public libraries will find the book useful for reference and as a beginning research point for students, parents, and caregivers."
— *American Reference Books Annual, 2001*

"The strength of this work is that it compiles many basic fact sheets and addresses for further information in one volume. It is intended and suitable for the general public. This sourcebook is relevant to any collection providing health information to the general public."
— *E-Streams, Nov '00*

"From preventing retardation to parenting and family challenges, this covers health, social and legal issues and will prove an invaluable overview."
— *Reviewer's Bookwatch, Jul '00*

Obesity Sourcebook

Basic Consumer Health Information about Diseases and Other Problems Associated with Obesity, and Including Facts about Risk Factors, Prevention Issues, and Management Approaches

Along with Statistical and Demographic Data, Information about Special Populations, Research Updates, a Glossary, and Source Listings for Further Help and Information

Edited by Wilma Caldwell and Chad T. Kimball. 376 pages. 2001. 0-7808-0333-7. $78.

"This is a very useful resource book for the lay public."
— *Doody's Review Service, Nov '01*

"Well suited for the health reference collection of a public library or an academic health science library that serves the general population." — *E-Streams, Sep '01*

"Recommended reference source."
— *Booklist, American Library Association, Apr '01*

" Recommended pick both for specialty health library collections and any general consumer health reference collection." — *The Bookwatch, Apr '01*

Ophthalmic Disorders Sourcebook

Basic Information about Glaucoma, Cataracts, Macular Degeneration, Strabismus, Refractive Disorders, and More

Along with Statistical and Demographic Data and Reports on Current Research Initiatives

Edited by Linda M. Ross. 631 pages. 1996. 0-7808-0081-8. $78.

Oral Health Sourcebook

Basic Information about Diseases and Conditions Affecting Oral Health, Including Cavities, Gum Disease, Dry Mouth, Oral Cancers, Fever Blisters, Canker Sores, Oral Thrush, Bad Breath, Temporomandibular Disorders, and other Craniofacial Syndromes

Along with Statistical Data on the Oral Health of Americans, Oral Hygiene, Emergency First Aid, In-

formation on Treatment Procedures and Methods of Replacing Lost Teeth

Edited by Allan R. Cook. 558 pages. 1997. 0-7808-0082-6. $78.

"Unique source which will fill a gap in dental sources for patients and the lay public. A valuable reference tool even in a library with thousands of books on dentistry. Comprehensive, clear, inexpensive, and easy to read and use. It fills an enormous gap in the health care literature." — Reference and User Services Quarterly, American Library Association, Summer '98

"Recommended reference source."
— Booklist, American Library Association, Dec '97

■

Osteoporosis Sourcebook

Basic Consumer Health Information about Primary and Secondary Osteoporosis and Juvenile Osteoporosis and Related Conditions, Including Fibrous Dysplasia, Gaucher Disease, Hyperthyroidism, Hypophosphatasia, Myeloma, Osteopetrosis, Osteogenesis Imperfecta, and Paget's Disease

Along with Information about Risk Factors, Treatments, Traditional and Non-Traditional Pain Management, a Glossary of Related Terms, and a Directory of Resources

Edited by Allan R. Cook. 584 pages. 2001. 0-7808-0239-X. $78.

"This would be a book to be kept in a staff or patient library. The targeted audience is the layperson, but the therapist who needs a quick bit of information on a particular topic will also find the book useful."
— Physical Therapy, Jan '02

"Recommended for all public libraries and general health collections, especially those supporting patient education or consumer health programs."
— E-Streams, Nov '01

"Will prove valuable to any library seeking to maintain a current, comprehensive reference collection of health resources. . . . From prevention to treatment and associated conditions, this provides an excellent survey."
— The Bookwatch, Aug '01

"Recommended reference source."
— Booklist, American Library Association, July '01

SEE ALSO Women's Health Concerns Sourcebook

■

Pain Sourcebook

Basic Information about Specific Forms of Acute and Chronic Pain, Including Headaches, Back Pain, Muscular Pain, Neuralgia, Surgical Pain, and Cancer Pain

Along with Pain Relief Options Such as Analgesics, Narcotics, Nerve Blocks, Transcutaneous Nerve Stimulation, and Alternative Forms of Pain Control, Including Biofeedback, Imaging, Behavior Modification, and Relaxation Techniques

Edited by Allan R. Cook. 667 pages. 1997. 0-7808-0213-6. $78.

"The text is readable, easily understood, and well indexed. This excellent volume belongs in all patient education libraries, consumer health sections of public libraries, and many personal collections."
— American Reference Books Annual, 1999

"A beneficial reference." — Booklist Health Sciences Supplement, American Library Association, Oct '98

"The information is basic in terms of scholarship and is appropriate for general readers. Written in journalistic style . . . intended for non-professionals. Quite thorough in its coverage of different pain conditions and summarizes the latest clinical information regarding pain treatment." — Choice, Association of College and Research Libraries, Jun '98

"Recommended reference source."
— Booklist, American Library Association, Mar '98

■

Pediatric Cancer Sourcebook

Basic Consumer Health Information about Leukemias, Brain Tumors, Sarcomas, Lymphomas, and Other Cancers in Infants, Children, and Adolescents, Including Descriptions of Cancers, Treatments, and Coping Strategies

Along with Suggestions for Parents, Caregivers, and Concerned Relatives, a Glossary of Cancer Terms, and Resource Listings

Edited by Edward J. Prucha. 587 pages. 1999. 0-7808-0245-4. $78.

"An excellent source of information. Recommended for public, hospital, and health science libraries with consumer health collections." — E-Streams, Jun '00

"Recommended reference source."
— Booklist, American Library Association, Feb '00

"A valuable addition to all libraries specializing in health services and many public libraries."
— American Reference Books Annual, 2000

■

Physical & Mental Issues in Aging Sourcebook

Basic Consumer Health Information on Physical and Mental Disorders Associated with the Aging Process, Including Concerns about Cardiovascular Disease, Pulmonary Disease, Oral Health, Digestive Disorders, Musculoskeletal and Skin Disorders, Metabolic Changes, Sexual and Reproductive Issues, and Changes in Vision, Hearing, and Other Senses

Along with Data about Longevity and Causes of Death, Information on Acute and Chronic Pain, Descriptions of Mental Concerns, a Glossary of Terms, and Resource Listings for Additional Help

Edited by Jenifer Swanson. 660 pages. 1999. 0-7808-0233-0. $78.

"This is a treasure of health information for the layperson." — Choice Health Sciences Supplement, Association of College & Research Libraries, May 2000

Podiatry Sourcebook

Basic Consumer Health Information about Foot Conditions, Diseases, and Injuries, Including Bunions, Corns, Calluses, Athlete's Foot, Plantar Warts, Hammertoes and Clawtoes, Clubfoot, Heel Pain, Gout, and More

Along with Facts about Foot Care, Disease Prevention, Foot Safety, Choosing a Foot Care Specialist, a Glossary of Terms, and Resource Listings for Additional Information

Edited by M. Lisa Weatherford. 380 pages. 2001. 0-7808-0215-2. $78.

Pregnancy & Birth Sourcebook

Basic Information about Planning for Pregnancy, Maternal Health, Fetal Growth and Development, Labor and Delivery, Postpartum and Perinatal Care, Pregnancy in Mothers with Special Concerns, and Disorders of Pregnancy, Including Genetic Counseling, Nutrition and Exercise, Obstetrical Tests, Pregnancy Discomfort, Multiple Births, Cesarean Sections, Medical Testing of Newborns, Breastfeeding, Gestational Diabetes, and Ectopic Pregnancy

Edited by Heather E. Aldred. 737 pages. 1997. 0-7808-0216-0. $78.

SEE ALSO *Congenital Disorders Sourcebook, Family Planning Sourcebook*

Prostate Cancer Sourcebook

Basic Consumer Health Information about Prostate Cancer, Including Information about the Associated Risk Factors, Detection, Diagnosis, and Treatment of Prostate Cancer

Along with Information on Non-Malignant Prostate Conditions, and Featuring a Section Listing Support and Treatment Centers and a Glossary of Related Terms

Edited by Dawn D. Matthews. 358 pages. 2001. 0-7808-0324-8. $78.

Public Health Sourcebook

Basic Information about Government Health Agencies, Including National Health Statistics and Trends, Healthy People 2000 Program Goals and Objectives, the Centers for Disease Control and Prevention, the Food and Drug Administration, and the National Institutes of Health

Along with Full Contact Information for Each Agency

Edited by Wendy Wilcox. 698 pages. 1998. 0-7808-0220-9. $78.

Reconstructive & Cosmetic Surgery Sourcebook

Basic Consumer Health Information on Cosmetic and Reconstructive Plastic Surgery, Including Statistical Information about Different Surgical Procedures, Things to Consider Prior to Surgery, Plastic Surgery Techniques and Tools, Emotional and Psychological Considerations, and Procedure-Specific Information

Along with a Glossary of Terms and a Listing of Resources for Additional Help and Information

Edited by M. Lisa Weatherford. 374 pages. 2001. 0-7808-0214-4. $78.

Rehabilitation Sourcebook

Basic Consumer Health Information about Rehabilitation for People Recovering from Heart Surgery, Spinal Cord Injury, Stroke, Orthopedic Impairments, Amputation, Pulmonary Impairments, Traumatic Injury, and More, Including Physical Therapy, Occupational Therapy, Speech/ Language Therapy, Massage Therapy, Dance Therapy, Art Therapy, and Recreational Therapy

Along with Information on Assistive and Adaptive Devices, a Glossary, and Resources for Additional Help and Information

Edited by Dawn D. Matthews. 531 pages. 1999. 0-7808-0236-5. $78.

Respiratory Diseases & Disorders Sourcebook

Basic Information about Respiratory Diseases and Disorders, Including Asthma, Cystic Fibrosis, Pneumonia, the Common Cold, Influenza, and Others, Featuring Facts about the Respiratory System, Statistical and Demographic Data, Treatments, Self-Help Management Suggestions, and Current Research Initiatives

Edited by Allan R. Cook and Peter D. Dresser. 771 pages. 1995. 0-7808-0037-0. $78.

"Designed for the layperson and for patients and their families coping with respiratory illness. . . . an extensive array of information on diagnosis, treatment, management, and prevention of respiratory illnesses for the general reader." — *Choice, Association of College and Research Libraries, Jun '96*

"A highly recommended text for all collections. It is a comforting reminder of the power of knowledge that good books carry between their covers." — *Academic Library Book Review, Spring '96*

"A comprehensive collection of authoritative information presented in a nontechnical, humanitarian style for patients, families, and caregivers." — *Association of Operating Room Nurses, Sep/Oct '95*

■

Sexually Transmitted Diseases Sourcebook, 1st Edition

Basic Information about Herpes, Chlamydia, Gonorrhea, Hepatitis, Nongonoccocal Urethritis, Pelvic Inflammatory Disease, Syphilis, AIDS, and More

Along with Current Data on Treatments and Preventions

Edited by Linda M. Ross. 550 pages. 1997. 0-7808-0217-9. $78.

■

Sexually Transmitted Diseases Sourcebook, 2nd Edition

Basic Consumer Health Information about Sexually Transmitted Diseases, Including Information on the Diagnosis and Treatment of Chlamydia, Gonorrhea, Hepatitis, Herpes, HIV, Mononucleosis, Syphilis, and Others

Along with Information on Prevention, Such as Condom Use, Vaccines, and STD Education; And Featuring a Section on Issues Related to Youth and Adolescents, a Glossary, and Resources for Additional Help and Information

Edited by Dawn D. Matthews. 538 pages. 2001. 0-7808-0249-7. $78.

"Every school and public library should have a copy of this comprehensive and user-friendly reference book." — *Choice, Association of College & Research Libraries, Sep '01*

"This is a highly recommended book. This is an especially important book for all school and public libraries." — *AIDS Book Review Journal, Jul-Aug '01*

"Recommended reference source." — *Booklist, American Library Association, Apr '01*

"Recommended pick both for specialty health library collections and any general consumer health reference collection." — *The Bookwatch, Apr '01*

■

Skin Disorders Sourcebook

Basic Information about Common Skin and Scalp Conditions Caused by Aging, Allergies, Immune Reactions, Sun Exposure, Infectious Organisms, Parasites, Cosmetics, and Skin Traumas, Including Abrasions, Cuts, and Pressure Sores

Along with Information on Prevention and Treatment

Edited by Allan R. Cook. 647 pages. 1997. 0-7808-0080-X. $78.

". . . comprehensive, easily read reference book." — *Doody's Health Sciences Book Reviews, Oct '97*

SEE ALSO Burns Sourcebook

■

Sleep Disorders Sourcebook

Basic Consumer Health Information about Sleep and Its Disorders, Including Insomnia, Sleepwalking, Sleep Apnea, Restless Leg Syndrome, and Narcolepsy

Along with Data about Shiftwork and Its Effects, Information on the Societal Costs of Sleep Deprivation, Descriptions of Treatment Options, a Glossary of Terms, and Resource Listings for Additional Help

Edited by Jenifer Swanson. 439 pages. 1998. 0-7808-0234-9. $78.

"This text will complement any home or medical library. It is user-friendly and ideal for the adult reader." — *American Reference Books Annual, 2000*

"A useful resource that provides accurate, relevant, and accessible information on sleep to the general public. Health care providers who deal with sleep disorders patients may also find it helpful in being prepared to answer some of the questions patients ask." — *Respiratory Care, Jul '99*

"Recommended reference source." — *Booklist, American Library Association, Feb '99*

■

Sports Injuries Sourcebook

Basic Consumer Health Information about Common Sports Injuries, Prevention of Injury in Specific Sports, Tips for Training, and Rehabilitation from Injury

Along with Information about Special Concerns for Children, Young Girls in Athletic Training Programs, Senior Athletes, and Women Athletes, and a Directory of Resources for Further Help and Information

Edited by Heather E. Aldred. 624 pages. 1999. 0-7808-0218-7. $78.

"While this easy-to-read book is recommended for all libraries, it should prove to be especially useful for public, high school, and academic libraries; certainly it should be on the bookshelf of every school gymnasium."   — E-Streams, Mar '00

"Public libraries and undergraduate academic libraries will find this book useful for its nontechnical language."   —American Reference Books Annual, 2000

■

Substance Abuse Sourcebook

Basic Health-Related Information about the Abuse of Legal and Illegal Substances Such as Alcohol, Tobacco, Prescription Drugs, Marijuana, Cocaine, and Heroin; and Including Facts about Substance Abuse Prevention Strategies, Intervention Methods, Treatment and Recovery Programs, and a Section Addressing the Special Problems Related to Substance Abuse during Pregnancy

Edited by Karen Bellenir. 573 pages. 1996. 0-7808-0038-9. $78.

"A valuable addition to any health reference section. Highly recommended."
— The Book Report, Mar/Apr '97

". . . a comprehensive collection of substance abuse information that's both highly readable and compact. Families and caregivers of substance abusers will find the information enlightening and helpful, while teachers, social workers and journalists should benefit from the concise format. Recommended."
— Drug Abuse Update, Winter '96/'97

SEE ALSO *Alcoholism Sourcebook, Drug Abuse Sourcebook*

■

Transplantation Sourcebook

Basic Consumer Health Information about Organ and Tissue Transplantation, Including Physical and Financial Preparations, Procedures and Issues Relating to Specific Solid Organ and Tissue Transplants, Rehabilitation, Pediatric Transplant Information, the Future of Transplantation, and Organ and Tissue Donation

Along with a Glossary and Listings of Additional Resources

Edited by Joyce Brennfleck Shannon. 628 pages. 2002. 0-7808-0322-1. $78.

■

Traveler's Health Sourcebook

Basic Consumer Health Information for Travelers, Including Physical and Medical Preparations, Transportation Health and Safety, Essential Information about Food and Water, Sun Exposure, Insect and Snake Bites, Camping and Wilderness Medicine, and Travel with Physical or Medical Disabilities

Along with International Travel Tips, Vaccination Recommendations, Geographical Health Issues, Disease Risks, a Glossary, and a Listing of Additional Resources

Edited by Joyce Brennfleck Shannon. 613 pages. 2000. 0-7808-0384-1. $78.

"Recommended reference source."
— Booklist, American Library Association, Feb '01

"This book is recommended for any public library, any travel collection, and especially any collection for the physically disabled."
—American Reference Books Annual, 2001

■

Women's Health Concerns Sourcebook

Basic Information about Health Issues That Affect Women, Featuring Facts about Menstruation and Other Gynecological Concerns, Including Endometriosis, Fibroids, Menopause, and Vaginitis; Reproductive Concerns, Including Birth Control, Infertility, and Abortion; and Facts about Additional Physical, Emotional, and Mental Health Concerns Prevalent among Women Such as Osteoporosis, Urinary Tract Disorders, Eating Disorders, and Depression

Along with Tips for Maintaining a Healthy Lifestyle

Edited by Heather E. Aldred. 567 pages. 1997. 0-7808-0219-5. $78.

"Handy compilation. There is an impressive range of diseases, devices, disorders, procedures, and other physical and emotional issues covered . . . well organized, illustrated, and indexed."   — Choice, Association of College and Research Libraries, Jan '98

SEE ALSO *Breast Cancer Sourcebook, Cancer Sourcebook for Women, 1st and 2nd Editions, Healthy Heart Sourcebook for Women, Osteoporosis Sourcebook*

■

Workplace Health & Safety Sourcebook

Basic Consumer Health Information about Workplace Health and Safety, Including the Effect of Workplace Hazards on the Lungs, Skin, Heart, Ears, Eyes, Brain, Reproductive Organs, Musculoskeletal System, and Other Organs and Body Parts

Along with Information about Occupational Cancer, Personal Protective Equipment, Toxic and Hazardous Chemicals, Child Labor, Stress, and Workplace Violence

Edited by Chad T. Kimball. 626 pages. 2000. 0-7808-0231-4. $78.

"As a reference for the general public, this would be useful in any library."   —E-Streams, Jun '01

"Provides helpful information for primary care physicians and other caregivers interested in occupational medicine. . . . General readers; professionals."
— Choice, Association of College & Research Libraries, May '01

Worldwide Health Sourcebook

Basic Information about Global Health Issues, Including Malnutrition, Reproductive Health, Disease Dispersion and Prevention, Emerging Diseases, Risky Health Behaviors, and the Leading Causes of Death

Along with Global Health Concerns for Children, Women, and the Elderly, Mental Health Issues, Research and Technology Advancements, and Economic, Environmental, and Political Health Implications, a Glossary, and a Resource Listing for Additional Help and Information

Edited by Joyce Brennfleck Shannon. 614 pages. 2001. 0-7808-0330-2. $78.

Health Reference Series

Adolescent Health Sourcebook

AIDS Sourcebook, 1st Edition

AIDS Sourcebook, 2nd Edition

Alcoholism Sourcebook

Allergies Sourcebook, 1st Edition

Allergies Sourcebook, 2nd Edition

Alternative Medicine Sourcebook, 1st Edition

Alternative Medicine Sourcebook, 2nd Edition

Alzheimer's, Stroke & 29 Other Neurological Disorders Sourcebook, 1st Edition

Alzheimer's Disease Sourcebook, 2nd Edition

Arthritis Sourcebook

Asthma Sourcebook

Attention Deficit Disorder Sourcebook

Back & Neck Disorders Sourcebook

Blood & Circulatory Disorders Sourcebook

Brain Disorders Sourcebook

Breast Cancer Sourcebook

Breastfeeding Sourcebook

Burns Sourcebook

Cancer Sourcebook, 1st Edition

Cancer Sourcebook (New), 2nd Edition

Cancer Sourcebook, 3rd Edition

Cancer Sourcebook for Women, 1st Edition

Cancer Sourcebook for Women, 2nd Edition

Cardiovascular Diseases & Disorders Sourcebook, 1st Edition

Caregiving Sourcebook

Colds, Flu & Other Common Ailments Sourcebook

Communication Disorders Sourcebook

Congenital Disorders Sourcebook

Consumer Issues in Health Care Sourcebook

Contagious & Non-Contagious Infectious Diseases Sourcebook

Death & Dying Sourcebook

Diabetes Sourcebook, 1st Edition

Diabetes Sourcebook, 2nd Edition

Diet & Nutrition Sourcebook, 1st Edition

Diet & Nutrition Sourcebook, 2nd Edition

Digestive Diseases & Disorder Sourcebook

Disabilities Sourcebook

Domestic Violence & Child Abuse Sourcebook

Drug Abuse Sourcebook

Ear, Nose & Throat Disorders Sourcebook

Eating Disorders Sourcebook

Emergency Medical Services Sourcebook

Endocrine & Metabolic Disorders Sourcebook

Environmentally Induced Disorders Sourcebook

Ethnic Diseases Sourcebook

Family Planning Sourcebook

Fitness & Exercise Sourcebook, 1st Edition

Fitness & Exercise Sourcebook, 2nd Edition

Food & Animal Borne Diseases Sourcebook

Food Safety Sourcebook

Forensic Medicine Sourcebook

Gastrointestinal Diseases & Disorders Sourcebook